bed 9pm.
wake 1am
leave 3am
on plane ~6 am

P9-DEB-842

Moorestown, N.J.
609-234-6276

Applied Probability and Statistics

BAILEY · The Elements of Stochastic Processes with Applications to the Natural Sciences

BAILEY · Mathematics, Statistics and Systems for Health

BARTHOLOMEW · Stochastic Models for Social Processes, *Second Edition*

BECK and ARNOLD · Parameter Estimation in Engineering and Science

BENNETT and FRANKLIN · Statistical Analysis in Chemistry and the Chemical Industry

BHAT · Elements of Applied Stochastic Processes

BLOOMFIELD · Fourier Analysis of Time Series: An Introduction

BOX · R. A. Fisher, The Life of a Scientist

BOX and DRAPER · Evolutionary Operation: A Statistical Method for Process Improvement

BOX, HUNTER, and HUNTER · Statistics for Experimenters: An Introduction to Design, Data Analysis, and Model Building

BROWN and HOLLANDER · Statistics: A Biomedical Introduction

BROWNLEE · Statistical Theory and Methodology in Science and Engineering, *Second Edition*

BURY · Statistical Models in Applied Science

CHAMBERS · Computational Methods for Data Analysis

CHATTERJEE and PRICE · Regression Analysis by Example

CHERNOFF and MOSES · Elementary Decision Theory

CHOW · Analysis and Control of Dynamic Economic Systems

CLELLAND, deCANI, BROWN, BURSK, and MURRAY · Basic Statistics with Business Applications, *Second Edition*

COCHRAN · Sampling Techniques, *Third Edition*

COCHRAN and COX · Experimental Designs, *Second Edition*

COX · Planning of Experiments

COX and MILLER · The Theory of Stochastic Processes, *Second Edition*

DANIEL · Application of Statistics to Industrial Experimentation

DANIEL · Biostatistics: A Foundation for Analysis in the Health Sciences, *Second Edition*

DANIEL and WOOD · Fitting Equations to Data

DAVID · Order Statistics

DEMING · Sample Design in Business Research

DODGE and ROMIG · Sampling Inspection Tables, *Second Edition*

DRAPER and SMITH · Applied Regression Analysis

DUNN · Basic Statistics: A Primer for the Biomedical Sciences, *Second Edition*

DUNN and CLARK · Applied Statistics: Analysis of Variance and Regression

ELANDT-JOHNSON · Probability Models and Statistical Methods in Genetics

FLEISS · Statistical Methods for Rates and Proportions

GALAMBOS · The Asymptotic Theory of Extreme Order Statistics

GIBBONS, OLKIN, and SOBEL · Selecting and Ordering Populations: A New Statistical Methodology

GNANADESIKAN · Methods for Statistical Data Analysis of Multivariate Observations

GOLDBERGER · Econometric Theory

GOLDSTEIN and DILLON · Discrete Discriminant Analysis

continued on back

BIOSTATISTICS: A FOUNDATION FOR ANALYSIS IN THE HEALTH SCIENCES

BIOSTATISTICS: A FOUNDATION FOR ANALYSIS IN THE HEALTH SCIENCES

SECOND EDITION

WAYNE W. DANIEL

Professor of Quantitative Methods
Georgia State University

JOHN WILEY & SONS

New York • Chichester • Brisbane • Toronto • Singapore

Copyright © 1974 and 1978 by John Wiley & Sons, Inc.

All rights reserved. Published simultaneously in Canada.

Reproduction or translation of any part of this work beyond that permitted by Sections 107 or 108 of the 1976 United States Copyright Act without the permission of the copyright owner is unlawful. Requests for permission or further information should be addressed to the Permissions Department, John Wiley & Sons, Inc.

Library of Congress Cataloging in Publication Data:

Daniel, Wayne W 1929-
Biostatistics

(Wiley series in probability and mathematical statistics)
Bibliography: p.
Includes index.
1. Medical statistics. I. Title.
RA409.D35 1978 519.5′02′4574 77-28253
ISBN 0-471-02591-7

Printed in the United States of America

10 9 8

To my wife, Mary, and my children, Jean, Carolyn, and John

PREFACE

This second edition of *Biostatistics: A Foundation for Analysis in the Health Sciences* should appeal to the same audience for which the first edition was written: the advanced undergraduate and beginning graduate student and the health professional in need of a reference book on statistical methodology.

The present edition improves on the first edition in three important areas. I have (1) included additional topics; (2) expanded, revised, and further clarified some of the topics appearing in the first edition; and (3) included additional student exercises.

Like the first edition, this edition requires few mathematical prerequisites. Only reasonable proficiency in algebra is required for an understanding of the concepts and methods underlying the calculations. The emphasis continues to be on an intuitive understanding of principles rather than an understanding based on mathematical sophistication

Since the publication of the first edition, the ready availability of inexpensive hand-held calculators has had a tremendous impact on the teaching of statistics, as it is the rare student who does not own one of these calculators. Now, more than ever, the statistics instructor can concentrate on teaching concepts and principles and devote less class time to tracking down computational errors made by students. Relieved of the tedium and labor associated with lengthy hand calculations, today's students have reason to view their course in statistics as a much more enjoyable experience than their predecessors.

The instructor who takes advantage of these facts may be able to cover more material during a term than previously. However, the material in the present edition should be sufficient for a one- or two-term course.

The following specific improvements have been incorporated in this second edition:

1. I have added more than 150 new exercises. Like the original exercises and examples, the new ones have been drawn from a wide variety of health disciplines, and, although they are all fictitious, they have been made as interesting and realistic as possible.

2. Most of the new exercises appear at the ends of the chapters to provide review material when chapters have been completed. As in the first edition, exercises also appear at the ends of sections within chapters to provide immediate reinforcement of techniques and concepts as they are taught.

3. Several new drawings have been added in the text to help clarify some of the more troublesome concepts.

4. In the chapter on analysis of variance, a discussion of Tukey's method for comparing individual pairs of means has been added. Examples and exercises to illustrate the procedure have also been included.

5. Also in the analysis of variance chapter the discussion of interaction has been considerably expanded and several drawings have been added to help clarify this topic.

6. The concept of *p*-values, treated rather cursorily in the first edition, receives a greatly expanded coverage in the present edition. Most of the examples illustrating a test of a hypothesis include the determination of the associated *p*-value. Also in the exercises requiring a hypothesis test, the student is asked to determine the *p*-value for the test.

7. To facilitate the use and understanding of the appendix tables, sketches have been added to illustrate the area given in the table of the tabulated distribution where appropriate.

8. The table of the cumulative Poisson distribution (Appendix Table E) has been changed so that it gives cumulative probabilities from the lower end (greater than or equal to) rather than from the upper end (less than or equal to) as in the first edition. In its present form the Poisson table is read in the same manner as the binomial table. I hope this will eliminate a source of confusion to the student.

9. The exercises in Chapters 5 and 6 of the first edition which required the student to refer back to previous exercises for data have been replaced by new exercises that are self-contained.

I would like to take this opportunity to express my gratitude to the many readers and users of my book as a textbook for their helpful suggestions for this second edition. In particular I would like to thank the following people who made detailed recommendations for this revision: *Professor Donald A. Pierce, Department of Statistics, Oregon State University. Professor John W. McCloskey, Chairman Department of Statistics, The University of Dayton.*

I would also like to thank Mr. Robert Armstrong, Chief, Mortality Statistics Branch of the National Center for Health Statistics, who made some valuable suggestions for the improvement of Chapter 12. For any remaining deficiencies in the book, however, I must accept full responsibility.

Finally, I am grateful for the help of my wife Mary, without whose skills as a typist, proofreader, and critic this book could not have been published.

Wayne W. Daniel

CONTENTS

BIOSTATISTICS:
A FOUNDATION FOR
ANALYSIS IN THE
HEALTH SCIENCES

1

ORGANIZING AND SUMMARIZING DATA

1.1 INTRODUCTION

The objectives of this book are twofold: (1) to teach the student to organize and summarize data, and (2) to teach the student how to reach decisions about a large body of data by examining only a small part of the data. The concepts and methods necessary for achieving the first objective are presented under the heading of *descriptive statistics* and the second objective is reached through the study of what is called *inferential statistics*. This chapter discusses descriptive statistics. Chapters 2 to 5 discuss topics that form the foundation of statistical inference, and most of the remainder of the book deals with inferential statistics.

Since this volume is designed for persons preparing for or already pursuing a career in the health field, the illustrative material and exercises reflect the problems and activities that these persons are likely to encounter in the performance of their duties.

1.2 SOME BASIC CONCEPTS

Let us first define some basic terms that will be encountered here.

Statistics. The meaning of *statistics* is implicit in the previous section. More concretely, however, we may say that *statistics is a field of study concerned with (1) the organization and summarization of data, and (2) the drawing of inferences about a body of data when only a part of the data are observed.*

Biostatistics. The tools of statistics are employed in many fields—business, education, psychology, agriculture, and economics, to mention only a few. When the data being analyzed are derived from the biological sciences and medicine, we use the term biostatistics to distinguish this particular application of statistical tools and concepts. This area of application is the concern of this book.

Variable. If, as we observe a characteristic, we find that it takes on different values in different persons, places, or things, we label the characteristic a *variable.* We do this for the simple reason that the characteristic is not the same when observed in different possessors of it. Some examples of variables include the heights of adult males, the weights of preschool children, and the ages of patients seen in a dental clinic.

Quantitative Variables. A *quantitative variable* is one that can be measured. We can, for example, obtain measurements on the heights of adult males, the weights of preschool children, and the ages of patients seen in a dental clinic. These are examples of *quantitative variables.*

Qualitative Variables. Some characteristics are not capable of being measured in the sense that height, weight, and age are measured. Many characteristics can be categorized only, as for example, when an ill person is given a medical diagnosis, a person is designated as being in a socioeconomic group, or when a person, place, or object is said to possess or not to possess some characteristic of interest. We refer to variables of this kind as *qualitative variables.*

Although, in the case of qualitative variables, measurement in the usual sense of the word is not achieved, we can count the number of persons, places, or things belonging to various categories. A hospital administrator, for example, can count the number of patients admitted during a day under each of the various admitting diagnoses.

Random Variable. Whenever we determine the height, weight, or age of an individual, the result is frequently referred to as a *value* of the respective variable. When the values obtained arise as a result of chance factors, the variable is called a *random variable.* Values resulting from measurement procedures are often referred to as *observations* or, simply, *measurements.*

Discrete Random Variable. Variables may be characterized further as to whether they are *discrete* or *continuous.* Since mathematically rigorous definitions of discrete and continuous variables are beyond the level of this book, we offer, instead, nonrigorous definitions and give an example of each.

A discrete random variable is characterized by gaps or interruptions in the values that it can assume. These gaps or interruptions indicate the absence of values between particular values that the variable can assume. Some examples illustrate the point. The number of daily admissions to a general hospital is a discrete random variable since the number of admissions each day must be represented by a whole number, such as 0, 1, 2, 3, and so on. The number of admissions on a given day cannot be a number such as 1.5, 2.997, or 3.3333. The number of decayed, missing, or filled teeth per child in an elementary school is another example of a discrete variable.

Continuous Random Variable. *A continuous random variable does not possess the gaps or interruptions characteristic of a discrete random variable.* A continuous random variable can assume any value within a specified interval of values assumed by the variable. Examples of continuous variables include the various measurements that can be made on individuals such as height, weight, and skull circumference. No matter how close together the observed heights of two people, for example, we can, theoretically, find another person whose height falls somewhere in between.

Because of the limitations of available measuring instruments, however, variables that are inherently continuous are often treated as if they were discrete. Height, for example, is usually recorded to the nearest one-quarter, one-half, or whole inch whereas, with a perfect measuring device, such a measurement could be made as precise as desired.

Population. The average person thinks of a population as a collection of entities, usually people. A population or collection of entities may, however, consist of animals, machines, plants, or cells. For our purposes, we define a *population of entities as the largest collection of entities for which we have an interest at a particular time.* If we take a measurement of some variable on each of the entities in a population, we generate a population of values of that variable. We may, therefore, define a *population of values as the largest collection of values of a random variable for which we have an interest at a particular time.* If, for example, we are interested in the weights of all the elementary children enrolled in a certain county school system, our population consists of all these weights. If our interest lies only in the weights of first grade students in the system, we have a different population—weights of first grade students enrolled in the school system. Hence, populations are determined or defined by our sphere of interest. Populations may be *finite* or *infinite.* If a population of values consists of a fixed number of these values, the population is said to be *finite.* If, on the other hand, a population consists of an endless succession of values, the population is an *infinite* one.

Sample. A sample may be defined simply as *a part of a population.* Suppose our population consists of the weights of all the elementary school children enrolled in a certain county school system. If we collect for analysis the weights of only a fraction of these children, we have only a part of our population of weights, that is, we have a *sample*. There are many kinds of samples that can be selected from a population. They are discussed in succeeding chapters.

1.3 THE ORDERED ARRAY

When measurements of a random variable are taken on the entities of a population, the resulting values usually come to the researcher or statistician as a mass of unordered data. Unless the number of observations is extremely small it will be unlikely that these data will impart much information until

Table 1.3.1

Ages (in Years) of Patients Admitted to a Chronic Disease Hospital During a Certain Month

Number	Age	Number	Age	Number	Age	Number	Age
1	10	26	48	51	63	76	53
2	22	27	39	52	53	77	33
3	24	28	6	53	88	78	3
4	42	29	72	54	48	79	85
5	37	30	14	55	52	80	8
6	77	31	36	56	87	81	51
7	89	32	69	57	71	82	60
8	85	33	40	58	51	83	58
9	28	34	61	59	52	84	9
10	63	35	12	60	33	85	14
11	9	36	21	61	46	86	74
12	10	37	54	62	33	87	24
13	7	38	53	63	85	88	87
14	51	39	58	64	22	89	7
15	2	40	32	65	5	90	81
16	1	41	27	66	87	91	30
17	52	42	33	67	28	92	76
18	7	43	1	68	2	93	7
19	48	44	25	69	85	94	6
20	54	45	22	70	61	95	27
21	32	46	6	71	16	96	18
22	29	47	81	72	42	97	17
23	2	48	11	73	69	98	53
24	15	49	56	74	7	99	70
25	46	50	5	75	10	100	49

they have been put in some kind of order. If the number of observations is not too large, a first step in organizing these data is the preparation of an *ordered array*. An *ordered array* is a listing of the values of a collection (either population or sample) in order of magnitude from the smallest value to the largest value.

Example 1.3.1

Table 1.3.1 consists of a list of the ages of patients admitted to a chronic disease hospital during a certain month. The table reflects the order in which the patients were admitted. As can be seen it requires considerable searching to ascertain such elementary information as the age of the youngest and oldest patient admitted. Table 1.3.2 presents the same data in the form of an ordered

Table 1.3.2

An Ordered Array of the Ages of Patients Admitted to a Chronic Disease Hospital During a Certain Month

Number	Age	Number	Age	Number	Age	Number	Age
1	1	26	14	51	37	76	58
2	1	27	15	52	39	77	60
3	2	28	16	53	40	78	61
4	2	29	17	54	42	79	61
5	2	30	18	55	42	80	63
6	3	31	21	56	46	81	63
7	5	32	22	57	46	82	69
8	5	33	22	58	48	83	69
9	6	34	22	59	48	84	70
10	6	35	24	60	48	85	71
11	6	36	24	61	49	86	72
12	7	37	25	62	51	87	74
13	7	38	27	63	51	88	76
14	7	39	27	64	51	89	77
15	7	40	28	65	52	90	81
16	7	41	28	66	52	91	81
17	8	42	29	67	52	92	85
18	9	43	30	68	53	93	85
19	9	44	32	69	53	94	85
20	10	45	32	70	53	95	85
21	10	46	33	71	53	96	87
22	10	47	33	72	54	97	87
23	11	48	33	73	54	98	87
24	12	49	33	74	56	99	88
25	14	50	36	75	58	100	89

array. If additional computations and organization of the data have to be done by hand, the work may be facilitated by working from the ordered array. If the data are to be analyzed by a computer, it may be undesirable to prepare an ordered array.

1.4 MEASURES OF CENTRAL TENDENCY

An ordered array leaves a lot to be desired with respect to summarization. What we need is the ability to summarize the data by means of just a few *descriptive measures.* Descriptive measures may be computed from the data of a sample or the data of a population. To distinguish between them we have the following definitions.

1. *A descriptive measure computed from the data of a sample is called a* ***statistic****.*
2. *A descriptive measure computed from the data of a population is called a* ***parameter****.*

There are several types of descriptive measures that can be computed from a set of data. In this chapter, however, we limit discussion to *measures of central tendency* and *measures of dispersion.* We consider measures of central tendency in this section and measures of dispersion in the following one.

In each of the measures of central tendency, of which we discuss three, we have a single value that is considered to be typical of the set of data as a whole. The three most commonly used measures of central tendency are the *mean*, the *median*, and the *mode.*

Arithmetic Mean. The most familiar measure of central tendency is the arithmetic mean. It is the descriptive measure most people have in mind when they speak of the "average." The adjective, arithmetic, distinguishes this mean from other means that can be computed. Since we are not covering these other means in this book, there should be no cause for confusion if we refer to the arithmetic mean simply as the *mean.* The mean is obtained by adding all the values in a population or sample and dividing by the number of values that are added. To obtain the mean age of the 100 patients represented in Table 1.3.1, we proceed as follows:

$$\text{mean age} = \frac{10 + 22 + \cdots + 70 + 49}{100} = \frac{3920}{100} = 39.20$$

The three dots in the numerator represent the values not shown to save space.

It will be convenient if we can generalize the procedure for obtaining the mean and, also, represent the procedure in a more compact notational form. Let us begin by designating the random variable of interest by the capital letter, X. In our present illustration we let X represent the random variable, age. Specific values of a random variable will be designated by the lowercase letter, x. To distinguish one value from another we attach a subscript to the x and let the subscript refer to the first, the second, the third value, and so on. For example, from Table 1.3.1 we have

$$x_1 = 10, \qquad x_2 = 22, \ldots, \qquad \text{and} \qquad x_{100} = 49$$

In general, a typical value of a random variable will be designated by x_i and the final value, in a finite population of values, by x_N. Finally we will use the Greek letter μ to stand for the population mean. We may now write the general formula for a finite population mean as follows:

$$\mu = \frac{\sum_{i=1}^{N} x_i}{N} \tag{1.4.1}$$

The symbol $\sum_{i=1}^{N}$ instructs us to add all values of the variable from the first to the last. This symbol, $\sum$, called the *summation sign*, will be used extensively in this book. When from the context it is obvious which values are to be added, the symbols above and below $\sum$ will be omitted.

When we compute the mean for a sample of values, the procedure just outlined is followed with some modifications in notation. We use $\bar{x}$ to designate the sample mean and n to indicate the number of values in the sample. The sample mean then is expressed as

$$\bar{x} = \frac{\sum_{i=1}^{n} x_i}{n} \tag{1.4.2}$$

Suppose we have available a sample consisting of the following five ($n = 5$) observations from Table 1.3.1. Substitution of our sample data into

Population Observation Number	Sample Observation Number	Value
x_{12}	x_1	10
x_{20}	x_2	54
x_{36}	x_3	21
x_{62}	x_4	33
x_{98}	x_5	53

Equation 1.4.2 gives

$$\bar{x} = \frac{\sum_{i=1}^{n} x_i}{n} = \frac{10 + 54 + 21 + 33 + 53}{5} = \frac{171}{5} = 34.2$$

The arithmetic mean possesses certain properties, some desirable and some not so desirable. These properties include the following.

1. Uniqueness. For a given set of data there is one and only one arithmetic mean.
2. Simplicity. The arithmetic mean is easily understood and easy to compute.
3. Since each and every value in a set of data enters into the computation of the mean, it is affected by each value. Extreme values, therefore, have an influence on the mean and, in some cases, can so distort it that it becomes undesirable as a measure of central tendency.

As an example of how extreme values may affect the mean, consider the following situation. Suppose the five physicians who practice in an area are surveyed to determine their charges for a certain procedure. Assume that they report these charges: \$5, \$5, \$5.50, \$5.50, and \$20. The mean charge for the five physicians is found to be \$8.20, a value that is not very representative of the set of data as a whole. The single atypical value had the effect of inflating the mean.

Median. The median of a finite set of values is that value which divides the set into two equal parts such that the number of values equal to or greater than the median is equal to the number of values equal to or less than the median. If the number of values is odd, the median will be the middle value when all values have been arranged in order of magnitude. When the number of observations is even, there is no single middle observation, but two middle observations. In this case the median is taken to be the mean of these two middle observations, when all observations have been arranged in the order of their magnitude.

Let us illustrate this by finding the median of the data in Table 1.3.2. Here the values are already ordered so we need only to find the two middle values These are observation numbers 50 and 51. The values are 36 and 37, and the median, therefore, is $(36 + 37)/2 = 36.5$.

Let us now obtain the median of the sample consisting of the values 10, 54, 21, 33, and 53. Arraying these in the order of their magnitude we have 10, 21, 33, 53, and 54. Since this is an odd number of values, the median is the middle value, or 33.

Properties of the median include the following:

1. Uniqueness. As is true with the mean, there is only one median for a given set of data.
2. Simplicity. The median is easy to calculate.
3. It is not as drastically affected by extreme values as is the mean.

The Mode. The mode of a set of values is that value which occurs most frequently. If all the values are different there is no mode; on the other hand, a set of values may have more than one mode. Again, looking at the data in Table 1.3.2 we find that 7, which occurs five times, is the most frequently occurring value, and, therefore, is the mode.

For an example of a set of values that has more than one mode, let us consider a laboratory with 10 employees whose ages are 20, 21, 20, 20, 34, 22, 24, 27, 27, and 27. We could say that these data have two modes, 20 and 27. The sample consisting of the values 10, 21, 33, 53, and 54 has no mode since all the values are different.

The mode may be used for describing qualitative data. For example, suppose the patients seen in a mental health clinic during a given year received one of the following diagnoses: mental retardation, organic brain syndrome, psychosis, neurosis, and personality disorder. The diagnosis occurring most frequently in the group of patients would be called the modal diagnosis.

Exercises

1.4.1. The following are the fasting blood glucose levels of 10 children.

Number	Value	Number	Value
1	56	6	65
2	62	7	65
3	63	8	68
4	65	9	70
5	65	10	72

Compute: (a) The mean.
(b) The median.
(c) The mode.

1.4.2. The following are the weights of 10 experimental animals following a surgical procedure.

Number	Weight (kg)	Number	Weight (kg)
1	13.2	6	14.4
2	15.4	7	13.6
3	13.0	8	15.0
4	16.6	9	14.6
5	16.9	10	13.1

Find: (a) The mean.
(b) The median.

1.4.3. Fifteen patients making initial visits to a county health department traveled these distances:

Patient	Distance (Miles)	Patient	Distance (Miles)
1	5	8	6
2	9	9	13
3	11	10	7
4	3	11	3
5	12	12	15
6	13	13	12
7	12	14	15
		15	5

Find: (a) The mean distance traveled by these patients.
(b) The median distance traveled.

1.4.4. The first 11 patients admitted for diagnosis and evaluation to a newly opened psychiatric ward of a general hospital experienced the following lengths of stay:

Number	Length of Stay (Days)	Number	Length of Stay (Days)
1	29	6	14
2	14	7	28
3	11	8	14
4	24	9	18
5	14	10	22
		11	14

Find: (a) The mean length of stay for these patients.
(b) The median.
(c) The mode.

1.4.5. Twenty patients on the convalescent wing of a general hospital were offered a choice of four meats for lunch. Their choices were as follows: chicken, fish, fish, liver, chicken, chicken, meat loaf, chicken, fish, meat loaf, liver, fish, meat loaf, chicken, chicken, chicken, liver, fish, meat loaf, chicken.
What was the modal choice?

1.5 MEASURES OF DISPERSION

The *dispersion* of a set of observations refers to the variety that the values of the observations exhibit. If all the values are the same, there is no dispersion; if they are not all the same, dispersion is present in the data. The amount of dispersion may be small, when the values, though different, are close together. If the values are widely scattered, the dispersion is greater. Other terms used synonymously with dispersion include *variation*, *spread*, and *scatter*.

The Range. One way to measure the variation in a set of values is to compute the *range*. The range is the difference between the smallest and largest value in a set of observations. If we denote the range by R, the largest value by x_L, and the smallest value by x_S, we compute the range as follows:

$$R = x_L - x_S \tag{1.5.1}$$

Using the data in Table 1.3.2 we have

$$R = 89 - 1 = 88$$

The usefulness of the range is limited. The fact that it takes into account only two values causes it to be a poor measure of dispersion. The main advantage in using the range is the simplicity of its computation.

The Variance. When the values of a set of observations lie close to their mean, the dispersion is less than when they are scattered over a wide range. Since this is true, it would be intuitively appealing if we could measure dispersion relative to the scatter of the values about their mean. Such a measure is realized in what is known as the *variance*. In computing the variance, we subtract the mean from each of the values, square the differences, and then add them up. This sum of the squared deviations of the values from their mean is divided by the sample size, minus 1, to obtain the variance. Letting s^2 stand for the sample variance, the procedure may be written in notational form as follows:

$$s^2 = \frac{\sum_{i=1}^{n} (x_i - \bar{x})^2}{n - 1} \tag{1.5.2}$$

Let us illustrate by computing the variance of our now familiar sample.

$$s^2 = \frac{(10 - 34.2)^2 + (54 - 34.2)^2 + (21 - 34.2)^2 + (33 - 34.2)^2 + (53 - 34.2)^2}{4}$$

$$= \frac{1506.8}{4} = 376.7$$

The reason for dividing by $n - 1$ rather than n, as we might have expected, is the theoretical consideration referred to as *degrees of freedom*. In computing the variance, we say that we have $n - 1$ *degrees of freedom.* We reason as follows. The sum of the deviations of the values from their mean is equal to zero, as can be shown. If, then, we know the values of $n - 1$ of the deviations from the mean, we know the nth one, since it is automatically determined because of the necessity of all n values to add to zero. The concept of degrees of freedom will be discussed again later. Students interested in pursuing the matter further at this time should refer to the article by Walker (1).

When the number of observations is large, the use of Equation 1.5.2 can be tedious. The following formula may prove to be less troublesome especially when a desk calculator or hand-held calculator is used.

$$s^2 = \frac{n \sum_{i=1}^{n} x_i^2 - \left(\sum_{i=1}^{n} x_i \right)^2}{n(n-1)} \tag{1.5.3}$$

When we compute the variance from a population of values, the procedures outlined above are followed except that usually we divide by N rather than $N - 1$. If we let σ^2 stand for the finite population variance, the definitional and computational formulas, respectively, are as follows:

$$\sigma^2 = \frac{\sum_{i=1}^{N} (x_i - \mu)^2}{N} \tag{1.5.4}$$

$$\sigma^2 = \frac{N \sum_{i=1}^{N} x_i^2 - \left(\sum_{i=1}^{N} x_i \right)^2}{N \cdot N} \tag{1.5.5}$$

The variance represents squared units and, therefore, is not an appropriate measure of dispersion when we wish to express this concept in terms of the original units. To obtain a measure of dispersion in original units, we merely take the square root of the variance. The result is called the *standard deviation.* In general, the standard deviation of a sample is given by

$$s = \sqrt{s^2} = \sqrt{\frac{\sum_{i=1}^{n} (x_i - \bar{x})^2}{n - 1}} \tag{1.5.6}$$

The standard deviation of a finite population is obtained by taking the square root of the quantity obtained by Equation 1.5.4.

The Coefficient of Variation. The standard deviation is useful as a measure of variation within a given set of data. When one desires to compare the dispersion in two sets of data, however, comparing the two standard deviations may lead to fallacious results. It may be that the two variables involved are measured in different units. For example, we may wish to know, for a certain population, whether serum cholesterol levels, measured in mg per 100 ml, are more variable than body weight, measured in pounds.

Furthermore, although the same unit of measurement is used, the two means may be quite different. If we compare the standard deviation of weights of first grade children with the standard deviation of weights of high school freshmen, we may find that the standard deviation of the latter is numerically larger than the former, because the weights themselves are larger, not because the dispersion is greater.

What is needed in situations like these is a measure of relative variation rather than absolute variation. Such a measure is found in the *coefficient of variation* which expresses the standard deviation as a percentage of the mean. The formula is given by

$$\text{C.V.} = \frac{s}{\bar{x}}(100) \tag{1.5.7}$$

We see that, since the mean and standard deviation are expressed in the same unit of measurement, the unit of measurement cancels out in computing the coefficient of variation. What we have, then, is a measure that is independent of the unit of measurement.

Suppose two samples of human males yield the following results.

	Sample 1	Sample 2
Age	25 years	11 years
Mean weight	145 pounds	80 pounds
Standard deviation	10 pounds	10 pounds

A comparison of the standard deviations might lead one to conclude that the two samples possess equal variability. If we compute the coefficients of variation, however, we have for the twenty-five-year-olds

$$\text{C.V.} = \tfrac{10}{145}(100) = 6.9$$

and for the eleven-year-olds

$$\text{C.V.} = \tfrac{10}{80}(100) = 12.5$$

If we compare these results we get quite a different impression.

The coefficient of variation is also useful in comparing the results obtained by different persons who are conducting investigations involving the same variable.

Exercises

1.5.1. Refer to Exercise 1.4.1 and compute:
(a) The range.
(b) The variance, s^2.
(c) The standard deviation, s.

1.5.2. Refer to Exercise 1.4.2. Compute:
(a) The range.
(b) The variance, s^2.
(c) The standard deviation, s.
(d) The coefficient of variation.

1.5.3. Refer to Exercise 1.4.3. Compute:
(a) The range.
(b) The variance, s^2.
(c) The standard deviation, s.
(d) The coefficient of variation.

1.5.4. Refer to Exercise 1.4.4. Compute:
(a) The range.
(b) The variance, s^2.
(c) The standard deviation, s.
(d) The coefficient of variation.

1.6 GROUPED DATA—THE FREQUENCY DISTRIBUTION

As we have seen, a set of observations can be made more comprehensible and meaningful by means of an ordered array. Further summarization may be achieved by grouping the data. To group a set of observations we select a set of contiguous, nonoverlapping intervals such that each value in the set of observations can be placed in one, and only one, of the intervals. These intervals are usually referred to as *class intervals*.

One of the first things to consider, when data are to be grouped, is how many intervals to include. Too few intervals are undesirable because of the resulting loss of information. On the other hand, if too many intervals are used, the objective of summarization will not be met. The best guide to this, as well as to other decisions to be made in grouping data, is your knowledge of the data. It may be that class intervals have been determined by precedent, as in the case of annual tabulations, when the class intervals of previous years are maintained for comparative purposes. Those who wish guidance in this matter may consult a formula given by Sturges (2). This formula gives $k = 1 + 3.322(\log_{10} n)$, where k stands for the number of class intervals and

n is the number of values in the data set under consideration. The answer obtained by applying *Sturges' rule* should not be regarded as final, but should be considered as a guide only. The number of class intervals specified by the rule should be increased or decreased for convenience and clear presentation.

Another question that must be decided regards the width of the class intervals. Although sometimes impossible, class intervals generally should be of the same width. This width may be determined by dividing the range by k, the number of class intervals. Symbolically, the class interval width is given by

$$w = \frac{R}{k} \tag{1.6.1}$$

As a rule this procedure yields a width that is inconvenient for use. Again, we may exercise our good judgment and select a width (usually close to the one given by Equation 1.6.1) that is more convenient.

Example 1.6.1

Table 1.6.1 contains air pollution data as reported for 57 large cities. To get an idea as to the number of class intervals to use, we can apply Sturges'

Table 1.6.1

Suspended Particulate Matter (Micrograms per Cubic Meter) in Samples of Air Taken at 57 Large Cities

City	Value	City	Value	City	Value	City	Value
1	68	16	65	31	12	46	22
2	63	17	43	32	32	47	43
3	42	18	25	33	49	48	27
4	27	19	74	34	38	49	49
5	30	20	51	35	42	50	28
6	36	21	36	36	27	51	23
7	28	22	42	37	31	52	19
8	32	23	28	38	50	53	46
9	79	24	31	39	38	54	30
10	27	25	28	40	21	55	43
11	22	26	25	41	16	56	49
12	23	27	45	42	24	57	12
13	24	28	12	43	69		
14	25	29	57	44	47		
15	44	30	51	45	23		

Source: Statistical Abstract of the United States, 1970, p. 174.

rule to obtain

$$\begin{aligned} k &= 1 + 3.322(\log 57) \\ &= 1 + 3.322(1.7559) \\ &\approx 7 \end{aligned}$$

Now let us divide the range by 7 to get some idea about the class interval width. We have

$$\frac{R}{k} = \frac{79 - 12}{7} = \frac{67}{7} = 9.6$$

It is apparent that a class interval width of 10 will be more convenient to use, as well as more meaningful to the reader. We may now construct our intervals. Since the smallest value in Table 1.6.1 is 12 and the largest value is 79, we may begin our intervals with 10 and end with 79. This gives the following intervals:

10–19
20–29
30–39
40–49
50–59
60–69
70–79

We see that there are seven of these intervals, the number suggested by Sturges' rule. Determining the number of values falling into each class

Table 1.6.2

Distribution of Suspended Particulate Matter (Micrograms per Cubic Meter) in Samples of Air Taken at 57 Large Cities

Class Interval		**Frequency**
10–19	~~////~~	5
20–29	~~////~~ ~~////~~ ~~////~~ ////	19
30–39	~~////~~ ~~////~~	10
40–49	~~////~~ ~~////~~ ///	13
50–59	////	4
60–69	////	4
70–79	//	2
Total		57

interval is merely a matter of looking at the values one by one and of placing a tally mark beside the appropriate interval. When we do this, we have Table 1.6.2.

A table of this kind is called a *frequency distribution.* This table shows the way in which the values of the variable are distributed among the specified class intervals. By consulting it, we can determine the frequency of occurrence of values within any one of the class intervals shown.

It may be useful at times to know the proportion, rather than the number, of values falling within a particular class interval. We obtain this information by dividing the number of values in the particular class interval by the total number of values. If, in our example, we wish to know the proportion of values between 30 and 39, inclusive, we divide 10 by 57 obtaining .18. Thus we say that 10 out of 57, or 10/57ths, or .18, of the values are between 30 and 39. Multiplying .18 by 100 gives us the percentage of values between 30 and 39. We can say, then, that 18 percent of the 57 values are between 30 and 39. We may refer to the proportion of values falling within a class interval as the *relative frequency of occurrence* of values in that interval.

In determining the frequency of values falling within two or more class intervals, we obtain the sum of the number of values falling within the class intervals of interest. Similarly, if we want to know the relative frequency of occurrence of values falling within two or more class intervals, we add the respective relative frequencies. We may *cumulate* the frequencies and relative frequencies to facilitate obtaining information regarding the frequency or relative frequency of values within two or more class intervals. Table 1.6.3

Table 1.6.3

Distribution of Suspended Particulate Matter (Micrograms per Cubic Meter) in Samples of Air Taken at 57 Large Cities

Class Intervals	Frequency	Cumulative Frequency	Relative Frequency	Cumulative Relative Frequency
10 to 19	5	5	.0877	.0877
20 to 29	19	24	.3333	.4210
30 to 39	10	34	.1754	.5964
40 to 49	13	47	.2281	.8245
50 to 59	4	51	.0702	.8947
60 to 69	4	55	.0702	.9649
70 to 79	2	57	.0351	1.0000
Total	57		1.0000	

shows the data of Table 1.6.2 along with the *cumulative frequencies*, the *relative frequencies*, and *cumulative relative frequencies.*

Suppose that we are interested in the relative frequency of values between 40 and 69. We use the cumulative relative frequency column of Table 1.6.3 and subtract .5964 from .9649, obtaining .3685.

The Histogram. We may display a frequency distribution (or a relative frequency distribution) graphically in the form of a *histogram* as shown in Figure 1.6.1. In constructing a histogram the values of the variable under consideration make up the horizontal axis, while the vertical axis has as its scale the frequency (or relative frequency if desired) of occurrence. Above each class interval on the horizontal axis a rectangular bar, or cell, as it is sometimes called, is erected so that the height corresponds to the respective

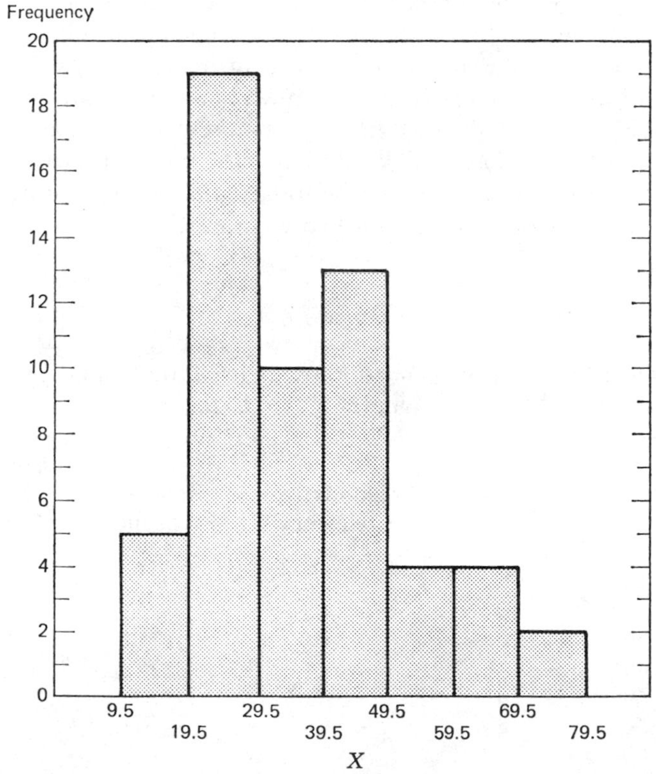

Figure 1.6.1. Histogram of suspended particulate matter (micrograms per cubic meter) in samples of air taken at 57 large cities.

Table 1.6.4

The Data of Table 1.6.2
Showing True Class Limits

True Class Limits	Frequency
9.5–19.5	5
19.5–29.5	19
29.5–39.5	10
39.5–49.5	13
49.5–59.5	4
59.5–69.5	4
69.5–79.5	2

frequency. The cells of a histogram must be joined and, to accomplish this, we must take into account the true boundaries of the class intervals to prevent gaps from occurring between the cells of our graph.

The level of precision observed in reported data that are measured on a continuous scale indicates some order of rounding. The order of rounding reflects either the reporter's personal preference or the limitations of the measuring instrument employed. When a frequency distribution is constructed from the data, the class interval limits usually reflect the degree of precision of the raw data. This has been done in our illustrative example. We know, however, that some of the values falling in the second class interval, for example, when measured precisely, would probably be a little less than 20 and some would be a little greater than 29. Considering the underlying continuity of our variable, and assuming that the data were rounded to the nearest whole number, we find it convenient to think of 19.5 and 29.5 as the *true limits* of this second interval. The true limits for each of the class intervals, then, we take to be as shown in Table 1.6.4.

If we draw a graph using these class limits as the base of our rectangles, no gaps will result, and we will have the histogram shown in Figure 1.6.1.

Note that each observation is allotted one unit of the area of the histogram. Since we have 57 observations, the histogram consists of a total of 57 units. Each cell contains a certain proportion of the total area, depending on the frequency. The second cell, for example, contains nineteen fifty-sevenths of the area. This, as we have learned, is the relative frequency of occurrence of values between 19.5 and 29.5. From this we see that subareas of the histogram defined by the cells correspond to the frequencies of occurrence of values between the horizontal scale boundaries of the areas. The ratio of a particular subarea to the total area of the histogram is equal to the relative frequency of occurrence of values between the corresponding points on the horizontal axis.

The Frequency Polygon. A frequency distribution can be portrayed graphically in yet another way by means of a *frequency polygon.* To draw a frequency polygon we connect the midpoints of the tops of the cells of the histogram by a straight line. In Figure 1.6.2 we have a frequency polygon corresponding to the histogram of Figure 1.6.1.

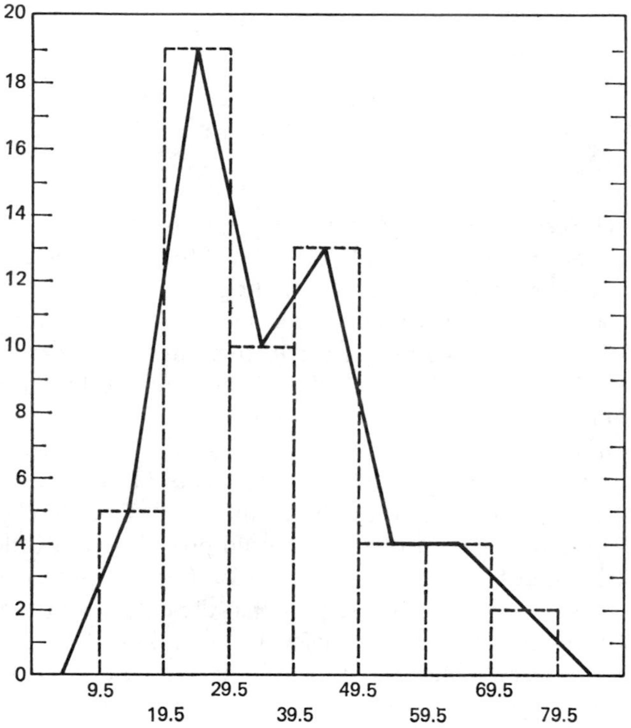

Figure 1.6.2. A frequency polygon. Suspended particulate matter (micrograms per cubic meter) in samples of air taken at 57 large cities.

Note that the polygon is brought down to the horizontal axis at the ends at points that would be the midpoints if there were an additional cell at each end of the corresponding histogram. This allows for the total area to be enclosed. The frequency polygon serves the same purpose as the histogram. The relative frequency of occurrence of observations between any two values is equal to the proportion of the total area between the two points. The total area under the frequency polygon is equal to the area under the histogram.

Exercises

1.6.1. The following are the fasting blood glucose levels of 100 children:

56	61	57	77	62	75	63	55	64	60
60	57	61	57	67	62	69	67	68	59
65	72	65	61	68	73	65	62	75	80
66	61	69	76	72	57	75	68	81	64
69	64	66	65	65	76	65	58	65	64
68	71	72	58	73	55	73	79	81	56
65	60	65	80	66	80	68	55	66	71
72	73	73	75	75	74	66	68	73	65
73	74	68	59	69	55	67	65	67	63
67	56	67	62	65	75	62	63	63	59

Prepare: (a) A frequency distribution.
(b) A histogram.
(c) A relative frequency distribution.
(d) A frequency polygon.

1.6.2. Using the data of Table 1.3.1, prepare:
(a) A frequency distribution.
(b) A relative frequency distribution.
(c) A histogram.
(d) A frequency polygon.

1.6.3. The following are scores made on an intelligence test by a group of children who participated in an experiment:

Child Number	Score	Child Number	Score	Child Number	Score	Child Number	Score
1	114	16	90	31	137	46	118
2	115	17	89	32	120	47	110
3	113	18	106	33	138	48	108
4	112	19	104	34	111	49	134
5	113	20	126	35	100	50	118
6	132	21	127	36	116	51	114
7	130	22	115	37	101	52	142
8	128	23	116	38	111	53	120
9	122	24	109	39	110	54	119
10	121	25	108	40	137	55	143
11	126	26	122	41	119	56	133
12	117	27	123	42	115	57	85
13	115	28	149	43	83	58	117
14	88	29	140	44	109	59	147
15	113	30	121	45	117	60	102

Construct: (a) A frequency distribution.
(b) A relative frequency distribution.
(c) A histogram.
(d) A frequency polygon.

1.6.4. Seventy-five employees of a general hospital were asked to perform a certain task. The time in minutes required for each employee to complete the task was recorded. The results were as shown below.

Employee Number	Time	Employee Number	Time	Employee Number	Time
1	1.3	26	2.2	51	3.2
2	1.5	27	2.3	52	3.0
3	1.4	28	2.6	53	3.4
4	1.5	29	2.8	54	3.4
5	1.7	30	2.1	55	3.2
6	1.0	31	2.3	56	4.5
7	1.3	32	2.4	57	4.6
8	1.7	33	2.0	58	4.9
9	1.2	34	2.8	59	4.1
10	1.8	35	2.2	60	4.6
11	1.1	36	2.5	61	4.2
12	1.0	37	2.9	62	4.0
13	1.8	38	2.0	63	4.3
14	1.6	39	2.9	64	4.8
15	2.1	40	2.5	65	4.5
16	2.1	41	3.6	66	5.1
17	2.1	42	3.1	67	5.7
18	2.1	43	3.5	68	5.1
19	2.4	44	3.7	69	5.4
20	2.9	45	3.7	70	5.7
21	2.7	46	3.4	71	6.7
22	2.3	47	3.1	72	6.8
23	2.8	48	3.5	73	6.6
24	2.0	49	3.6	74	6.0
25	2.7	50	3.5	75	6.1

From these data construct: (a) A frequency distribution.
(b) A relative frequency distribution.
(c) A histogram.
(d) A frequency polygon.

1.7 MEASURES OF CENTRAL TENDENCY COMPUTED FROM GROUPED DATA

After data have been grouped, it may be desirable to compute some of the descriptive measures, such as the mean and variance. Frequently an investigator does not have access to the raw data in which he or she is interested, but does have a frequency distribution. Data frequently are published in the form of a frequency distribution without an accompanying list of individual values or descriptive measures. Readers interested in a measure of central tendency or a measure of dispersion for these data must compute their own.

When data are grouped the individual observations lose their identity. By looking at a frequency distribution we are able to determine the number of observations falling into the various class intervals, but the actual values cannot be determined. Because of this we must make certain assumptions about the values when we compute a descriptive measure from grouped data. As a consequence of making these assumptions our results are only approximations to the true values.

The Mean Computed from Grouped Data. In calculating the mean from grouped data, we assume that all values falling into a particular class interval are located at the *midpoint* of the interval. The midpoint of a class interval is obtained by computing the mean of the upper and lower limits of the interval. The midpoint of the first class interval of the distribution shown in Table 1.6.3, is equal to $(10 + 19)/2 = 29/2 = 14.5$. The midpoints of successive class intervals may be found by adding the class interval width to the previous midpoint. The midpoint of the second class interval in Table 1.6.3, for example, is equal to $14.5 + 10 = 24.5$.

To find the mean we multiply each midpoint by the corresponding frequency, sum these products, and divide by the sum of the frequencies. If the data represent a sample of observations, the computation of the mean may be shown symbolically as

$$\bar{x} = \frac{\sum_{i=1}^{k} m_i f_i}{\sum_{i=1}^{k} f_i} \tag{1.7.1}$$

where $k =$ the number of class intervals, $m_i =$ the midpoint of the ith class interval, and $f_i =$ the frequency of the ith class interval.

When we compute the mean from grouped data, it is convenient to prepare a work table such as Table 1.7.1, which has been prepared for the data of Table 1.6.3.

Table 1.7.1

Work Table for Computing the Mean from the Grouped Data of Table 1.6.3

Class Interval	Class Midpoint m_i	Class Frequency f_i	$m_i f_i$
10–19	14.5	5	72.5
20–29	24.5	19	465.5
30–39	34.5	10	345.0
40–49	44.5	13	578.5
50–59	54.5	4	218.0
60–69	64.5	4	258.0
70–79	74.5	2	149.0
Total		57	2086.5

We may now compute the mean.

$$\bar{x} = \frac{\sum_{i=1}^{k} m_i f_i}{\sum_{i=1}^{k} f_i} = \frac{2086.5}{57} = 36.6$$

Computing a mean from a population of values grouped into a finite number of classes is carried out in exactly the same manner.

The Median—Grouped Data. We have previously defined the median, computed from ungrouped data, as the value above and below which one-half of the observations lie when they have been arranged in order of magnitude. We retain this definition when considering the computation of the median from grouped data. We must, however, make an assumption regarding the distribution of values within the class intervals. Whereas, in computing the mean from grouped data, we assumed the values within a class interval to be located at the midpoint; in computing the median, we assume that the values within a class interval are evenly distributed through the interval.

The first step in computing the median from grouped data is to locate the class interval in which it is located. Referring to the air pollution data again for illustrative purposes, we recall that there are 57 observations. The value of the middle observation, the 29th, is the median. Looking at Table 1.6.3 we see that the first two class intervals account for 24 of the observations, and that 34 observations are accounted for by the first three class intervals. The 29th observation, therefore, is in the third class interval. It is somewhere between 29.5 and 39.5 if we consider the true class limits. The question now is: How far must we proceed into this interval before reaching the median? Under the assumption that the values are evenly distributed through the interval, it seems reasonable that we should move a distance equal to 5/10 of the total distance of the class interval, since after reaching the lower limit of the class interval containing the median we need five more observations, and there are a total of 10 observations in the interval. The value of the median then is equal to the value of the lower limit of the interval containing the median plus 5/10 of the interval width. For the data of Table 1.6.3 we compute the median to be $29.5 + (5/10)(10) = 34.5$.

In general, the median may be computed from grouped data by the following formula:

$$\text{median} = L_i + \frac{j}{f_i}(U_i - L_i) \tag{1.7.2}$$

where L_i = the true lower limit of the interval containing the median, U_i = the true upper limit of the interval containing the median, j = the number of observations still lacking to reach the median, after the lower limit of the interval containing the median has been reached, and f_i = the frequency of the interval containing the median.

When working with grouped data, and n is even, the median is taken to be the $n/2$th value.

The Mode—Grouped Data. We have defined the mode of a set of values as the value that occurs most frequently. When designating the mode of grouped data, we usually refer to the *modal class*, where the modal class is the class interval with the highest frequency. In our air pollution data the modal class would be the second class, 20–29, or 19.5–29.5, using the true class limits. If a single value for the mode of grouped data must be specified, it is taken as the midpoint of the modal class. In the present example this is 24.5. The assumption is made that all values in the interval fall at the midpoint.

1.8 THE VARIANCE AND STANDARD DEVIATION—GROUPED DATA

In calculating the variance and standard deviation from grouped data we assume that all values falling into a particular class interval are located at the midpoint of the interval. This, it will be recalled, is the assumption made in computing the mean and the mode. The variance of a sample, then, is given by

$$s^2 = \frac{\sum_{i=1}^{k} (m_i - \bar{x})^2 f_i}{\sum_{i=1}^{k} f_i - 1} \tag{1.8.1}$$

where the symbols have the definitions given in Equation 1.7.1.

The following computing formula for the sample variance on occasion may be preferred:

$$s^2 = \frac{n \sum_{i=1}^{k} m_i^2 f_i - \left(\sum_{i=1}^{k} m_i f_i \right)^2}{n(n-1)} \tag{1.8.2}$$

where

$$n = \sum_{i=1}^{k} f_i$$

The definitional formula for σ^2 is the same as for s^2 except that μ replaces $\bar{x}$ and the denominator is $\sum_{i=1}^{k} f_i$. The computational formula for σ^2 has $N \cdot N$ in the denominator rather than $n(n-1)$.

Let us now illustrate the computation of the variance and standard deviation, by both the definitional and the computational formula, using the data of Table 1.6.3. To do this, another work table such as Table 1.8.1 will be useful.

Dividing the total of column 6 by the total of column 3, less 1, we have

$$s^2 = \frac{\sum_{i=1}^{k} (m_i - \bar{x})^2 f_i}{\sum_{i=1}^{k} f_i - 1} = \frac{13347.37}{56} = 238.3459$$

The standard deviation is

$$s = \sqrt{238.3459} = 15.44$$

If we use the computing formula of Equation 1.8.2, we have

$$s^2 = \frac{57(89724.25) - (2086.5)^2}{57(56)} = 238.3459$$

Table 1.8.1

Work Table for Computing the Variance and Standard Deviation from the Grouped Data of Table 1.6.3

(1) Class Interval	(2) Class Midpoint m_i	(3) Class Frequency f_i	(4) $(m_i - \bar{x})$	(5) $(m_i - \bar{x})^2$	(6) $(m_i - \bar{x})^2 f_i$	(7) m_i^2	(8) $m_i^2 f_i$
10–19	14.5	5	−22.1	488.41	2442.05	210.25	1051.25
20–29	24.5	19	−12.1	146.41	2781.79	600.25	11404.75
30–39	34.5	10	−2.1	4.41	44.10	1190.25	11902.50
40–49	44.5	13	7.9	62.41	811.33	1980.25	25743.25
50–59	54.5	4	17.9	320.41	1281.64	2970.25	11881.00
60–69	64.5	4	27.9	778.41	3113.64	4160.25	16641.00
70–79	74.5	2	37.9	1436.41	2872.82	5550.25	11100.50
Total		57		3236.87	13347.37		89724.25
$\bar{x} = 36.6$							

Exercises

1.8.1. See Exercise 1.6.1. Find: (a) the mean, (b) the median, (c) the modal class, (d) the variance, and (e) the standard deviation.

1.8.2. See Exercise 1.6.2. Find (a) the mean, (b) the median, (c) the modal class, (d) the variance, and (e) the standard deviation.

1.8.3. See Exercise 1.6.3. Find (a) the mean, (b) the median, (c) the modal class, (d) the variance, and (e) the standard deviation.

1.8.4. See Exercise 1.6.4. Find (a) the mean, (b) the median, (c) the modal class, (d) the variance, and (e) the standard deviation.

1.9 COMPUTERS AND BIOSTATISTICAL ANALYSIS

The relatively recent widespread use of computers has had a tremendous impact on health sciences research in general and biostatistical analysis in particular. The necessity to perform long and tedious arithmetic computations as part of the statistical analysis of data lives only in the memory of those researchers and practitioners whose careers antedate the so-called "computer revolution." Computers can perform more calculations faster and far more accurately than can human technicians. The use of computers makes it possible for investigators to devote more time to the improvement of the quality of raw data and the interpretation of the results.

Canned computer programs are available for performing most of the descriptive and inferential statistical procedures that the average investigator is likely to need. Two widely used "packages" of statistical procedures are *BMDP: Biomedical Computer Programs* (3) and *SPSS Statistical Package for the Social Sciences* (4). Dixon and Jennrich (5), in a review article, describe 38 different packaged statistical programs. They provide information regarding the machines on which the programs may be run, core memory requirements, program languages, available documentation, and sources of additional information. The calculations for many of the exercises in this book can be performed by the programs in these and other statistical program packages.

The usefulness of the computer in the health sciences is not limited to statistical analysis. The reader interested in learning more about the use of computers in biology, medicine, and the other health sciences will find the books by Krasnoff (6), Ledley (7), Lindberg (8), Sterling and Pollack (9), and Taylor (10) helpful.

Current developments in the use of computers in biology, medicine, and related fields are reported in several periodicals devoted to the subject. Three such periodicals are *Computers in Biology and Medicine*, *Computers and Biomedical Research*, and *International Journal of Bio-Medical Computing*.

1.10 SUMMARY

In this chapter we define statistics as an area of study that is concerned with describing data and making inferences. Early in the chapter a basic statistics vocabulary is provided. Various descriptive statistical procedures are explained. These include the organization of data by means of the ordered array, the frequency distribution, the relative frequency distribution, the histogram, and the frequency polygon. The concepts of central tendency and variation are described, along with methods for computing their more common measures: the mean, median, mode, range, variance, and standard deviation. The concepts and methods are presented in a way that makes possible the handling of both grouped and ungrouped data.

Review Questions and Exercises

1. Explain what is meant by descriptive statistics.
2. Explain what is meant by inferential statistics.
3. Define:
   (a) Statistics
   (b) Biostatistics
   (c) Variable
   (d) Quantitative Variable
   (e) Qualitative Variable
   (f) Random Variable
   (g) Population
   (h) Finite Population
   (i) Infinite Population
   (j) Sample
   (k) Discrete Variable
   (l) Continuous Variable
4. What is an ordered array?
5. Define and compare the characteristics of the mean, the median, and the mode.
6. What are the advantages and limitations of the range as a measure of dispersion?
7. What is a frequency distribution?
8. What is a relative frequency distribution?
9. Describe from your field of study a population of data where knowledge of the central tendency and dispersion would be useful. Obtain real or realistic synthetic values from this population and compute the mean, median, mode, variance, and standard deviation, using the techniques for ungrouped data.
10. Collect a set of real, or realistic, data from your field of study and construct a frequency distribution, a relative frequency distribution, a histogram and a frequency polygon.

11. Compute the mean, median, modal class, variance, and standard deviation for the data in Exercise 10, using the techniques for grouped data.
12. Find an article in a journal from your field of study in which some measure of central tendency and dispersion have been computed.
13. In a study designed to investigate the effectiveness of a potential local anesthetic, various doses were administered to 15 laboratory animals. A record was made of the duration (in minutes) of response. The results were as follows:

Animal Number	Duration of Response	Animal Number	Duration of Response
1	31	9	22
2	14	10	20
3	19	11	32
4	17	12	19
5	34	13	27
6	25	14	11
7	17	15	23
8	35		

Compute the mean, median, variance, and standard deviation for these data.

14. The following table shows the daily fat intake (grams) of 150 adult males in a developing country. Prepare a frequency distribution and histogram for these data. Compute the mean, median, variance, and standard deviation.

22	62	77	84	91	102	117	129	137	141
42	56	78	73	96	105	117	125	135	143
37	69	82	93	93	100	114	124	135	142
30	77	81	94	97	102	119	125	138	142
46	89	88	99	95	100	116	121	131	152
63	85	81	94	93	106	114	127	133	155
51	80	88	98	97	106	119	122	134	151
52	70	76	95	107	105	117	128	144	150
68	79	82	96	109	108	117	120	147	153
67	75	76	92	105	104	117	129	148	164
62	85	77	96	103	105	116	132	146	168
53	72	72	91	102	101	128	136	143	164
65	73	83	92	103	118	127	132	140	167
68	75	89	95	107	111	128	139	148	168
68	79	82	96	109	108	117	130	147	153

15. The following are the hemoglobin values (g/100 ml) of 10 children receiving treatment for hemolytic anemia:

9.1	8.3
10.0	9.9
11.4	9.1
12.4	7.5
9.8	6.7

Compute the mean, median, variance, and standard deviation.

16. Twenty postmenopausal women who had undergone a hysterectomy during their premenopausal years received synthetic estrogen therapy daily for four months. After treatment the following estrogen values were recorded:

61	58	54	54
81	56	81	75
61	80	92	59
63	83	71	58
82	92	69	94

Compute the mean, median, variance, and standard deviation.

17. The following table shows the age distribution of cases of a certain disease reported during a year in a particular state.

Age	Number of Cases
5–14	5
15–24	10
25–34	20
35–44	22
45–54	13
55–64	5
Total	75

Compute the mean, median, variance, and standard deviation.

References

References cited

1. Helen M. Walker, "Degrees of Freedom," *The Journal of Educational Psychology*, *31* (1940), 253–269.
2. H. A. Sturges, "The Choice of a Class Interval," *Journal of the American Statistical Association*, *21* (1926), 65–66.

3. W. J. Dixon, Editor, *BMDP: Biomedical Computer Programs*, University of California Press, Berkeley, 1975.
4. Norman H. Nie, C. Hadlai Hull, Jean G. Jenkins, Karin Steinbrenner, and Dale H. Bent, *SPSS Statistical Package for the Social Sciences*, Second Edition, McGraw-Hill, New York, 1975.
5. W. J. Dixon, and R. L. Jennrich, "Scope, Impact, and Status of Packaged Statistical Programs," *Annual Review of Biophysics and Bioengineering*, *1* (1972), 505–528.
6. Sidney O. Krasnoff, *Computers in Medicine*, Charles C. Thomas, Springfield, Ill., 1967.
7. Robert Steven Ledley, *Use of Computers in Biology and Medicine*, McGraw-Hill, New York, 1965.
8. Donald A. B. Lindberg, *The Computer and Medical Care*, Charles C. Thomas, Springfield, Ill., 1968.
9. Theodor D. Sterling and Seymour V. Pollack, *Computers and the Life Sciences*, Columbia University Press, New York, 1965.
10. Thomas R. Taylor, *The Principles of Medical Computing*, Blackwell Scientific Publications, Oxford, 1967.

Other References, Books

1. Wilfred J. Dixon and Frank J. Massey, Jr., *Introduction to Statistical Analysis*, Third Edition, McGraw-Hill, New York, 1969.
2. A. Bradford Hill, *Principles of Medical Statistics*, Eighth Edition, Oxford University Press, New York, 1967.
3. George W. Snedecor and William G. Cochran, *Statistical Methods*, Sixth Edition, The Iowa State University Press, Ames, 1967.
4. George H. Weinberg and John A. Schumaker, *Statistics: An Intuitive Approach*, Second Edition, Wadsworth, Belmont, Cal., 1969.
5. Bernard G. Greenberg, "Biostatistics," in Hugh Rodman Leavell, and E. Gurney Clark, *Preventive Medicine*, McGraw-Hill, New York, 1965.

Other References, Journal Articles

1. I. Altman and A. Ciocco, "Introduction to Occupational Health Statistics I," *Journal of Occupational Medicine*, *6* (1964), 297–301.
2. A. R. Feinstein, "Clinical Biostatistics I, A New Name and Some Other Changes of the Guard," *Clinical Pharmacology and Therapeutics*, (1970), 135–138.
3. Alva R. Feinstein, "Clinical Biostatistics VI, Statistical Malpractice—and the Responsibility of a Consultant," *Clinical Pharmacology and Therapeutics*, *11* (1970), 898–914.

4. Lyon Hyams, "The Practical Psychology of Biostatistical Consultation," *Biometrics*, *27* (1971), 201–211.

5. Johannes Ipsen, "Statistical Hurdles in the Medical Career," *American Statistician*, *19* (June 1965), 22–24.

6. Richard K. Means, "Interpreting Statistics: An Art," *Nursing Outlook* *13* (May 1965), 34–37.

7. E. S. Pearson, "Studies in the History of Probability and Statistics. XIV Some Incidents in the Early History of Biometry and Statistics, 1890–94," *Biometrika*, *52* (1965), 3–18.

8. Harold M. Schoolman, "Statistics in Medical Research," *The New England Journal of Medicine*, *280* (1969), 218–19.

9. Stanley Schor and Irving Karten, "Statistical Evaluation of Medical Journal Manuscripts," *Journal of the American Medical Association*, *195* (1966), 1123–1128.

10. H. C. Selvin and A. Stuart "Data—Dredging Procedures in Surgery Analysis," *American Statistician*, *20* (June 1966), 20–22.

11. Robert L. Stearman, "Statistical Concepts in Microbiology," *Bacteriological Reviews*, *19* (1955), 160–215.

12. Harry E. Ungerleider and Courtland C. Smith, "Use and Abuse of Statistics," *Geriatrics*, *22* (Feb. 1967), 112–120.

13. James P. Zimmerman, "Statistical Data and Their Use," *Physical Therapy*, *49* (1969), 301–302.

14. Robert I. Rollwagen, "Statistical Methodology in Medicine," *Canadian Medical Association Journal*, *112* (1975), 677.

15. Editorial, "Limitations of Computers in Medicine," *Canadian Medical Association Journal*, *104* (1971), 234–235.

16. Carol M. Newton, "Biostatistical Computing," *Federation Proceeding, Federation of American Societies for Experimental Biology*, *33* (1974), 2317–2319.

2

SOME BASIC PROBABILITY CONCEPTS

2.1 INTRODUCTION

The theory of probability provides the foundation for statistical inference. However, this theory, which is a branch of mathematics, is not the main concern of this book and, consequently, only its fundamental concepts are discussed here. Students who desire to pursue this subject should refer to the books on probability by Bates (1), Dixon (2), Mosteller et al. (3), Earl et al. (4), Berman (5), Hausner (6), and Mullins and Rosen (7). They will also find helpful the books on mathematical statistics by Freund (8), Hogg and Craig (9), and Mood and Graybill (10). For those interested in the history of probability, the books by Todhunter (11) and David (12) are recommended. From the latter, for example, we learn that the first mathematician to calculate a theoretical probability correctly was the Italian, Girolamo Cardano, who lived from 1501 to 1576. The objectives of this chapter are to help the students gain some mathematical ability in the area of probability and to assist them in developing an understanding of the more important concepts. Progress along these lines will contribute immensely to their success in understanding the statistical inference procedures presented later in this book.

The concept of probability is not foreign to health workers and is frequently encountered in everyday communication. For example, we may hear a physician say that a patient has a 50-50 chance of surviving a certain operation. Another physician may say that she is 95 percent certain that a patient has a particular disease. A public health nurse may say that nine times out of ten a certain client will break an appointment. Thus we are accustomed to measuring the probability of the occurrence of some event by a number between zero and one. The more likely the event, the closer the number is to one; and the more unlikely the event, the closer the number is to zero. An event that cannot occur has a probability of zero, and an event that is certain to occur has a probability of one.

2.2 TWO VIEWS OF PROBABILITY—OBJECTIVE AND SUBJECTIVE

Until fairly recently probability was thought of by statisticians and mathematicians only as an *objective* phenomenon derived from objective processes.

The concept of *objective probability* may be categorized further under the headings of (1) *classical*, or *a priori*, *probability* and (2) the *relative frequency*, or *a posteriori*, concept of probability.

The classical treatment of probability dates back to the seventeenth century and the work of two mathematicians, Pascal and Fermat (11, 12). Much of this theory developed out of attempts to solve problems related to games of chance, such as the rolling of dice. Examples from games of chance illustrate very well the principles involved in classical probability. For example, if a fair 6-sided die is rolled, the probability that a 1 will be observed is equal to 1/6 and is the same for the other five faces. If a card is picked at random from a well-shuffled deck of ordinary playing cards, the probability of picking a heart is 13/52. Probabilities such as these are calculated by the processes of abstract reasoning. It is not necessary to roll a die or draw a card to compute the above probabilities. In the rolling of the die we say that each of the six sides is *equally likely* to be observed if there is no reason to favor any one of the six sides. Similarly, if there is no reason to favor the drawing of a particular card from a deck of cards we say that each of the 52 cards is equally likely to be drawn. We may define probability in the classical sense as follows.

Definition

If an event can occur in N *mutually exclusive and equally likely ways, and if* m *of these possess a characteristic,* E, *the probability of the occurrence of* E *is equal to* m/N.

If we read $P(E)$ as "the probability of E," we may express the above definition as

$$P(E) = \frac{m}{N} \tag{2.2.1}$$

The relative frequency approach to probability depends on the repeatability of some process and the ability to count the number of repetitions, as well as the number of times that some event of interest occurs. In this context we may define the probability of observing some characteristic, E, of an event as follows.

Definition

If some process is repeated a large number of times, n, *and if some resulting event with the characteristic,* E, *occurs* m *times, the relative frequency of occurrence of* E, m/n, *will be approximately equal to the probability of* E.

To express this definition in compact form we write

$$P(E) = \frac{m}{n} \tag{2.2.2}$$

We must keep in mind, however, that strictly speaking, m/n is only an estimate of $P(E)$.

In the early 1950s L. J. Savage (13) gave considerable impetus to what is called the "personalistic" concept of probability. This view holds that probability measures the confidence that a particular individual has in the truth of a particular proposition. This concept does not rely on the repeatability of any process. In fact, by applying this concept of probability, one may evaluate the probability of an event that can only happen once, for example, the probability that a cure for cancer will be discovered within the next 10 years.

Although this view of probability has enjoyed increased attention over the years, it has not been fully accepted by statisticians who have traditional orientations.

2.3 ELEMENTARY PROPERTIES OF PROBABILITY

In 1933 the axiomatic approach to probability was formalized by the Russian mathematician, A. N. Kolmogorov (14). The basis of this approach is embodied in three properties from which a whole system of probability theory is constructed through the use of mathematical logic. The three properties are as follows.

1. Given some process (or experiment) with n *mutually exclusive outcomes, (called events),* $E_1, E_2, \ldots, E_n$, *the probability of any event,* E_i, *is assigned a nonnegative number.* That is,

$$P(E_i) \geqq 0 \tag{2.3.1}$$

In other words, all events must have a probability greater than or equal to zero; a reasonable requirement, in view of the difficulty of conceiving of negative probability. A key concept in the statement of this property is the concept of *mutually exclusive* outcomes. Two events are said to be mutually exclusive if they cannot occur simultaneously.

2. *The sum of the probabilities of all mutually exclusive outcome is equal to 1.*

$$P(E_1) + P(E_2) + \cdots + P(E_n) = 1 \tag{2.3.2}$$

This is the property of *exhaustiveness* and refers to the fact that the observer of a probabilistic process must allow for all possible events, and when all are taken together, their total probability is 1. The requirement that the events be mutually exclusive is specifying that the events $E_1, E_2, \ldots, E_n$ do not overlap.

3. *Consider any two mutually exclusive events,* E_i *and* E_j. *The probability of the occurrence of either* E_i *or* E_j *is equal to the sum of their individual probabilities.*

$$P(E_i \quad \text{or} \quad E_j) = P(E_i) + P(E_j) \tag{2.3.3}$$

Suppose the two events were not mutually exclusive, that is, suppose they could occur at the same time. In attempting to compute the probability of the occurrence of either E_i or E_j the problem of overlapping would be discovered, and the procedure could become quite complicated.

Before we use these properties to calculate the probability of an event, it is useful to review some basic ideas of set theory and counting techniques. These topics are covered in the next two sections.

2.4 SET THEORY AND SET NOTATION (BASIC NOTIONS)

George Cantor (1845–1918) introduced set theory in the latter part of the nineteenth century. It is an important mathematical tool that is useful in many branches of mathematics, including probability. For this reason, set theory is included in the present chapter. However, only a minimum of its basic concepts will be covered. The books by Breuer (15), Stoll (16), and Maher (17), among others, may be consulted for a more complete treatment.

A *set* is a collection of definite, distinct *objects.* The objects that constitute a set are called the *elements* or *members* of the set. We will use capital letters to designate a set.

A set may be described in either one of the following ways.

1. By listing all the elements in the set.

Examples:

Set — *All Elements in the Set*

A = {patient number 1, patient number 2, patient number 3}

B = {drug A, drug B, drug C, drug D}

C = {animal 1, animal 2, . . . , animal n}

D = {Mrs. Smith, Ms. Jones, Mr. Johnson, Ms. King}

2. By describing the type of element of which the set is composed.
   Examples:
   Set   *Type of Element*
   $A = \{$all patients in critical condition on fourth floor$\}$
   $B = \{$all drugs used in a certain experiment$\}$
   $C = \{$all animals used in a certain experiment$\}$
   $D = \{$all public health nurses employed in a certain clinic$\}$

Some additional concepts relating to sets are given, without proof, below.

1. A *unit set* is a set composed of only one element.
2. A set that contains no elements is called the *empty set*, or *null set*, and is designated by the symbol $\varnothing$.
3. The set of all elements for which there is interest in a given discussion is called the *universal set*. We will designate the universal set by the capital letter, U.
4. If the set A contains one or more elements from the set B, and if every element of A is an element of B, then A is said to be a *subset* of B.
5. The null set is a subset of every other set, by definition.
6. Two sets are equal if, and only if, they contain the same elements.

The following are some useful set operations. Where appropriate the various relationships among the sets will be portrayed visually by a device called a *Venn diagram*, which represents a set as a portion of a plane.

1. The *Union* of two sets, A and B, is another set and consists of all elements belonging to either A or B or both A and B. The symbol, $\cup$, will be used to designate the union of two sets.

Example: Suppose that in a mental health clinic a social worker's case load consists of the set of patients A, where

$A = \{$patients 1, 2, 3, 4, 5, 6$\}$ = all assigned patients who are receiving drug therapy

and the set of patients B, where

$B = \{$patients 2, 4, 7, 8, 9, 10, 11$\}$ = all assigned patients who are receiving group psychotherapy

The Union of these two sets may be written

$A \cup B = \{1, 2, 3, 4, 5, 6, 7, 8, 9, 10, 11\}$ = all assigned patients who are receiving drug therapy, group psychotherapy, or both

The two sets, A and B, are said to be *conjoint* because they have at least one element in common. In this case, the common elements are patients 2 and 4.

The three sets are shown with the use of Venn diagrams in Figure 2.4.1. Note that $A \cup B$ is the total shaded area in the rectangle on the right.

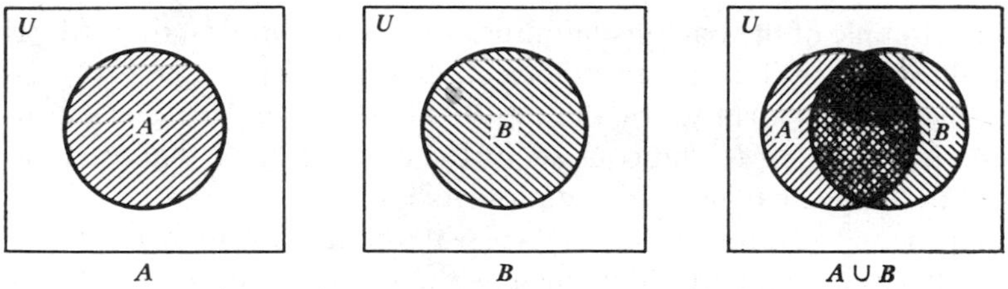

Figure 2.4.1. The union of two conjoint sets.

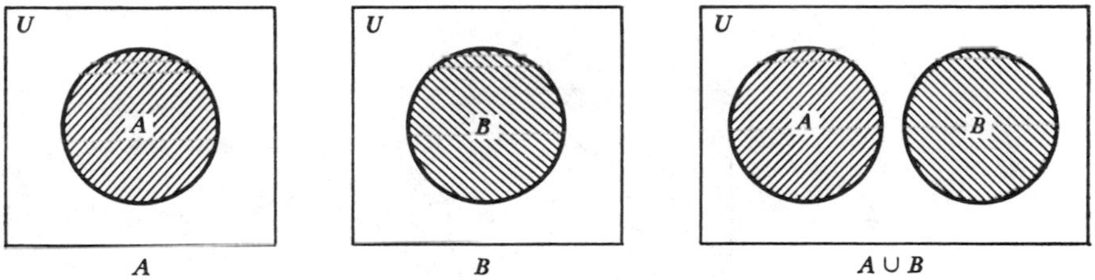

Figure 2.4.2. The union of two disjoint sets.

If two sets have no elements in common they are said to be *disjoint*. For example, suppose 15 patients, of whom 10 were over 30, and 5 were under 30 years of age, were admitted to a general hospital on March 10, 1978. Let us define the following sets:

$$A = \{\text{all patients over 30 admitted on March 10, 1978}\}$$
$$B = \{\text{all patients under 30 admitted on March 10, 1978}\}$$
$$A \cup B = \{\text{all patients admitted on March 10, 1978}\}$$

The sets A and B here are disjoint, since a patient cannot be both under 30 and over 30 years of age at the same time. The union of two disjoint sets is shown in Figure 2.4.2.

2. The *intersection* of two sets, A and B, is another set, and consists of all elements that are in both A and B. The symbol, $\cap$, will be used to designate the intersection of two sets.

In the previous example, which referred to patients in a mental health clinic, the intersection of sets A and B would consist of all patients receiving both drug and group psychotherapy, that is, patients 2 and 4. In set notation we write this as $A \cap B = \{\text{all patients receiving both drug and group psychotherapy}\}$. In Figure 2.4.1, $A \cap B$ is shown as the double shaded area, representing the overlapping of sets A and B.

The example of the patients admitted to a general hospital on March 10, 1978, illustrates the fact that the intersection of two disjoint sets is the null set.

3. If the set A is a subset of the universal set, U, the *complement* of A is another subset of U and consists of the elements in U that are not in A. Let us designate the complement of A as $\bar{A}$.

Suppose, of 50 women receiving private prenatal care, 4 have type AB blood. If we designate the 50 women as the universal set, U, and the subset of 4 with type AB blood as the set A, then the complement of A is the set $\bar{A}$ consisting of the 46 women who have some other blood type. The complement of a set is illustrated in Figure 2.4.3.

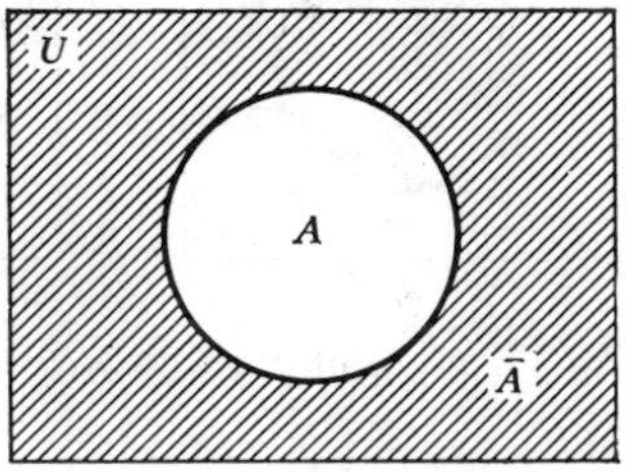

Figure 2.4.3. Venn diagram showing the sets A *and* $\bar{A}$.

Table 2.4.1

Professional and Technical Employees of a Group of Hospitals Classified by Age and Job Category

Job Category	A_1 ≤ 25	A_2 26–30	A_3 31–35	A_4 >35	Total
B_1 Physicians	0	5	25	75	105
B_2 Clinical laboratory services	20	30	35	35	120
B_3 Dietary services	3	6	6	10	25
B_4 Medical record services	7	15	8	12	42
B_5 Nursing services	200	375	442	203	1220
B_6 Pharmacy	1	12	8	3	24
B_7 Radiologic technology	4	10	19	12	45
B_8 Therapeutic services	5	25	15	10	55
B_9 Other professional and technical services	20	35	50	25	130
Total	260	513	608	385	1766

Example 2.4.1

It is frequently useful to be able to identify sets and subsets represented by cross-tabulated data, as in Table 2.4.1 which shows the professional and technical personnel of a group of hospitals tabulated by age and job category. Let us denote the number of elements in a set, say set A, as $n(A)$ and use set notation to identify some of the subsets defined in the table.

In Table 2.4.1, sets A_1 to A_4 consist of personnel falling into the specified age groups and the sets B_1 to B_9 consist of personnel falling into the specified job categories. We may specify other sets by employing the concepts of intersection, union, and complement. For example, the set $B_1 \cap A_4$ consists of physicians who are over 35 years of age, and $n(B_1 \cap A_4) = 75$. The set, $B_2 \cup A_2$ consists of clinical laboratory personnel or personnel between the ages of 26 and 30 or both, and $n(B_2 \cup A_2) = 120 + 513 - 30 = 603$. In calculating $n(B_2 \cup A_2)$, the number (30), who are both clinical laboratory personnel and between the ages of 26 and 30, has to be subtracted because it has been counted twice, that is, it is included in both the figure 120 and the figure 513. The complement of A_4, $\bar{A}_4$, consists of all personnel 35 years old or younger, and $n(\bar{A}_4) = 1766 - 385 = 1381$.

Exercises

2.4.1. The following table shows the patients admitted to a psychiatric hospital during a year. The data are cross-tabulated by diagnosis and age.

	Age (Years)							
Diagnosis	A_1 <15	A_2 15 to 24	A_3 25 to 34	A_4 35 to 44	A_5 45 to 54	A_6 55 to 64	A_7 65 and older	Total
B_1 Involutional psychotic reaction	0	0	0	7	27	20	4	58
B_2 Manic depressive reaction	0	1	1	4	9	5	4	24
B_3 Schizophrenia	5	90	140	160	103	44	7	549
B_4 Psychoneurotic reactions	0	26	44	47	29	13	3	162
B_5 Alcohol addiction	0	7	41	77	68	26	5	224
B_6 Drug addiction	0	2	2	4	2	2	1	13
Total	5	126	228	299	238	110	24	1030

Based on the above table, explain in words the following sets and give the number of patients in each:

(a) $A_4 \cap B_3$ (d) $A_6 \cup B_5$

(b) $B_5 \cap A_6$ (e) $\bar{A}_1$

(c) $B_3 \cup A_4$ (f) $(A_4 \cup A_5) \cap B_3$

2.5 COUNTING TECHNIQUES—PERMUTATIONS AND COMBINATIONS

In this section we present some useful techniques for counting the number of events satisfying some set of conditions. These techniques are helpful in computing the probability of an event when the total number of possible events is large.

Factorials. Given the positive integer n, the product of all the whole numbers from n down through 1 is called *n factorial* and is written $n!$

The following are some examples of factorials:

$$10! = 10 \cdot 9 \cdot 8 \cdot 7 \cdot 6 \cdot 5 \cdot 4 \cdot 3 \cdot 2 \cdot 1$$

$$5! = 5 \cdot 4 \cdot 3 \cdot 2 \cdot 1$$

$$2! = 2 \cdot 1$$

and, in general,

$$n! = n(n-1)(n-2)(n-3) \cdot \ldots \cdot 1$$

By definition, $0! = 1$.

It should also be noted that

$$10! = 10 \cdot 9!$$

$$5! = 5 \cdot 4!$$

$$n! = n(n-1)!$$

Example 2.5.1

By means of factorials we are able to answer questions regarding the number of ways objects can be arranged in a line. For example, suppose we have four containers of culture media each of which is inoculated with a different organism. In how many ways can they be placed in a line on a shelf? The answer is $4! = 4 \cdot 3 \cdot 2 \cdot 1 = 24$ ways. A graphic aid, called a tree diagram, is helpful in visualizing the possibilities. Let us designate the positions as the first, second, third, and fourth positions and the four media as A, B, C, and D. The tree diagram in Figure 2.5.1 represents the possible arrangements.

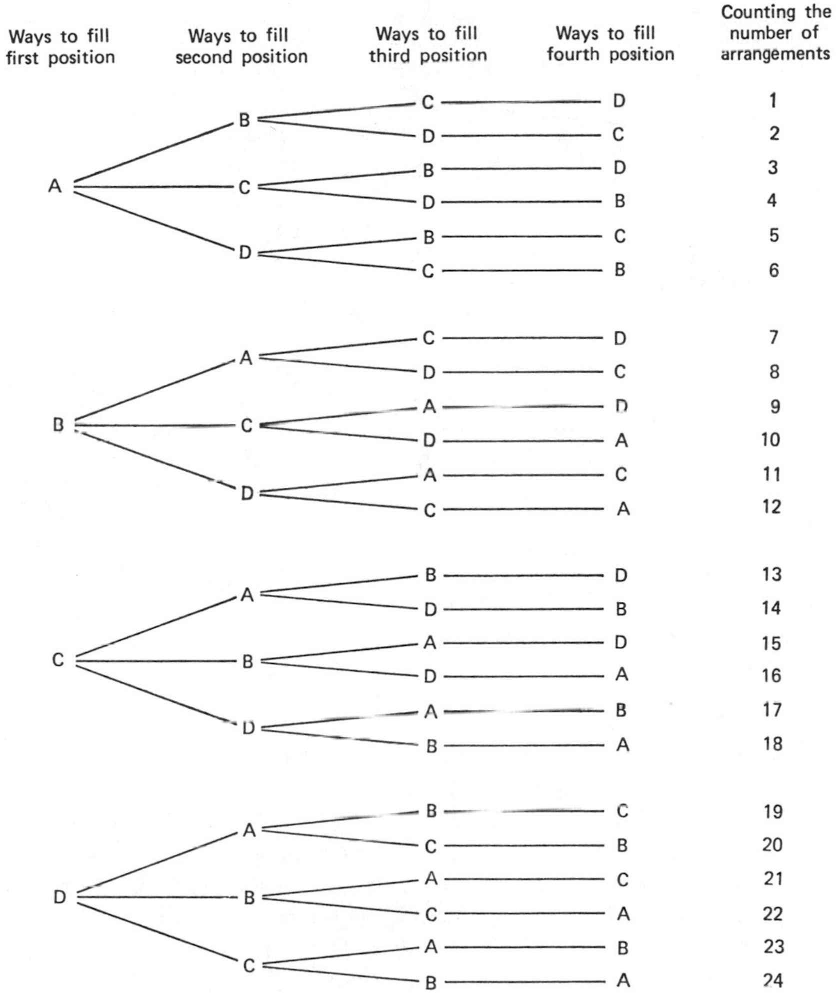

Figure 2.5.1. Tree diagram showing possible arrangements of four objects placed in a line.

Permutations. A *permutation* is an ordered arrangement of objects.

The 24 arrangements of culture media shown in Figure 2.5.1 are the possible permutations of four objects taken four at a time. At times we may have more objects than we have positions to fill. Suppose, in the preceding example, we have only two positions available on the shelf. In how many ways can we fill these two positions using the four culture media? To answer this question we must determine the number of possible permutations of four things taken two at a time. We have four objects, A, B, C, or D, with which to fill the first position. Once that position has been filled we have three

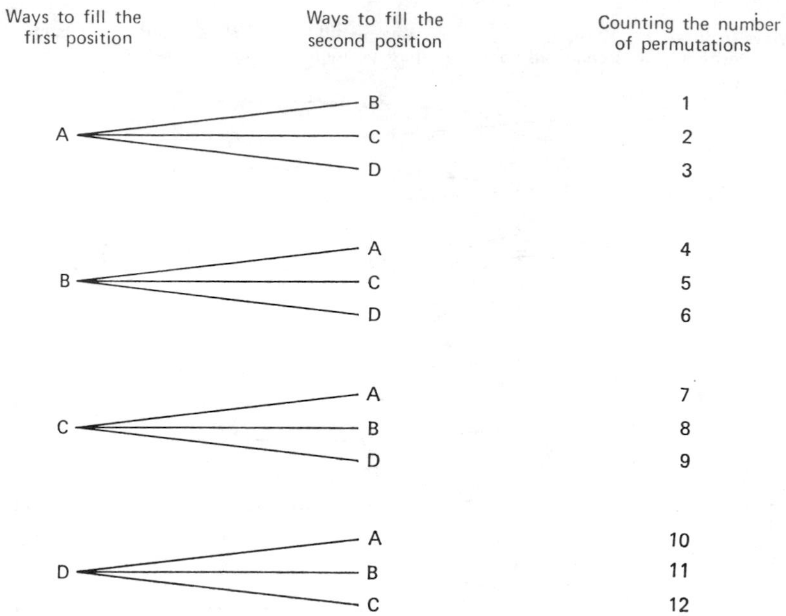

Figure 2.5.2. Tree diagram showing the permutations of four things taken two at a time.

objects, only, with which to fill the second position. Again, let us use a tree diagram (Figure 2.5.2) to illustrate.

We see from Figure 2.5.2 that there are $4 \cdot 3 = 12$ possible permutations of four things taken two at a time. Let us designate by n the number of distinct objects from which an ordered arrangement is to be derived, and by r the number of objects in the arrangement. The number of possible such ordered arrangements is referred to as the number of permutations of n things taken r at a time and may be written as ${}_nP_r$. In general,

$$ {}_nP_r = n(n-1)(n-2)\cdots(n-r+1) \qquad (2.5.1) $$

We may also evaluate ${}_nP_r$ by means of a fraction involving factorials as follows:

$$ {}_nP_r = \frac{n!}{(n-r)!} \qquad (2.5.2) $$

Expanding Equation 2.5.2 gives

$$ {}_nP_r = \frac{n(n-1)(n-2)\cdots(n-r+1)(n-r)(n-r-1)\cdots 1}{(n-r)(n-r-1)\cdots 1} $$

The denominator and terms in the numerator beyond $(n-r+1)$ cancel, leaving the right side of Equation 2.5.1.

Let us illustrate the evaluation of permutations by means of another example.

Example 2.5.2

In a county health department there are five adjacent offices to be occupied by five nurses, A, B, C, D, and E. In how many ways can the five nurses be assigned to the offices? The answer is obtained by evaluating ${}_5P_5$ which is

$$ {}_5P_5 = \frac{5!}{(5-5)!} = 5 \cdot 4 \cdot 3 \cdot 2 \cdot 1 = 120 $$

Suppose that there were six nurses to be assigned to four adjacent offices. Here we need to determine the number of permutations of six things taken four at a time which is

$$ {}_6P_4 = \frac{6!}{(6-4)!} = \frac{6 \cdot 5 \cdot 4 \cdot 3 \cdot 2!}{2!} = 360 $$

Combinations. A *combination* is an arrangement of objects without regard to order. We write the number of combinations of n things taken r at a time as $\binom{n}{r}$.

In Figure 2.5.2 the permutations of four things taken two at a time consisted of the following 12 arrangements:

AB
AC
AD
BA
BC
BD
CA
CB
CD
DA
DB
DC

We note that in the list above there are several pairs of arrangements that are alike except for the order in which the letters occur. We may match these pairs to obtain

AB	AC	AD	BC	BD	CD
BA	CA	DA	CB	DB	DC

In certain cases we may not want to make a distinction between arrangement AB and arrangement BA, for example. We may want to consider them as the same subset, in which case we say that *order does not count*, and refer to the arrangements as combinations. Whereas, in the culture media example we have 12 permutations, we have only six combinations. In other words, we have two permutations of each combination. In general, we will have $r!$ permutations for each combination of n things taken r at a time, or putting it another way, we will, in general, have $r!$ times as many permutations as combinations. That is,

$$_nP_r = r!\binom{n}{r} \tag{2.5.3}$$

If we solve Equation 2.5.3 for $\binom{n}{r}$, we have

$$\binom{n}{r} = \frac{_nP_r}{r!}$$

By rewriting the numerator in accordance with Equation 2.5.2, we have the formula for the number of combinations of n things taken r at a time:

$$\binom{n}{r} = \frac{n!}{r!(n-r)!} \tag{2.5.4}$$

Now let us show that when we use Equation 2.5.4 to obtain the number of combinations of four things taken two at a time we get six:

$$\binom{4}{2} = \frac{4!}{2!2!} = \frac{4 \cdot 3 \cdot 2!}{2 \cdot 1 \cdot 2!} = 6$$

Example 2.5.3

As a further example, suppose that a group therapy leader in a mental health clinic has 10 patients from whom to form a group of six. How many combinations of patients are possible? We find the answer to be

$$\binom{10}{6} = \frac{10!}{6!4!} = \frac{10 \cdot 9 \cdot 8 \cdot 7 \cdot 6!}{6!4 \cdot 3 \cdot 2 \cdot 1} = 210$$

Permutations of Objects That Are Not All Different. In discussing permutations, we have considered the case where all objects being permuted are different. In some situations we may have, in a set of objects to be permuted, some one or more subsets of items that are indistinguishable. The question of how many permutations are possible under these circumstances now arises. It seems logical that the number would be smaller than when all objects are different.

Example 2.5.4

Let us illustrate by referring to the case of five nurses, A, B, C, D, and E who are to be assigned adjacent offices. Suppose two of the nurses want their offices painted white, two yellow, and the remaining nurse wants the office painted green. How many sequences of colors are possible? We assume that with respect to color the two white offices are indistinguishable and the two yellow offices are indistinguishable. The possible color sequences for the five adjacent offices are as follows:

WWYYG	YYWWG	YWWYG
WWYGY	YYWGW	YWWGY
WWGYY	YYGWW	YWGWY
WGWYY	YGYWW	YGWWY
GWWYY	GYYWW	GYWWY
WYWYG	YWYWG	WYYWG
WYWGY	YWYGW	WYYGW
WYGWY	YWGYW	WYGYW
WGYWY	YGWYW	WGYYW
GWYWY	GYWYW	GWYYW

As we can see, there are 30 possible sequences. If each nurse had wanted a different color, so that with respect to color all offices were different, there would be ${}_5P_5 = 5! = 120$ possible color sequences.

Suppose the two whites are distinguishable, say one is an off-white; and the yellows are distinguishable, say dark and light. Let us indicate the differences by subscripts as follows: W_1, W_2, Y_1, Y_2. We can take any one of the previously given sequences and obtain three additional sequences by permuting the subscripts. We do this by permuting the two subscripts for white, while we leave the yellows unchanged. There are 2! such permutations. We can obtain 2! additional sequences by permuting the subscripts of the yellows leaving the whites unchanged. Since there is only one green, we don't have to be concerned with its effect on the number of permutations, simply noting that there are 1! permutations of the single green. If, however, there were two distinguishable greens we would have to take into account the resulting 2! possible permutations. Let us take the first sequence and illustrate. The four possible sequences, when we distinguish between the whites and yellows, are

$$W_1W_2Y_1Y_2G$$
$$W_2W_1Y_1Y_2G$$
$$W_1W_2Y_2Y_1G$$
$$W_2W_1Y_2Y_1G$$

Since we can do this for any of the 30 previous sequences, we see that there are $30 \cdot 2! \cdot 2! \cdot 1! = 120$ sequences when all objects are different. This, of course, is equal to ${}_5P_5 = 120$ which was found previously.

If we let ${}_nP_{n_1,n_2,\ldots,n_k}$ equal the number of distinguishable sequences that can be formed from n objects taken n at a time, when n_1 are of one type, n_2 are of a second type, . . . , and n_k are of a kth type, and $n = n_1 + n_2 + \cdots + n_k$, we can generalize the above results by writing

$$n! = ({}_nP_{n_1,n_2,\ldots,n_k})n_1!n_2! \cdots n_k!$$

If we solve for ${}_nP_{n_1,n_2,\ldots,n_k}$ we obtain

$${}_nP_{n_1,n_2,\ldots,n_k} = \frac{n!}{n_1!n_2! \cdots n_k!} \tag{2.5.5}$$

Using the current example to illustrate, we have

$${}_5P_{2,2,1} = \frac{5!}{2!2!1!} = \frac{120}{4} = 30$$

which is the number of sequences listed previously.

Example 2.5.5

Let us illustrate with another example. Suppose the food service department of a hospital on a certain day is serving two white, two green, and two yellow vegetables. How many distinguishable arrangements of these vegetables can be made on the serving line if we are interested only in distinguishing between vegetables on the basis of color? By Equation 2.5.5 we find the answer to be

$${}_6P_{2,2,2} = \frac{6!}{2!2!2!} = \frac{720}{8} = 90$$

An important special case of Equation 2.5.5 occurs when only two types of objects are present, that is, when r are of one type and $n - r$ are of another type. In this case we have

$${}_nP_{r,n-r} = \frac{n!}{r!(n-r)!} = \binom{n}{r} \tag{2.5.6}$$

From this we see that the number of distinct permutations of n things of which r are of one type and $n - r$ are of another type is equal to the number of combinations of n different things, taken r at a time.

Exercises

2.5.1. Evaluate the following:

(a) ${}_6P_2$ (d) $\binom{6}{2}$ (g) $\binom{8}{5}$

(b) ${}_7P_3$ (e) $\binom{7}{3}$ (h) $\binom{9}{5}$

(c) ${}_{10}P_5$ (f) $\binom{10}{5}$ (i) $\binom{5}{2}$

2.5.2. A public health nurse is preparing a program for a meeting with expectant mothers. She has four topics to cover, and they may be covered in any order.

(a) How many different programs is it possible for her to prepare?
(b) Suppose at the last minute she finds that she has time for only three topics. How many different programs is it possible for her to present if she considers all four of equal importance?

2.5.3. For lunch a patient in a hospital may choose one of four meats, two of five vegetables, and one of three desserts. How many different meals does the patient have from which to choose if he selects the specified number from each group?

2.5.4. A physical therapist planning his day's schedule, finds that he has seven activities to perform that day.

(a) If he may perform these activities in any order he wishes, how many different schedules can he prepare?
(b) If he decides to take the afternoon off so that he has time for only three of his activities, how many schedules can he prepare?

2.5.5. A health educator has three posters to display in a row on the lobby wall of a health center. How many different displays can he prepare?

2.5.6. Suppose in a certain laboratory there are four jobs to be done on a particular afternoon and five people to do the jobs. In how many ways can the five people be assigned to the four jobs?

2.5.7. A researcher has four drugs she wishes to test, but she has only enough experimental animals to test three of the drugs. How many combinations of drugs can she test?

2.5.8. A health educator has engaged four community leaders, two men and two women, to appear on a panel discussion program. In how many ways can she arrange the panel in a row facing the audience if she wishes to distinguish among the panelists only on the basis of sex?

2.5.9. Eight experimental animals have been inoculated with a certain drug; three with type A, three with type B, and two with type C. Each animal is to be placed in one of eight adjacent cages for observation. If the animals are distinguishable only on the basis of the type of drug received, how many different arrangements are possible?

2.6 CALCULATING THE PROBABILITY OF AN EVENT

We now make use of the concepts and techniques of the previous sections in calculating the probabilities of specific events. Additional ideas will be introduced as needed.

Example 2.6.1

For illustrative purposes let us refer to Example 2.4.1 and the data given in Table 2.4.1. Suppose an employee is picked at random from all employees represented, what is the probability that this person will be 25 years of age or younger? We consider the likelihood of selecting any one employee to be equal to the likelihood of selecting any other employee and define the probability of interest as the number of favorable outcomes divided by the total number of possible outcomes. The answer to our question then is

$$P(A_1) = \frac{n(A_1)}{n(U)} = \frac{260}{1766} = .15$$

Conditional Probability. On occasion, the set of "all possible outcomes" may constitute a subset of the universal set. In other words, the population of interest may be reduced by some set of conditions not applicable to the total population. When probabilities are calculated with a subset of the universal set as the denominator, the result is a *conditional probability*.

We may illustrate the concept of conditional probability by referring again to Table 2.4.1. Suppose we are interested in calculating the probability that an employee selected at random from the 1766 employees is a physician. This is an unconditional probability since no conditions have been placed on the set of all possible outcomes, and we compute it as follows.

$$P(B_1) = \frac{n(B_1)}{n(U)} = \frac{105}{1766} = .06$$

Suppose, however, that we reduce the set of all possible outcomes to those employees who are over 35 years of age (set A_4). Now, what is the probability that an employee is a physician, given that he or she is picked at random from the set of employees over 35 years old? We see in Table 2.4.1 that there are 385 members of set A_4, employees over 35 years of age. We also see that, of these, 75 are physicians and that these 75 are the number of members of the set $B_1 \cap A_4$. Thus we find the answer to our question to be

$$P(B_1 | A_4) = \frac{n(B_1 \cap A_4)}{n(A_4)}$$

$$= \tfrac{75}{385} = .19$$

The vertical line in $P(B_1 | A_4)$ is read "given."

We may obtain the conditional probability, $P(B_1 | A_4)$ in another way. Suppose that we divide the numerator and denominator by $n(U)$, the number in the universal set, the total number of employees. This gives

$$P(B_1 | A_4) = \frac{\dfrac{n(B_1 \cap A_4)}{n(U)}}{\dfrac{n(A_4)}{n(U)}}$$

The numerator of this last expression is the probability that an employee picked at random from all employees will be both a physician and over 35 years of age, and may be written $P(B_1 \cap A_4)$. The denominator is the probability that an employee picked at random will be over 35 years of age and may be written as $P(A_4)$. The entire expression may be written as

$$P(B_1 | A_4) = \frac{P(B_1 \cap A_4)}{P(A_4)} = \frac{\frac{75}{1766}}{\frac{385}{1766}} = \frac{.0425}{.2180} = .19$$

This result suggests the following general definition of a conditional probability.

Definition

The conditional probability of A *given* B *is equal to the probability of* A $\cap$ B *divided by the probability of* B, *provided the probability of* B *is not zero.* That is

$$P(A | B) = \frac{P(A \cap B)}{P(B)}, \qquad p(B) \neq 0 \qquad (2.6.1)$$

When we ask the question, what is the probability that an employee picked at random from all employees (Table 2.4.1) is over 35 years old, we are asking for a *marginal probability*. This marginal probability provides the denominator for our conditional probability, $P(B_1 | A_4)$. Our interest centers on a probability associated with a marginal total, and we disregard any other criterion of classification. In computing

$$P(A_4) = \tfrac{385}{1766} = .2180$$

a lack of interest in the B classification is implied. Similarly, if we are interested in the probability that an employee picked at random is a physician for example, we compute this probability using the marginal total, 105, and ignore the age classifications.

In general, then, we may say that when one or more criteria of classification are ignored in computing a probability, the resulting probability is called a *marginal probability*.

Now let us look at the numerator of $P(B_1 \mid A_4)$. This numerator is the probability of the *joint* occurrence of B_1 and A_4, that is, it is the condition of being simultaneously a physician and over 35 years of age. It has already been pointed out that if two events, A and B, cannot occur simultaneously, that is, if $A \cap B = \varnothing$, then A and B are mutually exclusive. When we refer to Table 2.4.1 we see that for this particular set of employees the events, being a physician and being 25 years of age or under are mutually exclusive, since $B_1 \cap A_1 = 0$.

The third property of probability given previously states that the probability of the occurrence of either one or the other of two mutually exclusive events is equal to the sum of their individual probabilities. In our example, then, the probability of being either a physician or 25 years of age or under is found to be

$$P(B_1) + P(A_1) = \tfrac{105}{1766} + \tfrac{260}{1766} = .06 + .15 = .21$$

What if two events are not mutually exclusive? This case is covered by what is known as the *addition rule*, which may be stated as follows.

Definition

Given two events A *and* B, *the probability that event* A, *or event* B, *or both occur is equal to the probability that event* A *occurs, plus the probability that event* B *occurs, minus the probability that both events occur simultaneously.* The addition rule may be written

$$P(A \cup B) = P(A) + P(B) - P(A \cap B) \tag{2.6.2}$$

Let us look once again at Table 2.4.1 and compute the probability that an employee picked at random will be either a physician, over 35 years of age, or both.

$$\begin{aligned} P(B_1 \cup A_4) &= P(B_1) + P(A_4) - P(B_1 \cap A_4) \\ &= \tfrac{105}{1766} + \tfrac{385}{1766} - \tfrac{75}{1766} \\ &= .23 \end{aligned}$$

Note that the 75 employees who are *both* physicians *and* over 35 years of age are included in the 105 who are physicians as well as in the 385 who are over 35 years of age. Since, in computing the probability, these 75 have been added into the numerator twice, they have to be subtracted out once to overcome the effect of duplication, or overlapping.

Another useful rule for computing the probability of an event is the *multiplication rule.* This rule is suggested by our definition of conditional probability and Equation 2.6.1:

$$P(A|B) = \frac{P(A \cap B)}{P(B)}, \qquad P(B) \neq 0$$

We can rewrite Equation 2.6.1 to obtain

$$P(A \cap B) = P(B)P(A|B) \tag{2.6.3}$$

Equation 2.6.3 tells us that the probability of the joint occurrence of events A and B is equal to the conditional probability of A given B times the marginal probability of B.

To illustrate, let us use Equation 2.6.3 to find the probability that an employee picked at random from all employees is both a physician and over 35 years of age.

$$\begin{aligned} P(B_1 \cap A_4) &= P(A_4)P(B_1|A_4) \\ &= \tfrac{385}{1766} \cdot \tfrac{75}{385} \\ &= \tfrac{75}{1766} \end{aligned}$$

This, of course, agrees with what we may compute directly from Table 2.4.1 by forming the ratio of the number of favorable outcomes, 75, to the total number of possible outcomes, 1766.

Let us look again at Equation 2.6.3.

$$P(A \cap B) = P(B)P(A|B)$$

Suppose the fact that we are given event B has no effect on the probability of A. In other words, suppose the probability of event A is the same whether event B occurs or does not occur. In such a case, $P(A|B) = P(A)$, and we say that A and B are *independent events.*

Example 2.6.2

Let us illustrate the concept of independence by means of the following example. In a certain high school class, consisting of 60 girls and 40 boys, it is observed that 24 girls and 16 boys wear eyeglasses. If a student is picked at random from this class, the probability that the student wears eyeglasses, $P(E)$, is 40/100, or .4. What is the probability that a student picked at random wears eyeglasses, given that the student is a boy. By using the formula for computing a conditional probability we find this to be

$$P(E|B) = \frac{P(E \cap B)}{P(B)} = \frac{16/100}{40/100} = .4$$

Thus the additional information that a student is a boy does not alter the probability that the student wears eyeglasses, and $P(E) = P(E|B)$. We say that the events being a boy, and wearing eyeglasses, for this group are independent. We may also show that the event of wearing eyeglasses, E, and *not* being a boy, $\bar{B}$, are also independent as follows:

$$P(E|\bar{B}) = \frac{P(E \cap \bar{B})}{P(\bar{B})} = \frac{24/100}{60/100} = \frac{24}{60} = .4$$

What is the probability of the joint occurrence of the events wearing eyeglasses and being a boy? Using the rule given in Equation 2.6.3, we have

$$P(E \cap B) = P(B)P(E|B)$$

but, since we have shown that events E and B are independent we may replace $P(E|B)$ by $P(E)$ to obtain

$$\begin{aligned} P(E \cap B) &= P(B)P(E) \\ &= (\tfrac{40}{100})(\tfrac{40}{100}) \\ &= .16 \end{aligned}$$

In general, then, when two events, A and B, are independent, and neither $P(A)$ nor $P(B)$ is equal to zero, the probability of their joint occurrence is equal to the product of their individual probabilities. That is

$$P(A \cap B) = P(A)P(B) \qquad (2.6.4)$$

if

$$P(A) \neq 0, \qquad P(B) \neq 0$$

Before we conclude this section, a reminder is appropriate. The probability of an event A is equal to 1 minus the probability of its complement, $\bar{A}$, and

$$P(\bar{A}) = 1 - P(A) \qquad (2.6.5)$$

This follows from the third property of probability since the event, A, and its complement, $\bar{A}$, are mutually exclusive.

Example 2.6.3

Suppose that of 1200 admissions to a general hospital during a certain period of time, 750 are private admissions. If we designate these as set A, then

$\bar{A}$ is equal to 1200 minus 750, or 450. We may compute

$$P(A) = 750/1200 = .625$$

and

$$P(\bar{A}) = 450/1200 = .375$$

and see that

$$P(\bar{A}) = 1 - P(A)$$
$$.375 = 1 - .625$$
$$.375 = .375$$

Exercises

2.6.1. Refer to Exercise 2.4.1 and compute:

(a) $P(A_4 \cap B_3)$ (c) $P(B_3 \cup A_4)$ (e) $P(\bar{A}_1)$
(b) $P(B_5 \cap A_6)$ (d) $P(A_6 \cup B_5)$ (f) $P[(A_4 \cup A_5) \cap B_3]$

2.6.2. The following table shows the first 1000 patients admitted to a clinic for retarded children by diagnostic classification and level of intelligence. For this group find:

(a) $P(A_3 \cap B_4)$.
(b) The probability that a patient picked at random is severely retarded.
(c) The probability that a patient picked at random is either not retarded or is borderline.
(d) The probability that a patient picked at random is profoundly retarded and has Down's syndrome.
(e) The probability that a patient is profoundly retarded, given that he or she has Down's syndrome.

	Level of Retardation						
Diagnostic Classification	A_1 Not Retarded	A_2 Pro-found	A_3 Severe	A_4 Moderate	A_5 Mild	A_6 Border-line	Total
B_1 Encephalopathies	33	38	57	114	103	55	400
B_2 Down's syndrome	2	4	34	88	27	5	160
B_3 Congenital cerebral defect	10	2	6	6	6	0	30
B_4 Mental retardation of unknown cause	0	0	9	36	62	35	142
B_5 Other	161	0	8	16	8	75	268
Total	206	44	114	260	206	170	1000

2.6.3. In a group of 502 persons it was determined that the distribution of blood groups was as follows:

Blood Group	Number
O	226
A	206
B	50
AB	20
Total	502

If a person is picked at random from this group what is the probability that he or she will have blood group:
(a) O? (b) A? (c) B? (d) AB?

2.6.4. Suppose that the data of Exercise 2.6.3 when classified by sex are as follows:

	Sex		
Blood Group	Male	Female	Total
O	113	113	226
A	103	103	206
B	25	25	50
AB	10	10	20
Total	251	251	502

For this group of persons would you say that sex and blood group are independent? Demonstrate by computing appropriate probabilities.

2.6.5. If the probability of left-handedness in a certain group of people is .05, what is the probability of right-handedness (assuming no ambidexterity)?

2.7 SUMMARY

In this chapter some of the basic ideas and concepts of probability are presented. The objective has been to provide enough of a "feel" for the subject so that the probabilistic aspects of statistical inference can be more readily understood and appreciated.

Review Questions and Exercises

1. Define the following:
   - (a) Probability
   - (b) Objective probability
   - (c) Subjective probability
   - (d) Classical probability
   - (e) The relative frequency concept of probability
   - (f) Mutually exclusive events
   - (g) Independence
   - (h) Marginal probability
   - (i) Joint probability
   - (j) Conditional probability
2. Name and explain the three properties of probability.
3. What is a set? Give three examples of sets.
4. Define the following:
   - (a) Unit set
   - (b) Empty set
   - (c) Universal set
   - (d) Subset
   - (e) Disjoint set
   - (f) Complement
5. Under what condition are two sets considered equal?
6. Define and give an example of the union of two sets.
7. Define and give an example of the intersection of two sets.
8. What is a Venn diagram?
9. Define and illustrate the following:
   - (a) Factorial
   - (b) Permutation
   - (c) Combination
   - (d) The addition rule
   - (e) The multiplication rule
10. Set C consists of the citizens of a certain town who voted "yes" for water fluoridation. Set D consists of the citizens of the same town who have preschool children. Define:
    - (a) $C \cup D$
    - (b) $A \cap D$
    - (c) $\bar{C}$
    - (d) $\bar{D}$
11. One hundred married women were asked to specify which type of birth control method they preferred. The following table shows the 100 responses cross-classified by educational level of the respondent.

Birth Control Method	Educational Level: High School (A)	College (B)	Graduate School (C)	Total
S	15	8	7	30
T	3	7	20	30
V	5	5	15	25
W	10	3	2	15
Total	33	23	44	100

Specify the number of members of each of the following sets:

(a) S (c) A (e) U (g) $T \cap B$

(b) $V \cup C$ (d) $\bar{W}$ (f) $\bar{B}$ (h) $\overline{(T \cap C)}$

12. A psychiatric social worker has ten clients to be visited in a week. The clients consist of three alcoholics, four drug addicts, two schizophrenic patients, and one manic-depressive. How many distinguishable visiting arrangements can the social worker prepare if she wishes to distinguish among the clients only on the basis of diagnosis?

13. A certain county health department has received 25 applications for an opening that exists for a public health nurse. Of these applicants ten are over 30 and fifteen are under 30. Seventeen hold bachelor's degrees only, and eight have master's degrees. Of those under 30, six have master's degrees. If a selection from among these 25 applicants is made at random, what is the probability that a person over 30 *or* a person with a master's degree will be selected?

14. The following table shows 1000 nursing school applicants classified according to scores made on a college entrance examination and the quality of the high school from which they graduated, as rated by a group of educators.

	Quality of High School			
Score	Poor (P)	Average (A)	Superior (S)	Total
Low (L)	105	60	55	220
Medium (M)	70	175	145	390
High (H)	25	65	300	390
Total	200	300	500	1000

(a) Calculate the probability that an applicant picked at random from this group
   1. Made a low score on the examination.
   2. Graduated from a superior high school.
   3. Made a low score on the examination and graduated from a superior high school.
   4. Made a low score on the examination given that he or she graduated from a superior high school.
   5. Made a high score or graduated from a superior high school.

(b) Calculate the following probabilities:
   1. $P(A)$ 3. $P(M)$ 5. $P(M \cap P)$
   2. $P(H)$ 4. $P(A|H)$ 6. $P(H|S)$

15. If the probability that a public health nurse will find a client at home is .7, what is the probability (assuming independence) that on two home visits made in a day both clients will be home?

16. The following table shows the outcome of 500 interviews completed during a survey to study the opinions about legalized abortion of residents of a certain city. The data are also classified by the area of the city in which the questionnaire was attempted.

Area of City	Outcome: For (F)	Against (Q)	Undecided (R)	Total
A	100	20	5	125
B	115	5	5	125
D	50	60	15	125
E	35	50	40	125
Total	300	135	65	500

(a) If a questionnaire is selected at random from the 500 what is the probability that
1. The respondent was for legalized abortion?
2. The respondent was against legalized abortion?
3. The respondent was undecided?
4. The respondent lived in Area A? B? D? E?
5. The respondent was for legalized abortion, given that he/she resided in Area B?
6. The respondent was undecided or resided in Area D?

(b) Calculate the following probabilities:

1. $P(A \cap R)$ 3. $P(\bar{D})$ 5. $P(B|R)$
2. $P(Q \cup D)$ 4. $P(Q|D)$ 6. $P(F)$

References

References cited

1. Grace E. Bates, *Probability*, Addison-Wesley, Reading, Mass., 1965.
2. John R. Dixon, *A Programmed Introduction to Probability*, Wiley, New York, 1964.
3. Frederick Mosteller, Robert E. K. Rourke, and George B. Thomas, Jr., *Probability With Statistical Applications*, Second Edition, Addison-Wesley, Reading, Mass., 1970.

4. Boyd Earl, William Moore, and Wendell I. Smith, *Introduction to Probability*, McGraw-Hill, New York, 1963.
5. Simeon M. Berman, *The Elements of Probability*, Addison-Wesley, Reading, Mass., 1969.
6. Melvin Hausner, *Elementary Probability Theory*, Harper and Row, New York, 1971.
7. E. R. Mullins, Jr., and David Rosen, *Concepts of Probability*, Bogden and Quigley, New York, 1972.
8. John E. Freund, *Mathematical Statistics*, Prentice-Hall, Englewood Cliffs, N.J., 1962.
9. Robert V. Hogg and Allen T. Craig, *Introduction to Mathematical Statistics*, Macmillan, New York, 1965.
10. Alexander M. Mood and Franklin A. Graybill, *Introduction to the Theory of Statistics*, Second Edition, McGraw-Hill, New York, 1963.
11. I. Todhunter, *A History of the Mathematical Theory of Probability*, G. E. Stechert, New York, 1931.
12. F. N. David, *Games, Gods and Gambling*, Hafner, New York, 1962.
13. L. J. Savage, *Foundations of Statistics*, Wiley, New York, 1954.
14. A. N. Kolmogorov, *Foundations of the Theory of Probability*, Chelsea, New York, 1964. (Original German edition published in 1933.)
15. Joseph Breuer, *An Introduction to the Theory of Sets*, Prentice-Hall, Englewood Cliffs, N.J., 1958 (Translated by Howard F. Fehr.)
16. Robert R. Stoll, *Set Theory and Logic*, W. H. Freeman, San Francisco, 1963.
17. Lawrence P. Maher, Jr., *Finite Sets, Theory, Counting, and Applications*, Charles E. Merrill, Columbus, Ohio, 1968.

3

PROBABILITY DISTRIBUTIONS

3.1 INTRODUCTION

In the preceding chapter we introduced the basic concepts of probability as well as methods for calculating the probability of an event. We build on these concepts in the present chapter and explore ways of calculating the probability of an event under somewhat more complex conditions.

3.2 PROBABILITY DISTRIBUTIONS OF DISCRETE VARIABLES

Let us begin our discussion of probability distributions by considering the probability distribution of a discrete variable, which we shall define as follows:

Definition

The probability distribution of a discrete random variable is a table, graph, formula, or other device used to specify all possible values of a discrete random variable along with their respective probabilities.

Example 3.2.1

A public health nurse has a case load of 50 families. Let us construct the probability distribution of X, the number of children per family for this population. We can do this with a table in which we list in one column, x,

Table 3.2.1

Probability Distribution of Number of Children per Family in a Population of 50 Families

x	**Frequency of Occurrence of x**	$P(X = x)$
0	1	1/50
1	4	4/50
2	6	6/50
3	4	4/50
4	9	9/50
5	10	10/50
6	7	7/50
7	4	4/50
8	2	2/50
9	2	2/50
10	1	1/50
	50	50/50

the possible values that X assumes, and in another column, $P(X = x)$, the probability with which X assumes a particular value, x. This has been done in Table 3.2.1.

Alternatively, we can present this probability distribution in the form of a graph as in Figure 3.2.1.

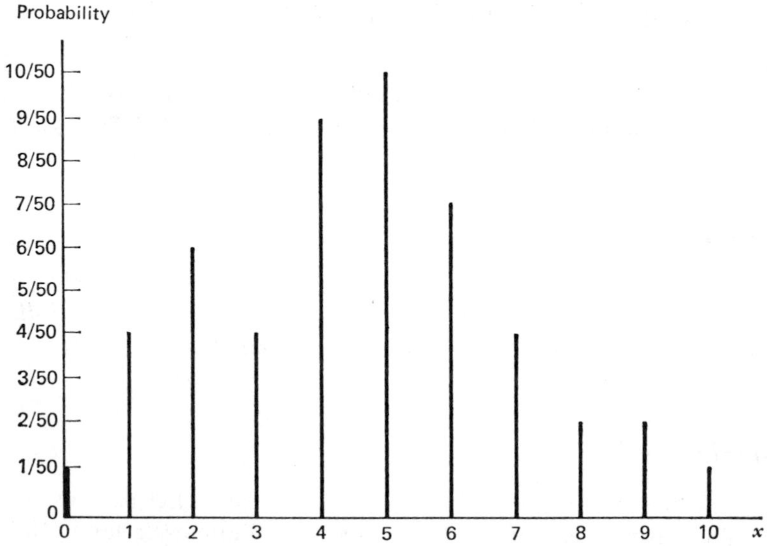

Figure 3.2.1. Graphical representation of the probability distribution of number of children per family for population of 50 families.

In Figure 3.2.1 the length of each vertical bar indicates the probability for the corresponding value of x.

It will be observed in the present example that the values of $P(X = x)$ are all positive, that they are all less than 1, and their sum is equal to 1. These are not phenomena peculiar to this particular example, but are characteristics of all probability distributions of discrete variables. We may then give the following two essential properties of a probability distribution of a discrete variable:

$$(1)\ 0 \leq P(X = x) \leq 1$$

$$(2)\ \sum P(X = x) = 1$$

The reader will also note that each of the probabilities in Table 3.2.1 is the *relative frequency of occurrence* of the corresponding value of X.

With its probability distribution available to us, we can make probability statements regarding the random variable X. Suppose the nurse, with the case load of 50 families, randomly picks a family to visit. What is the probability that the family will have three children? From Table 3.2.1 we see that the answer is $4/50 = .08$, that is, $P(X = 3) = .08$. What is the probability that a family chosen at random will have either three or four children? To answer this question we make use of the addition rule. Since the probability of three children is .08, and the probability of four children is .18, the probability of choosing a family having three or four children is $.08 + .18 = .26$. We may express this more compactly as

$$P(X = 3 \text{ or } X = 4) = P(X = 3) + P(X = 4) = .26$$

Cumulative Distributions. Sometimes it will be more convenient to work with the *cumulative probability distribution* of a random variable. The cumulative probability distribution for the discrete variable whose probability distribution is given in Table 3.2.1 may be obtained by successively adding the probabilities, $P(X = x)$, given in the last column. The resulting cumulative probability distribution is shown in Table 3.2.2.

By consulting the cumulative probability distribution we may answer questions like the following.

1. What is the probability that a family picked at random from the 50 will have less than 5 children? What is needed to answer the question is $P(X < 5)$, and this is obtained by determining the value of the cumulative probability for values of $X = 0$ through $X = 4$. From the table we see that this is $24/50 = .48$.
2. What is the probability that a randomly picked family will have 5 or more children? We may answer this question by means of the concept of the complement. The set of families with 5 or more children is the complement set of the set of families with fewer than 5 children. Their sum is equal to the universal set of 50 families. Since the total probability is 1, and we have found that $P(X < 5) = .48$; the desired probability, $P(X \geq 5)$, is equal to $1 - P(X < 5) = 1 - .48 = .52$.

Table 3.2.2

Cumulative Probability Distribution of Number of Children per Family in a Population of 50 Families

x	**Frequency of Occurrence of x**	$P(X = x)$	$P(X \leq x)$
0	1	1/50	1/50
1	4	4/50	5/50
2	6	6/50	11/50
3	4	4/50	15/50
4	9	9/50	24/50
5	10	10/50	34/50
6	7	7/50	41/50
7	4	4/50	45/50
8	2	2/50	47/50
9	2	2/50	49/50
10	1	1/50	50/50
	50	50/50	

3. What is the probability that a randomly selected family will have between 3 and 6 children, inclusive? What is needed is $P(3 \leq X \leq 6)$, which is equal to $P(X \leq 6) - P(X < 3)$. The probability that X is less than or equal to 6 is the cumulative probability through $X = 6$, or $41/50 = .82$; and the probability that X is less than 3 is the cumulative probability through $X = 2$, or $11/50 = .22$. Thus, we see that $P(3 \leq X \leq 6) = .82 - .22 = .60$.

The probability distribution given in Table 3.2.1 was developed out of actual experience, and to find another variable following this distribution would be coincidental. The probability distributions of many variables of interest, however, can be determined or assumed on the basis of theoretical considerations. In the following sections, we study in detail three of these theoretical probability distributions, the *binomial*, the *Poisson*, and the *normal*.

3.3 THE BINOMIAL DISTRIBUTION

The *binomial distribution* is one of the most widely encountered probability distributions in applied statistics. The distribution is derived from a process known as a *Bernoulli trial*, named in honor of the Swiss mathematician, James Bernoulli (1654–1705), who made significant contributions in the field of probability including, in particular, the binomial distribution. When a single trial of some process or experiment can result in only one of two mutually exclusive outcomes, such as dead or alive, sick or well, male or female, the trial is called a Bernoulli trial.

A sequence of Bernoulli trials forms a *Bernoulli process* under the following conditions.

1. Each trial results in one of two possible, mutually exclusive, outcomes. One of the possible outcomes is denoted (arbitrarily) as a success, and the other is denoted a failure.
2. The probability of a success, denoted by p, remains constant from trial to trial. The probability of a failure, $1 - p$, is denoted by q.
3. The trials are independent, that is, the outcome of any particular trial is not affected by the outcome of any other trial.

Example 3.3.1

We are interested in being able to compute the probability of x successes in n Bernoulli trials. For example, suppose that in a certain population 52 percent of all recorded births are males. We interpret this to mean that the probability of a recorded male birth is .52. If we randomly select five birth records from this population, what is the probability that exactly three of the records will be for male births? Let us designate the occurrence of a record for a male birth as a "success," and hasten to add that this is an arbitrary designation for purposes of clarity and convenience, and does not reflect an opinion regarding the relative merits of male versus female births. The occurrence of a birth record for a male will be designated a success, since we are looking for birth records of males. If we were looking for birth records of females, these would be designated successes, and birth records of males would be designated failures.

It will also be convenient to assign a value of 1 to a success (record for a male birth) and a value of 0 to a failure (record of a female birth).

The process that eventually results in a birth record we consider to be a Bernoulli process.

Suppose the five birth records selected resulted in this sequence of sexes:

MFMMF

In coded form we would write this as

10110

Since the probability of a success is denoted by p and the probability of a failure is denoted by q, the probability of the above sequence of outcomes is found by means of the multiplication rule to be

$$P(1, 0, 1, 1, 0) = pqppq = q^2p^3$$

The multiplication rule is appropriate for computing this probability since we are seeking the probability of a male, and a female, and a male, and a male, and a female, in that order or, in other words, the joint probability of the five events. For simplicity, commas, rather than intersection notation, have been used to separate the outcomes of the events in the probability statement above.

The resulting probability is that of obtaining the specific sequence of outcomes in the order shown. We are not, however, interested in the order of occurrence of records for male and female births but, instead, as has been stated already, the probability of the occurrence of exactly three records of male births out of five randomly selected records. Instead of occurring in the sequence shown above (call it sequence number 1), three successes and two failures could occur in any one of the following additional sequences as well:

Number	*Sequence*
2	11100
3	10011
4	11010
5	11001
6	10101
7	01110
8	00111
9	01011
10	01101

Each of these sequences has the same probability of occurring, and this probability is equal to q^2p^3, the probability computed for the first sequence mentioned.

When we draw a single sample of size five from the population specified, we obtain only one sequence of successes and failures. The question now becomes that of what is the probability of getting sequence number 1 or sequence number 2 $\cdots$ or sequence number 10? From the addition rule we know that this probability is equal to the sum of the individual probabilities. In the present example we need to add up the ten q^2p^3's or, equivalently, multiply q^2p^3 by ten. We may now answer our original question: What is the probability, in a random sample of size 5, drawn from the specified population, of observing three successes (record of a male birth) and two failures (record of a female birth)? Since in the population, $p = .52$, $q = (1 - p) = (1 - .52) = .48$, the answer to the question is

$$10(.48)^2(.52)^3 = 10(.2304)(.140608) = .32$$

We can easily anticipate that, as the size of the sample increases, listing the number of sequences becomes more and more difficult and tedious. What is needed is an easy method of counting the number of sequences. Such a method is provided by Equation 2.5.6, since we have n things some of which are of one type and the remainder are of another type. The number of sequences in our present example is found by Equation 2.5.6 to be $\binom{5}{2} = 5!/2!3! = 120/12 = 10$. In general, if we let n equal the total number of objects, x the number of objects of one type, and $n - x$ the number of objects of the other type, the number of sequences is equal to $\binom{n}{x} = n!/x!\,(n-x)!$, which is equal to the number of combinations of n things taken x at a time.

In our example we may let $x = 3$, the number of successes, so that $n - x = 2$, the number of failures. We then may write the probability of obtaining exactly x successes in n trials as

$$f(x) = \binom{n}{x} q^{n-x} p^x \qquad \text{for} \qquad x = 0, 1, 2, \ldots, n$$
$$= 0, \quad \text{elsewhere} \tag{3.3.1}$$

This expression is called the binomial distribution. In Equation 3.3.1 $f(x) = P(X = x)$ where X is the random variable, number of successes in n trials. We use $f(x)$ rather than $P(X = x)$ because of its compactness and because of its almost universal use.

We may present the binomial distribution in tabular form as in Table 3.3.1.

Table 3.3.1

The Binomial Distribution

Number of Successes, x	**Probability, $f(x)$**
0	$\binom{n}{0} q^{n-0} p^0$
1	$\binom{n}{1} q^{n-1} p^1$
2	$\binom{n}{2} q^{n-2} p^2$
$\vdots$	$\vdots$
x	$\binom{n}{x} q^{n-x} p^x$
$\vdots$	$\vdots$
n	$\binom{n}{n} q^{n-n} p^n$
Total	1

We establish the fact that Equation 3.3.1 is a probability distribution by showing that

1. $f(x) \geq 0$ for all real values of x. This follows from the fact that n and p are both nonnegative and, hence, $\binom{n}{x}$, p^x, and $(1 - p)^{n-x}$ are all nonnegative and, therefore, their product is greater than or equal to zero.
2. $\sum f(x) = 1$. This is seen to be true if we recognize that $\sum \binom{n}{x} q^{n-x}p^x$ is equal to $[(1 - p) + p]^n = 1^n = 1$, the familiar binomial expansion. If the binomial $(q + p)^n$ is expanded we have

$$(q + p)^n = q^n + nq^{n-1}p^1 + \frac{n(n-1)}{2} q^{n-2}p^2 + \cdots + nq^1p^{n-1} + p^n$$

If we compare the terms in the above expansion, term for term, with the $f(x)$ in Table 3.3.1 we see that they are, term for term, equivalent, since

$$\begin{aligned} f(0) &= \binom{n}{0} q^{n-0}p^0 \\ f(1) &= \binom{n}{1} q^{n-1}p^1 = nq^{n-1}p^1 \\ f(2) &= \binom{n}{2} q^{n-2}p^2 = \frac{n(n-1)}{2} q^{n-2}p^2 \\ &\vdots \\ f(n) &= \binom{n}{n} q^{n-n}p^n = p^n \end{aligned}$$

Example 3.3.2

As another example of the use of the binomial distribution, suppose that it is known that 30 percent of a certain population are immune to some disease. If a random sample of size 10 is selected from this population, what is the probability that it will contain exactly four immune persons? We take the probability of an immune person to be .3. Using Equation 3.3.1 we find

$$\begin{aligned} f(4) &= \binom{10}{4}(.7)^6(.3)^4 \\ &= \frac{10!}{4!6!}(.1176)(.0081) \\ &= .20 \end{aligned}$$

The calculation of a probability using Equation 3.3.1 can be a rather tedious undertaking if the sample size is large. Fortunately, probabilities for different values of n, p, and x have been tabulated, so that we need only to consult an appropriate table to obtain the desired probability. Table C of the Appendix is one of many such tables available. It gives the probability that x is greater than or equal to some specified value. That is, the table gives the cumulative probabilities from $x =$ some specified value up through n.

Let us illustrate the use of the table by using the example above where it was desired to find the probability that $x = 4$ when $n = 10$ and $p = .3$. Drawing on our knowledge of cumulative probability distributions from the previous section, we know that $P(x = 4)$ may be found by subtracting $P(X \geq 5)$ from $P(X \geq 4)$. If in the table we locate $p = .3$ for $n = 10$ we find that $P(X \geq 4) = .3504$ and $P(X \geq 5) = .1503$. Subtracting the latter from the former gives $.3504 - .1503 = .2001$, which agrees with our hand calculation to the third decimal place.

Let us look again at the example about the birth records. The objective was to determine the probability of observing exactly three records of male births when $n = 5$ and $p = .52$. To use the table we first locate $n = 5$. We discover, however, that the table does not contain an entry for $p = .52$. A little reflection will convince us that we can obtain the desired results if we restate the question as follows: What is the probability of observing exactly two records of female births if the probability of a record of a female birth is .48 and $n = 5$?

We can find $p = .48$ in the table for $n = 5$, and we see that $P(X \geq 2) = .7865$ and $P(X \geq 3) = .4625$. Subtraction gives $.7865 - .4625 = .324$, which agrees with the figure obtained previously.

Frequently we are interested in determining probabilities, not for specific values of X, but for intervals such as the probability that X is between, say, 5 and 10. Let us illustrate with an example.

Example 3.3.3

Suppose it is known that in a certain population 10 percent of the population is colorblind. If a random sample of 25 people is drawn from this population use Table C in the Appendix to find the probability that

1. Five or more will be colorblind.

   Solution. This probability is an entry in the table. No addition or subtraction is necessary. $P(X \geq 5) = .0980$.

2. Four or fewer will be colorblind.

   Solution. This set is the complement of the set specified in 1, therefore, $P(X \leq 4) = 1 - P(X \geq 5) = 1 - .0980 = .9020$.

3. Between six and nine inclusive will be colorblind.

   Solution. We find this by subtracting the probability that X is greater than or equal to 10 from the probability that X is greater than or equal to 6. That is,

$$P(6 \leq X \leq 9) = P(X \geq 6) - P(X \geq 10) = .0334 - .0001 = .0333$$

4. Two, three, or four will be colorblind.

Solution. This is the probability that X is between 2 and 4 inclusive.

$$P(2 \leq X \leq 4) = P(X \geq 2) - P(X \geq 5) = .7288 - .0980 = .6308$$

The binomial distribution has two parameters, n and p. They are parameters in the sense that they are sufficient to specify a binomial distribution. The binomial distribution is really a family of distributions with each possible value of n and p designating a different member of the family. The mean and variance of the binomial distribution are $\mu = np$ and $\sigma^2 = np(1 - p)$, respectively.

Strictly speaking the use of the binomial distribution is applicable in those situations where sampling is from an infinite population or from a finite population with replacement. Since in actual practice samples are usually drawn without replacement from finite populations, the question naturally arises as to the appropriateness of the binomial distribution under these circumstances. Whether or not the binomial is appropriate depends on how drastic is the effect of these conditions on the constancy of p from trial to trial. It is generally agreed that when n is small relative to N, the binomial model is appropriate. Some writers say that n is small relative to N if N is at least 10 times as large as n.

Exercises

In each of the following exercises, assume that N is sufficiently large relative to n, so that the binomial distribution may be used to find the desired probabilities.

3.3.1. Suppose that 24 percent of a certain population have blood group B. For a sample of size 20 drawn from this population find the probability that

(a) Exactly three persons with blood group B will be found.
(b) Three or more persons with the characteristic of interest will be found.
(c) Fewer than three will be found.
(d) Exactly five will be found.

3.3.2. In a large population, 16 percent of the members are left-handed. In a random sample of size 10 find:

(a) The probability that exactly two will be left-handed.
(b) $P(X \geq 2)$.
(c) $P(X < 2)$.
(d) $P(1 \leq X \leq 4)$.

3.3.3. Suppose it is known that the probability of recovery for a certain disease is .4. If 15 people are stricken with the disease (assume this to be a random sample), what is the probability that

(a) Three or more will recover?
(b) Four or more?
(c) Five or more?
(d) Fewer than three?

3.3.4. Suppose the mortality rate for a certain disease is .10, and suppose 10 people in a community contract the disease. What is the probability that

(a) None will survive?
(b) Fifty percent will die?
(c) At least three will die?
(d) Exactly three will die?

3.4 THE POISSON DISTRIBUTION

The next discrete distribution that we consider is the *Poisson distribution*, named for the French mathematician, Simeon Denis Poisson (1781–1840), who is generally credited for publishing its derivation in 1837 (1, 2). This distribution has been used extensively in biology and medicine. Haight (2) has prepared a farily extensive catalog of such applications in Chapter 7 of his book.

If x is the number of occurrences of some random event in an interval of time or space (or some volume of matter), the probability that x will occur is given by

$$f(x) = \frac{e^{-\lambda}\lambda^x}{x!}, \qquad x = 0, 1, 2, \ldots \qquad (3.3.1)$$

The Greek letter λ (lambda) is called the parameter of the distribution and is the average number of occurrences of the random event in the interval (or volume). The symbol e is the constant (to four decimals) 2.7183.

It can be shown that $f(x) \geq 0$ for every x and that $\sum_x f(x) = 1$, so that the distribution satisfies the requirements for a probability distribution.

The Poisson Process. We have seen that the binomial distribution results from a set of assumptions about an underlying process yielding a set of numerical observations. Such, also, is the case with the Poisson distribution. The following statements describe what is known as the *Poisson process.*

1. The occurrences of the events are independent. The occurrence of an event in an interval[1] of space or time has no effect on the probability of a second occurrence of the event in the same, or any other, interval.

[1] For simplicity the Poisson is discussed in terms of intervals, but other units such as a volume of matter are implied.

2. Theoretically, an infinite number of occurrences of the event must be possible in the interval.
3. The probability of the single occurrence of the event in a given interval is proportional to the length of the interval.
4. In any infinitesimally small portion of the interval the probability of more than one occurrence of the event is negligible.

An interesting feature of the Poisson distribution is the fact that the mean and variance are equal.

The Poisson distribution is employed when counts are made of events or entities that are distributed at random in space or time. One may suspect that a certain process obeys the Poisson law, and under this assumption probabilities of the occurrence of events or entities within some unit of space or time may be calculated. For example, under the assumption that the distribution of some parasite among individual host members follows the Poisson law, one may, with knowledge of the parameter λ, calculate the probability that a randomly selected individual host will yield x number of parasites. In a later chapter we will learn how to decide whether the assumption that a specified process obeys the Poisson law is plausible.

To illustrate the use of the Poisson distribution for computing probabilities, let us consider the following example.

Example 3.4.1

A hospital administrator, who has been studying daily emergency admissions over a period of several years, has concluded that they are distributed according to the Poisson law. Hospital records reveal that emergency admissions have averaged three per day during this period. If the administrator is correct in assuming a Poisson distribution find the probability that

1. Exactly two emergency admissions will occur on a given day.

Solution. We let λ be 3 and X be a random variable denoting the number of daily emergency admissions. Then, if X follows the Poisson distribution.

$$P(X = 2) = f(2) = \frac{e^{-3}3^2}{2!}$$

$$= \frac{.050(9)}{2 \cdot 1}$$

$$= .225$$

Table D of the Appendix lists values of e^x.

2. No emergency admissions will occur on a particular day.

Solution.

$$f(0) = \frac{e^{-3}3^0}{0!}$$
$$= \frac{.050(1)}{1}$$
$$= .05$$

3. Either three or four emergency cases will be admitted on a particular day.

Solution. Since the two events are mutually exclusive, we use the addition rule to obtain

$$f(3) + f(4) = \frac{e^{-3}3^3}{3!} + \frac{e^{-3}3^4}{4!}$$
$$= \frac{.05(27)}{3 \cdot 2 \cdot 1} + \frac{.05(81)}{4 \cdot 3 \cdot 2 \cdot 1}$$
$$= .225 + .16875$$
$$= .39$$

In the foregoing example the probabilities were evaluated directly from the equation. We may, however, use Appendix Table E which gives cumulative probabilities for various values of λ and X.

Example 3.4.2

In the study of a certain aquatic organism, a large number of samples were taken from a pond, and the number of organisms in each sample was counted. The average number of organisms per sample was found to be two. Assuming the number of organisms to be Poisson distributed, find the probability that

1. The next sample taken will contain one or more organisms.

Solution. In Table E we see that when $\lambda = 2$, the probability that $X \geq 1$ is .865. That is, $P(X \geq 1|2) = .865$.

2. The next sample taken will contain exactly three organisms.

Solution.

$$P(X = 3|2) = P(X \geq 3) - P(X \geq 4) = .323 - .143 = .180$$

3. The next sample taken will contain fewer than five organisms.

Solution. Since the set of fewer than five organisms does not include five we are asking for the probability that four or fewer organisms will be observed. This is the cumulative probability from 0 through 4, and we have

$$P(X \leq 4|2) = 1 - P(X \geq 5) = 1 - .053 = .947$$

Exercises

3.4.1. Suppose it is known that in a certain area of a large city the average number of rats per quarter block is five. Assuming that the number of rats is Poisson distributed, find the probability that in a randomly selected quarter block:

(a) There are exactly five rats.
(b) There are more than five rats.
(c) There are fewer than five rats.
(d) There are between five and seven rats, inclusive.

3.4.2. Suppose that over a period of several years the average number of deaths from a certain noncontagious disease has been ten. If the number of deaths from this disease follows the Poisson distribution, what is the probability that during the current year:

(a) Exactly seven people will die from the disease?
(b) Ten or more people will die from the disease?
(c) There will be no deaths from the disease?

3.4.3. If the mean number of serious accidents per year in a large factory (where the number of employees remains constant) is five, find the probability that in the current year:

(a) There will be exactly seven accidents.
(b) Ten or more accidents.
(c) No accidents.
(d) Fewer than five accidents.

didn't do

3.4.4. In a study of the effectiveness of an insecticide against a certain insect a large area of land was sprayed. Later the area was examined for live insects by randomly selecting squares and counting the number of live insects per square. Past experience has shown the average number of live insects per square after spraying to be .5. If the number of live insects per square is Poisson distributed, what is the probability that a selected square will contain:

(a) Exactly one live insect?
(b) No live insects?
(c) Exactly four live insects?
(d) One or more live insects?

3.5 CONTINUOUS PROBABILITY DISTRIBUTIONS

The probability distributions considered thus far, the binomial and the Poisson, are distributions of discrete variables. Let us now consider distributions of continuous random variables. In Chapter 1 we stated that a continuous variable is one that can assume any value within a specified interval of values assumed by the variable. Consequently, between any two values assumed by a continuous variable, there exist an infinite number of values.

To help us understand the nature of the distribution of a continuous random variable, let us consider the data presented in Table 1.6.1 and Figure 1.6.1. In the table we have 57 values of the random variable, suspended particulate matter (measured in micrograms per cubic meter) in samples of air. The histogram of Figure 1.6.1 was constructed by locating specified points on a line representing the measurement of interest and erecting a series of rectangles, whose widths were the distances between two specified points on the line, and whose heights represented the number of values of the variable falling between the two specified points. The intervals defined by any two, consecutive, specified points we called class intervals. As was noted in Chapter 1, subareas of the histogram correspond to the frequencies of occurrence of values of the variable between the horizontal scale boundaries of these subareas. This provides a way whereby the relative frequency of occurrence of values between any two specified points can be calculated: merely determine the proportion of the histogram's total area falling between the specified points. This can be more conveniently done by consulting the relative frequency or cumulative relative frequency columns of Table 1.6.3.

Imagine now the situation where the number of values of our random variable is very large and the width of our class intervals is made very small. The resulting histogram could look like that shown in Figure 3.5.1.

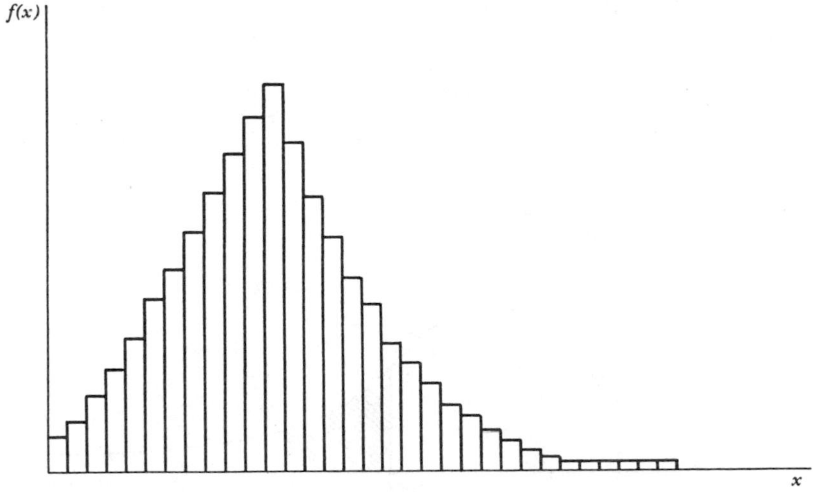

Figure 3.5.1. A histogram resulting from a large number of values and small class intervals.

If we were to connect the midpoints of the cells of the histogram in Figure 3.5.1 to form a frequency polygon, clearly we would have a much smoother figure than the frequency polygon of Figure 1.6.2. It should not be difficult to believe that, in general, as the number of observations, n, approaches infinity, and the width of the class intervals approaches zero, the frequency polygon approaches a smooth curve such as is shown in Figure 3.5.2. Such smooth curves are used to represent graphically the distributions of continuous random variables. This has some important consequences when we deal with probability distributions. First, the total area under the curve is equal to one as was true with the histogram, and the relative frequency of occurrence of values between any two points on the x-axis is equal to the total area bounded by the curve, the x-axis, and perpendicular lines erected at the

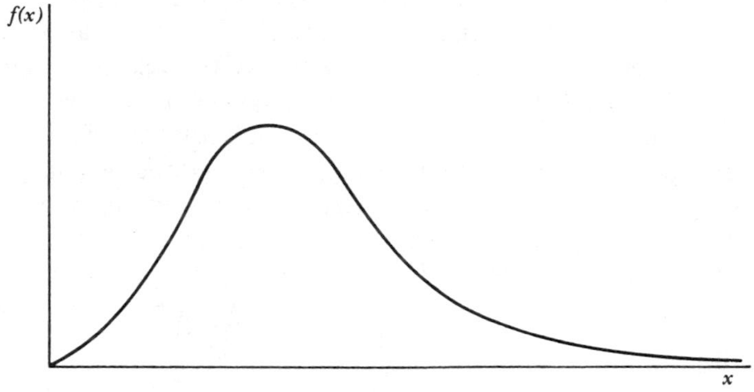

Figure 3.5.2. Graphical representation of a continuous distribution.

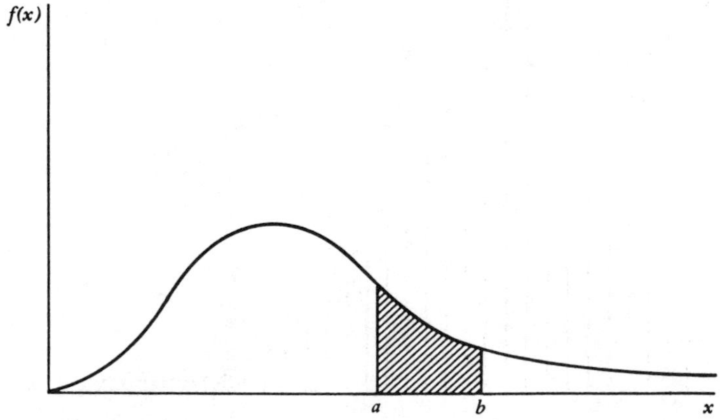

Figure 3.5.3. Graph of a continuous distribution showing area between a *and* b.

two points on the x-axis. See Figure 3.5.3. The probability of *any specific value* of the random variable is *zero*. This seems logical, since a specific value is represented by a point on the x-axis and the area above a point is zero.

With a histogram, as we have seen, subareas of interest can be found by adding areas represented by the cells. We have no cells in the case of a smooth curve so that we must seek an alternative method of finding subareas. Such a method is provided by the integral calculus. To find the area under a smooth curve between any two points, a and b, the *density function* is integrated from a to b. A *density function* is a formula used to represent the distribution of a continuous random variable. Integration is the limiting case of summation, but we shall not perform any integrations, since the mathematics involved are beyond the scope of this book. As we shall see later, for all the continuous distributions we shall consider, there will be an easier way to find areas under their curves.

Although the definition of a probability distribution for a continuous random variable has been implied in the above discussion, by way of summary, we present it in a more compact form as follows.

Definition

A function f(x) *is called a probability distribution (sometimes called probability density function) of the continuous random variable* X *if the total area bounded by its curve and the* x*-axis is equal to* 1, *and if the subarea under the curve bounded by the curve, the* x *axis and perpendiculars erected at any two points* a *and* b *gives the probability that* X *is between the points* a *and* b.

3.6 THE NORMAL DISTRIBUTION

We come now to the most important distribution in all of statistics—the *normal distribution.* The formula for this distribution was first published by Abraham De Moivre (1667–1754) on November 12, 1733 (3). Many other mathematicians figure prominently in the history of the normal distribution, including Carl Friedrich Gauss (1777–1855). The distribution is frequently called the *Gaussian distribution* in recognition of his contributions.

The normal density is given by

$$f(x) = \frac{1}{\sqrt{2\pi}\sigma} e^{-(x-\mu)^2/2\sigma^2}, \qquad -\infty < x < \infty \tag{3.6.1}$$

In Equation 3.6.1, π and e are the familiar constants, 3.14159 and 2.71828, respectively, which are frequently encountered in mathematics. The two

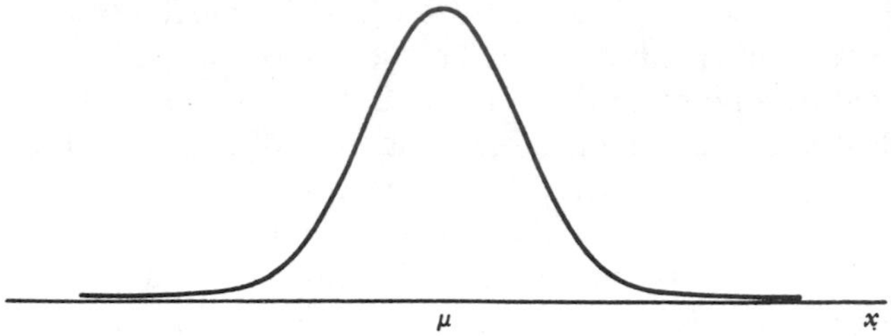

Figure 3.6.1. Graph of a normal distribution.

parameters of the distribution are μ, the mean, and σ, the standard deviation. For our purposes we may think of μ and σ of a normal distribution, respectively, as measures of central tendency and dispersion as discussed in Chapter 1. Since, however, a normally distributed random variable is continuous and takes on values between $-\infty$ and $+\infty$, its mean and standard deviation may be more rigorously defined; but such definitions cannot be given without using calculus. The graph of the normal distribution produces the familiar bell-shaped curve shown in Figure 3.6.1.

The following are some important characteristics of the normal distribution.

1. It is symmetrical about its mean, μ. As is shown in Figure 3.6.1 the curve on either side of μ is a mirror image of the other side.
2. The mean, the median, and the mode are all equal.
3. The total area under the curve above the x-axis is one square unit. This characteristic follows from the fact that the normal distribution is a probability distribution. Because of the symmetry already mentioned, 50 percent of the area is to the right of a perpendicular erected at the mean, and 50 percent is to the left.
4. If we erect perpendiculars a distance of one standard deviation from the mean in both directions, the area enclosed by these perpendiculars, the x-axis and the curve will be approximately 68 percent of the total area. If we extend these lateral boundaries a distance of two standard deviations on either side of the mean, approximately 95 percent of the area will be enclosed, and extending them a distance of three standard deviations will cause approximately 99.7 percent of the total area to be enclosed. These approximate areas are illustrated in Figure 3.6.2.
5. The normal distribution is completely determined by the parameters μ and σ. In other words, a different normal distribution is specified for each different value of μ and σ. Different values of μ shift the graph of the distribution along the x-axis as is shown in Figure 3.6.3. Different values of σ determine the degree of flatness or peakedness of the graph of the distribution as is shown in Figure 3.6.4.

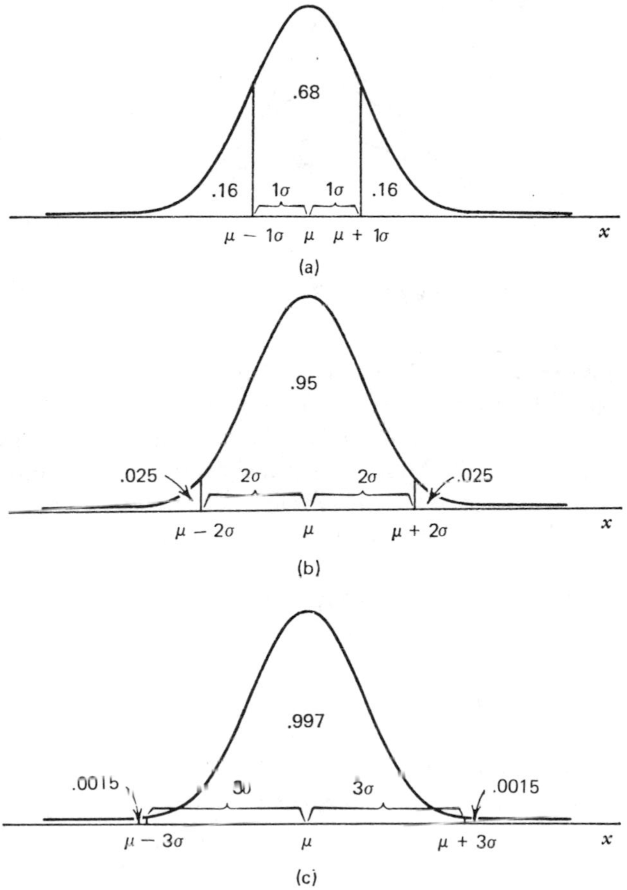

Figure 3.6.2. Subdivision of the area under the normal curve (areas are approximate).

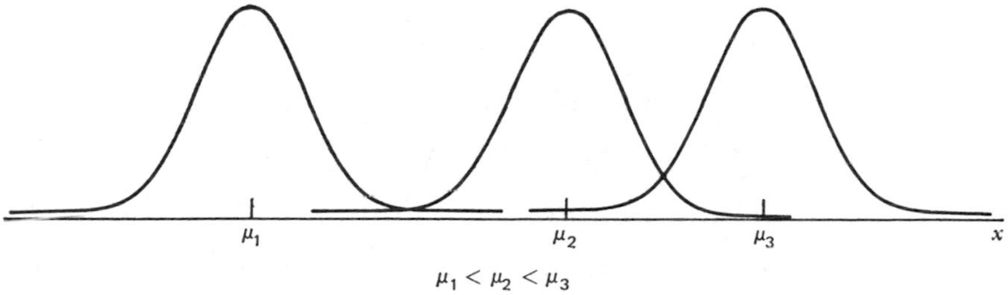

Figure 3.6.3. Three normal distributions with different means.

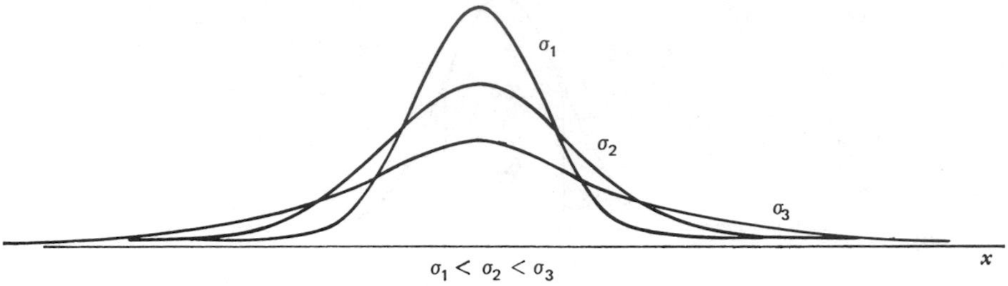

Figure 3.6.4. Three normal distributions with different standard deviations.

The Unit Normal or Standard Normal Distribution. The last-mentioned characteristic of the normal distribution implies that the normal distribution is really a family of distributions in which one member is distinguished from another on the basis of the values of μ and σ. The most important member of this family is the *unit normal or standard normal distribution*, so called because it has a mean of zero and a standard deviation of one. It may be obtained from Equation 3.6.1 by letting $\mu = 0$ and $\sigma = 1$. The random variable that results, $(x - \mu)/\sigma$, is usually designated by the letter z so that the equation for the unit normal distribution is written

$$f(z) = \frac{1}{\sqrt{2\pi}} e^{-z^2/2}, \qquad -\infty < z < \infty \tag{3.6.2}$$

The graph of the unit normal distribution is shown in Figure 3.6.5.

To find the probability that z takes on a value between any two points on the z-axis, say z_0 and z_1, we must find the area bounded by perpendiculars erected at these points, the curve and the horizontal axis. As we mentioned previously, areas under the curve of a continuous distribution are found by integrating the function between two values of the variable. In the case of the unit normal, then, to find the area between z_0 and z_1, we need to evaluate the following integral:

$$\int_{z_0}^{z_1} \frac{1}{\sqrt{2\pi}} e^{-z^2/2}\, dz$$

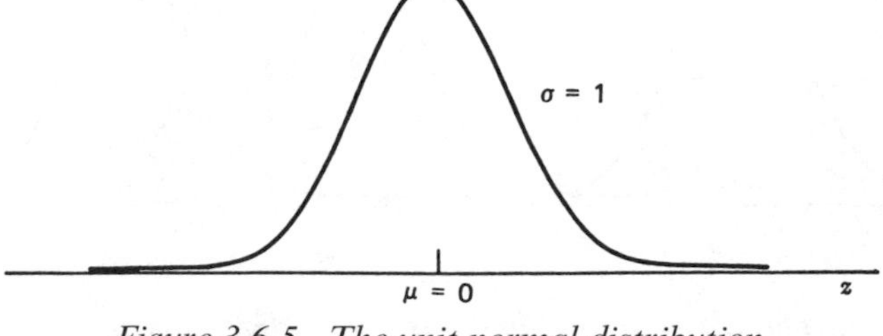

Figure 3.6.5. The unit normal distribution.

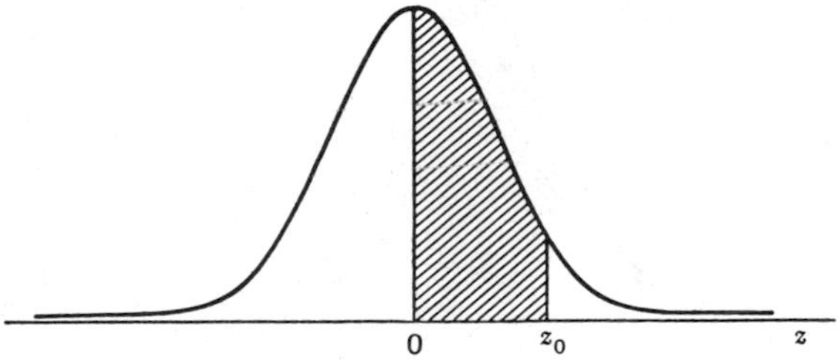

Figure 3.6.6. Area given by Appendix Table F.

Fortunately, we do not have to perform this integration, since there are tables available that provide the results of all such integrations in which we might be interested. Table F of the Appendix is an example of these tables. In the body of Table F are found the areas under the curve between 0 (the mean) and the values of z shown in the left-most column of the table. The shaded area in Figure 3.6.6 represents the area listed in the table as being between 0 and $z = z_0$.

We now illustrate the use of Table F by several examples.

Example 3.6.1

Given the unit normal distribution, find the area under the curve, above the z-axis between 0 and $z = 2$.

Solution. It will be helpful to draw a picture of the unit normal distribution and shade the desired area as in Figure 3.6.7. If we locate $z = 2$ in Table F and read the corresponding entry in the body of the table, we find the desired area to be .4772. We may interpret this area in several ways. We may interpret it as the probability that a z picked at random from the population of z's will have a value between 0 and 2. We may also interpret it as the relative frequency of occurrence (or proportion) of values of z between 0 and 2, or we may say that 47.72 percent of the z's have a value between 0 and 2.

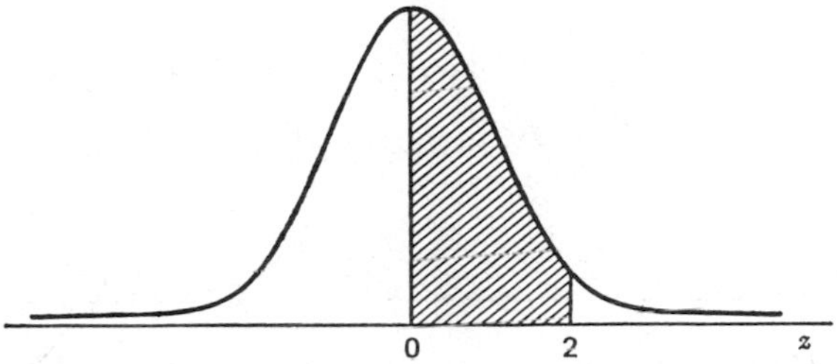

Figure 3.6.7. The unit normal distribution showing area between z = 0 and z = 2.

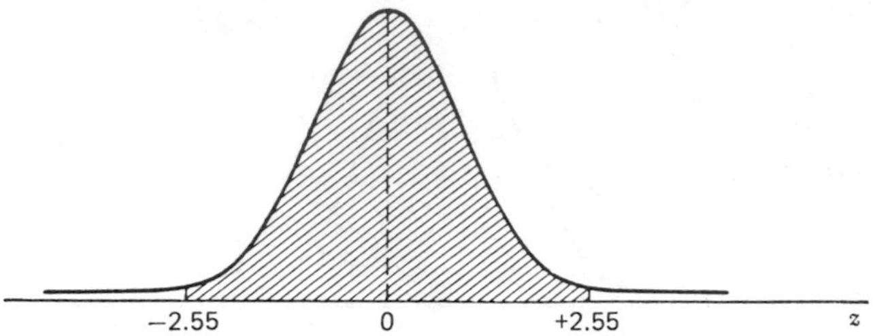

Figure 3.6.8. Unit normal curve showing P($-2.55 < z < 2.55$).

Example 3.6.2

What is the probability that a z picked at random from the population of z's will have a value between -2.55 and $+2.55$?

Solution. Figure 3.6.8 shows the area desired. Table F gives us the area between 0 and 2.55, which is found by locating 2.5 in the left-most column of the table and then moving across until we come to the entry in the column headed by .05. We find this area to be .4946. If we look at the picture we draw, we see that this is only part of the area desired, and if we recall that the normal distribution is symmetric about the mean, we realize that we have found exactly one half of the desired area. To obtain the total area desired we double .4946 to get .9892.

Example 3.6.3

What proportion of z values are between -2.74 and 1.53?

Solution. Figure 3.6.9 shows the area desired. We find in Table F that the area between 0 and 1.53 is .4370. Because of symmetry we know that the area between 0 and -2.74 is the same as the area between 0 and $+2.74$ which from the table, we find is .4969. To obtain the total area desired we add these two areas to get $.4370 + .4969 = .9339$.

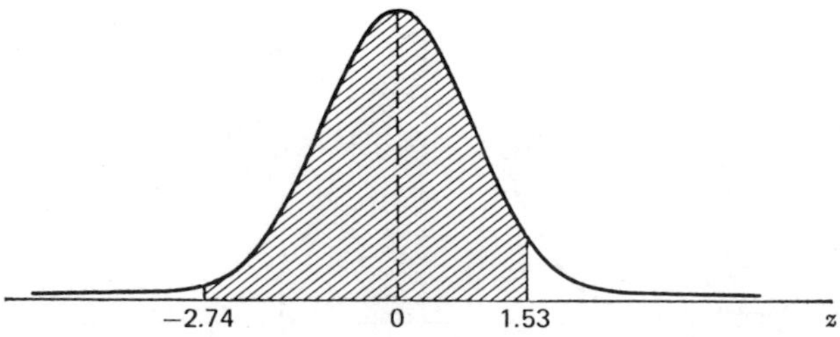

Figure 3.6.9. Unit normal curve showing proportion of z *values between* $z = -2.74$ *and* $z = 1.53$.

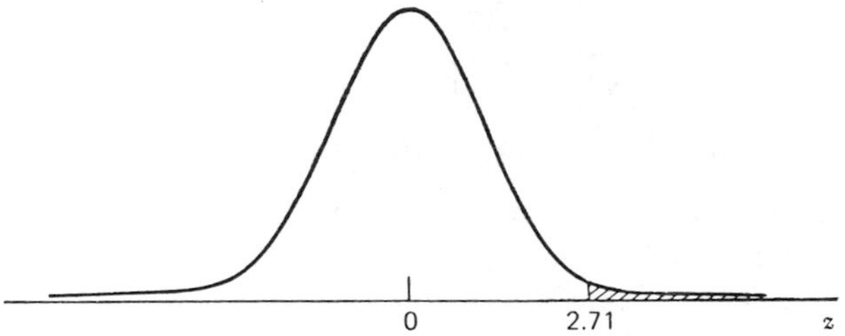

Figure 3.6.10. Unit normal distribution showing P(z ≥ *2.71*).

Example 3.6.4

Given the unit normal distribution find $P(z \geq 2.71)$.

Solution. The area desired is shown in Figure 3.6.10. We obtain the area to the right of $z = 2.71$ by subtracting the area between 0 and 2.71 from .5. Thus

$$\begin{aligned} P(z \geq 2.71) &= .5 - P(0 < z < 2.71) \\ &= .5 - .4966 \\ &= .0034 \end{aligned}$$

Example 3.6.5

Given the unit normal distribution find $P(.84 \leq z \leq 2.45)$.

Solution. The area we are looking for is shown in Figure 3.6.11. We first obtain the area between 0 and 2.45, and from that subtract the area between 0 and .84. In other words,

$$\begin{aligned} P(.84 \leq z \leq 2.45) &= P(0 \leq z \leq 2.45) - P(0 \leq z \leq .84) \\ &= .4929 - .2995 \\ &= .1934 \end{aligned}$$

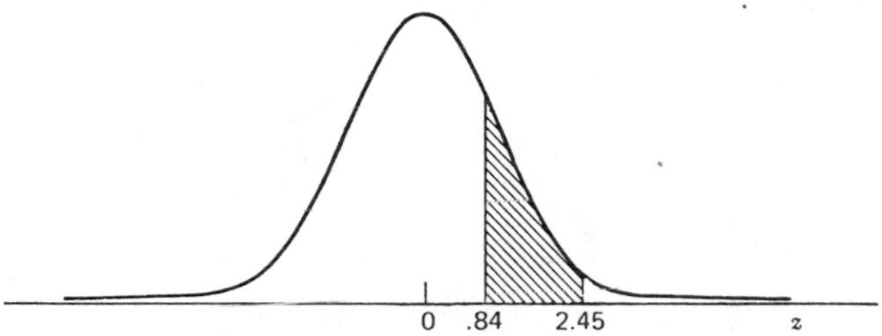

Figure 3.6.11. Unit normal curve showing P(*.84* ≤ z ≤ *2.45*).

Exercises

Given the unit normal distribution find:

3.6.1. The area under the curve between $z = 0$ and $z = 1.43$.

3.6.2. The probability that a z picked at random will have a value between $z = -2.87$ and $z = 2.64$.

3.6.3. $P(z \geq .55)$.

3.6.4. $P(z \geq -.55)$.

3.6.5. $P(z < -2.33)$.

3.6.6. $P(z < 2.33)$.

3.6.7. $P(-1.96 \leq z \leq 1.96)$.

3.6.8. $P(-2.58 \leq z \leq 2.58)$.

3.6.9. $P(-1.65 \leq z \leq 1.65)$.

3.6.10. $P(z = .74)$.

Applications. Although its importance in the field of statistics is indisputable, one should realize that the normal distribution is not a law that is adhered to by all measurable characteristics occurring in nature. It is true, however, that many of these characteristics are approximately normally distributed. Human stature and human intelligence are frequently cited as examples. On the other hand, Elveback et al. (4) and Nelson et al. (5) have pointed out that many distributions relevant to the health field cannot be described adequately by a normal distribution. Whenever it is known that a random variable is approximately normally distributed or when, in the absence of complete knowledge, it is considered reasonable to make this assumption, the statistician is aided tremendously in his or her efforts to solve practical problems relative to this variable.

There are several other reasons why the normal distribution is so important in statistics, and these will be considered in due time. For now, let us see how we may answer simple probability questions about random variables when we know, or are willing to assume, that they are, at least, approximately normally distributed.

Example 3.6.6

A physical therapist feels that scores on a certain manual dexterity test are approximately normally distributed with a mean of 10 and a standard deviation of 2.5. If a randomly selected individual takes the test, what is the probability that he or she will make a score of 15 or better?

Solution. First let us draw a picture of the distribution and shade the area corresponding to the probability of interest. This has been done in Figure 3.6.12.

If our distribution were the unit normal distribution with a mean of 0 and standard deviation of 1, we could make use of Table F and find the probability with little effort. Fortunately, it is possible for any normal distribution to be transformed easily to the unit normal. What we do is transform all values of X to corresponding values of z. This means that the mean of X must become 0, the mean of z. In Figure 3.6.13, both distributions are shown. We

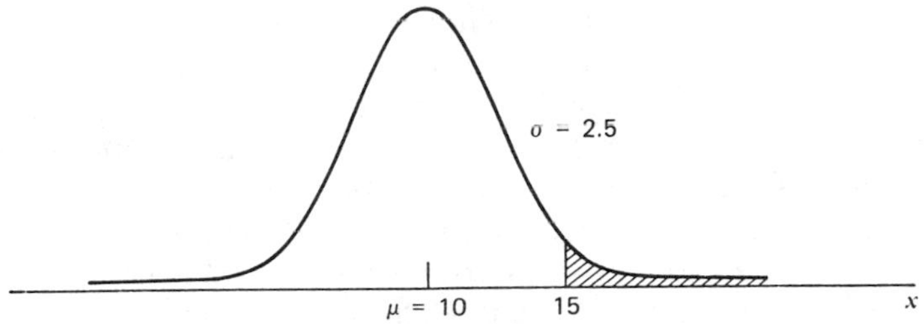

Figure 3.6.12. Normal distribution to approximate distribution of scores on a manual dexterity test

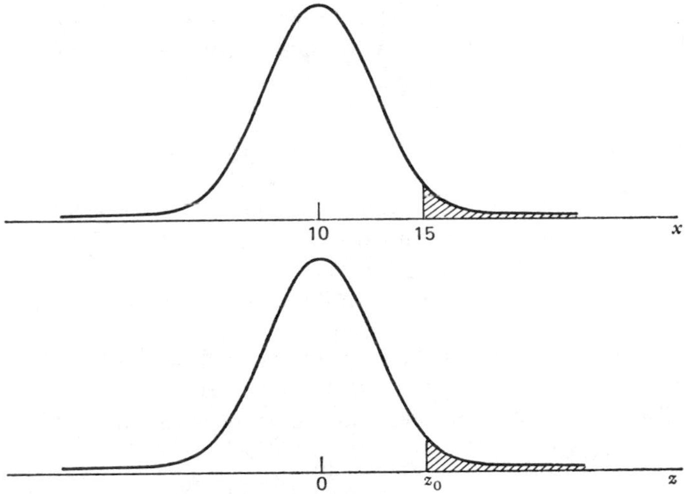

Figure 3.6.13. Normal distribution of manual dexterity scores (x) *and the unit normal distribution* (z).

must determine what value of z, say z_0, corresponds to an x of 15. This is done by the following formula:

$$z = \frac{x - \mu}{\sigma} \tag{3.6.3}$$

which transforms any value of x in any normal distribution to the corresponding value of z in the unit normal distribution. For the present example we have

$$z = \frac{15 - 10}{2.5} = \frac{5}{2.5} = 2$$

The value of z_0 we seek, then, is 2.

Let us examine these relationships more closely. It is seen that the distance from the mean, 10, to the x-value of interest, 15, is $15 - 10 = 5$, which is a distance of 2 standard deviations. When we transform x values to z values, the distance of the z value of interest from its mean, 0, is equal to the distance of the corresponding x value from its mean, 10, in standard deviation units. We have seen that this latter distance is 2 standard deviations. In the z distribution a standard deviation is equal to one, and consequently the point on the z scale located a distance of 2 standard deviations from 0 is $z = 2$, the result obtained by employing the formula. By consulting Table F, we find that the area to the right of $z = 2$ is .0228. We may summarize the above discussion as follows:

$$P(x \geq 15) = P\left(z \geq \frac{15 - 10}{2.5}\right) = P(z \geq 2) = .0228$$

To answer our original question, we say that the probability that a randomly chosen individual taking the test will make a score of 15 or better is .0228.

Example 3.6.7

Suppose it is known that the weights of a certain group of individuals are approximately normally distributed with a mean of 140 pounds and a standard deviation of 25 pounds. What is the probability that a person picked at random from this group will weigh between 100 and 170 pounds?

Solution. In Figure 3.6.14 are shown the distribution of weights and the z distribution to which we transform the original values to determine the desired probabilities. We find the z value corresponding to an x of 100 by

$$z = \frac{100 - 140}{25} = -1.6$$

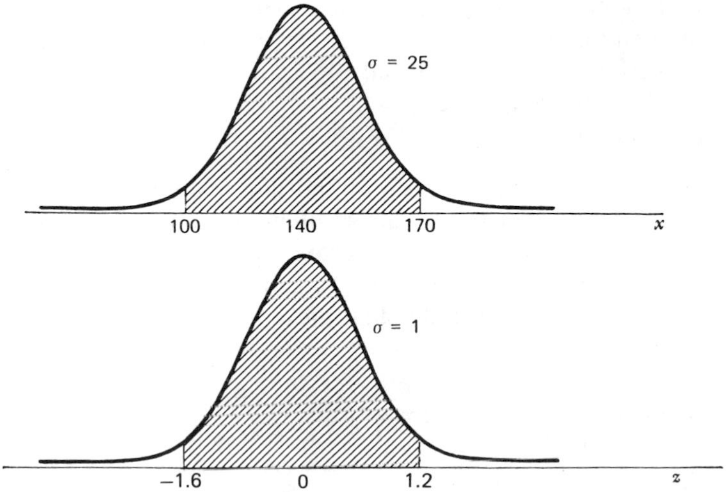

Figure 3.6.14. Distribution of weights (x) *and the corresponding unit normal distribution* (z).

Similarly for $x = 170$ we have

$$z = \frac{170 - 140}{25} = 1.2$$

From Table F we find the area between 0 and -1.6 to be .4452, and the area between 0 and 1.2 to be .3849. The area desired is the sum of these, .4452 + .3849 = .8301. To summarize

$$\begin{aligned} P(100 \le x \le 170) &= P\left(\frac{100 - 140}{25} \le z \le \frac{170 - 140}{25}\right) \\ &= P(-1.6 \le z \le 1.2) \\ &= P(-1.6 \le z \le 0) + P(0 \le z \le 1.2) \\ &= .4452 + .3849 \\ &= .8301 \end{aligned}$$

The probability asked for in our original question, then, is .8301.

Exercises

3.6.11. Suppose the ages at time of onset of a certain disease are approximately normally distributed with a mean of 11.5 years and a standard deviation of 3 years. A child has just come down with the disease. What is the probability that the child is:

(a) Between the ages of $8\frac{1}{2}$ and $14\frac{1}{2}$ years?
(b) Over 10 years of age?
(c) Under 12?

3.6.12. In the study of fingerprints an important quantitative characteristic is the total ridge count for the 10 fingers of an individual. Suppose that the total ridge counts of individuals in a certain population are approximately normally distributed with a mean of 140 and a standard deviation of 50. Find the probability that an individual picked at random from this population will have a ridge count:

(a) Of 200 or more.
(b) Less than 100.
(c) Between 100 and 200
(d) Between 200 and 250.

3.6.13. If the capacities of the cranial cavity of a certain population are approximately normally distributed with a mean of 1400 cc and a standard deviation of 125, find the probability that a person randomly picked from this population will have a cranial cavity capacity:

(a) Greater than 1450 cc.
(b) Less than 1350 cc.
(c) Between 1300 cc and 1500 cc.

3.6.14. Suppose the average length of stay in a chronic disease hospital of a certain type of patient is 60 days with a standard deviation of 15. If it is reasonable to assume an approximately normal distribution of lengths of stay, find the probability that a randomly selected patient from this group will have a length of stay

(a) Greater than 50 days.
(b) Less than 30 days.
(c) Between 30 and 60 days.
(d) Greater than 90 days.

3.6.15. If the total cholesterol values for a certain population are approximately normally distributed with a mean of 200 mg/100 ml and a standard deviation of 20 mg/100 ml, find the probability that an individual picked at random from this population will have a cholesterol value:

(a) Between 180 and 200 mg/100 ml.
(b) Greater than 225 mg/100 ml.
(c) Less than 150 mg/100 ml.
(d) Between 190 and 210 mg/100 ml.

3.6.16. Given a normally distributed population with a mean of 75 and a variance of 625, find:

(a) $P(50 \leq x \leq 100)$.
(b) $P(x > 90)$.
(c) $P(x < 60)$.
(d) $P(x \geq 85)$.
(e) $P(30 \leq x \leq 110)$.

3.7 SUMMARY

In the present chapter the concepts of probability described in the preceding chapter are further developed. The concepts of discrete and continuous random variables and their probability distributions are discussed. In particular, two discrete probability distributions, the binomial and the Poisson, and one continuous probability distribution, the normal, are examined in considerable detail. We have seen how these theoretical distributions allow us to make probability statements about certain random variables that are of interest to the health professional.

Review Questions and Exercises

1. What is a discrete random variable? Give three examples that are of interest to the health professional.
2. What is a continuous random variable? Give three examples of interest to the health professional.
3. Define the probability distribution of a discrete random variable.
4. Define the probability distribution of a continuous random variable.
5. What is a cumulative probability distribution?
6. What is a Bernoulli trial?
7. Describe the binomial distribution.
8. Give an example of a random variable which you think follows a binomial distribution.
9. Describe the Poisson distribution.
10. Give an example of a random variable that you think is distributed according to the Poisson law.
11. Describe the normal distribution.
12. Describe the unit normal distribution and tell how it is used in statistics.
13. Give an example of a random variable that you think is, at least, approximately normally distributed.
14. Using the data of your example 13 above, demonstrate the use of the unit normal distribution in answering probability questions relating to the variable selected.

15. The usual method for teaching a particular self-care skill to retarded persons is effective in 50 percent of the cases. A new method is tried with 10 persons. If the new method is no better than the standard, what is the probability that seven or more will learn the skill?

16. Personnel records of a large hospital show that 10 percent of housekeeping and maintenance employees quit within one year after being hired. If 10 new employees have just been hired,
    (a) what is the probability that exactly half of them will still be working after one year?
    (b) what is the probability that all will be working after one year?
    (c) what is the probability that three of the 10 will quit before the year is up.

17. In a certain developing country, 30 percent of the children are undernourished. In a random sample of 25 children from this area, what is the probability that the number of undernourished will be
    (a) exactly 10?
    (b) less than five?
    (c) five or more?
    (d) between three and five inclusive?
    (e) less than seven, but more than 4?

18. On the average, two students per hour report for treatment to the first aid room of a large elementary school.
    (a) What is the probability that during a given hour three students come to the first aid room for treatment?
    (b) What is the probability that during a given hour 2 or fewer students will report to the first aid room?
    (c) What is the probability that between 3 and 5 students, inclusive, will report to the first aid room during a given hour?

19. On the average, five smokers pass a certain street corner every ten minutes. What is the probability that during a given ten-minute period the number of smokers passing will be
    (a) six or fewer?
    (b) seven or more?
    (c) exactly eight?

20. In a certain metropolitan area there is an average of one suicide per month. What is the probability that during a given month the number of suicides will be
    (a) greater than one?
    (b) less than one?
    (c) greater than three?

21. The IQs of individuals admitted to a state school for the mentally retarded are approximately normally distributed with a mean of 60 and a standard deviation of 10.

(a) Find the proportion of individuals with IQs greater than 75.
(b) What is the probability that an individual picked at random will have an IQ between 55 and 75?
(c) Find $P(50 \leq X \leq 70)$.

22. A nurse supervisor has found that staff nurses, on the average, complete a certain task in 10 minutes. If the times required to complete the task are approximately normally distributed with a standard deviation of 3 minutes, find
    (a) the proportion of nurses completing the task in less than four minutes.
    (b) the proportion of nurses requiring more than five minutes to complete the task.
    (c) the probability that a nurse who has just been assigned the task will complete it within three minutes.
23. Scores made on a certain aptitude test by nursing students are approximately normally distributed with a mean of 500 and a variance of 10,000.
    (a) What proportion of those taking the test score below 200?
    (b) A person is about to take the test, what is the probability that he or she will make a score of 650 or more?
    (c) What proportion of scores fall between 350 and 675?
24. Given a binomial variable with a mean of 20 and a variance of 16, find n and p.
25. Suppose a variable X is normally distributed with a standard deviation of 10. Given that .0985 of the values of X are greater than 70, what is the mean value of X?

References

References cited

1. Norman L. Johnson and Samuel Kotz, *Discrete Distributions*, Houghton-Mifflin, Boston, 1969.
2. Frank A. Haight, *Handbook of the Poisson Distribution*, Wiley, New York, 1967.
3. Helen M. Walker, *Studies in the History of Statistical Method*, The Williams and Wilkins Company, Baltimore, 1931.
4. Lila R. Elveback, Claude L. Gulliver, and F. Raymond Deating, Jr., "Health, Normality and the Ghost of Gauss," *The Journal of the American Medical Association, 211* (1970), 69–75.
5. Jerald C. Nelson, Elizabeth Haynes, Rodney Willard, and Jan Kuzma, "The Distribution of Euthyroid Serum Protein-Bound Iodine Levels," *The Journal of the American Medical Association, 216* (1971), 1639–1641.

Other references

1. Sam Duker, "The Poisson Distribution in Educational Research," *Journal of Experimental Education, 23* (1955), 265–269.
2. M. S. Lafleur, P. R. Hinrichsen, P. C. Landry, and R. B. Moore, "The Poisson Distribution: An Experimental Approach to Teaching Statistics," *Physics Teacher, 10* (1972), 314–321.

4

SOME IMPORTANT SAMPLING DISTRIBUTIONS

4.1 INTRODUCTION

Before we examine the subject matter of the present chapter, let us review the high points of what we have covered thus far. In Chapter 1, the organization and summarization of data are emphasized. It is here that we encounter the concepts of central tendency and dispersion and learn how to compute their descriptive measures. In Chapter 2, we are introduced to the fundamental ideas of probability, and in Chapter 3, we consider the concept of a probability distribution. These concepts are fundamental to an understanding of statistical inference, the topic that comprises the major portion of this book.

The present chapter serves as a bridge between the preceding material, which is essentially descriptive in nature, and most of the remaining topics, which have been selected from the area of statistical inference.

4.2 SIMPLE RANDOM SAMPLING

Broadly speaking, there are two types of sampling, *probability sampling* and *nonprobability sampling*, but we consider only the former in this book. The reason is that only for probability sampling are there statistically sound procedures that allow us to infer, from the sample drawn, to the population of interest.

Definition

A probability sample is a sample drawn from a population in such a way that every member of the population has a known probability of being included in the sample.

From any finite population of size N, one may draw a number of different samples of size n. (This statement is made on the assumption that N is large enough to warrant sampling. As a rule, small populations, for obvious reasons, are not sampled.)

Definition

If a sample of size n *is drawn from a population of size* N *in such a way that every possible sample of size* n *has the same probability of being selected, the sample is called a* **simple random sample**.

The mechanics of drawing a sample to satisfy the definition of a simple random sample is called *simple random sampling.*

We shall demonstrate the procedure of simple random sampling shortly, but first let us consider the problem of whether to sample *with replacement* or *without replacement*. When sampling with replacement is employed, every member of the population is available at each draw. For example, suppose that we are drawing a sample from a population of former hospital patients as part of a study of length of stay. Let us assume that the sampling involves selecting from the shelves in the medical record department a sample of charts of discharged patients. In sampling with replacement we would proceed as follows: select a chart to be in the sample, record the length of stay, and return the chart to the shelf. The chart is back in the "population" and may be drawn again on some subsequent draw, in which case, the length of stay will again be recorded. In sampling without replacement, we would not replace a drawn chart to the shelf after recording the length of stay, but would lay it aside until the entire sample is drawn. Following this procedure, a given chart could appear in the sample only once. As a rule, in practice, sampling is always done without replacement. The significance and consequences of this will be explained later, but first let us see how one goes about selecting a simple random sample. To insure true randomness of selection we will need to follow some objective procedure. We certainly will want to avoid using our own judgment to decide which members of the population constitute a random sample.

Example 4.2.1

One way of selecting a simple random sample is to use a table of random numbers like that shown in Appendix Table G. Suppose our population of interest consists of the 150 fasting blood sugar values shown in Table 4.2.1.

From this population let us draw a simple random sample of size 10 using the random numbers in Table G. As the first step we locate a random

Table 4.2.1

Fasting Blood Sugar Values of 150 Apparently Normal Individuals

Subject Number	Value	Subject Number	Value	Subject Number	Value	Subject Number	Value	Subject Number	Value
1	91	31	107	61	87	91	91	121	90
2	94	32	94	62	104	92	104	122	105
3	115	33	101	63	109	93	109	123	100
4	85	34	95	64	93	94	92	124	89
5	89	35	80	65	95	95	85	125	90
6	107	36	104	66	107	96	108	126	106
7	94	37	94	67	88	97	99	127	94
8	105	38	102	68	107	98	103	128	100
9	94	39	89	69	113	99	81	129	92
10	103	40	98	70	95	100	96	130	91
11	104	41	106	71	102	101	105	131	87
12	105	42	85	72	94	102	91	132	105
13	88	43	93	73	99	103	115	133	102
14	107	44	103	74	87	104	108	134	101
15	90	45	119	75	102	105	102	135	111
16	95	46	90	76	105	106	101	136	91
17	104	47	82	77	80	107	94	137	92
18	93	48	90	78	90	108	93	138	98
19	109	49	113	79	108	109	102	139	81
20	87	50	104	80	105	110	119	140	117
21	92	51	97	81	90	111	96	141	103
22	117	52	101	82	115	112	104	142	96
23	98	53	90	83	82	113	85	143	101
24	89	54	88	84	90	114	108	144	88
25	105	55	108	85	102	115	103	145	100
26	101	56	95	86	91	116	90	146	100
27	81	57	100	87	103	117	105	147	95
28	108	58	103	88	107	118	99	148	103
29	94	59	108	89	107	119	88	149	101
30	104	60	85	90	97	120	103	150	90

starting point in the table. This can be done in a number of ways, one of which is to look away from the page while touching it with the point of a pencil. The random starting point is the digit closest to where the pencil touched the page. Let us assume that following this procedure led to a random starting point in Table G at the intersection of row 21 and column 28. The digit at this point is 5. Since we have 150 values to choose from, we can use only the random numbers 1 through 150. It will be convenient to pick three-digit numbers so that the numbers 001 through 150 will be the only eligible numbers. The first three-digit number, beginning at our random starting point, is 532, a number we cannot use. Let us move down past

Table 4.2.2

Sample of 10 Fasting Blood Sugar Values Drawn from Data in Table 4.2.1

Random Number	Sample Subject Number	Value
137	1	92
114	2	108
028	3	108
085	4	102
018	5	93
042	6	85
053	7	90
108	8	93
144	9	88
126	10	106

196, 372, 654, and 928 until we come to 137, a number we can use. The 137th value from Table 4.2.1 is 92, the first value in our sample. We record the random number, and the corresponding fasting blood sugar value, in Table 4.2.2. We record the random number to keep track of the random numbers selected. Since we want to sample without replacement, we do not want to include the same individual's value twice. Proceeding in the manner just described leads us to the remaining nine random numbers and their corresponding blood sugar values shown in Table 4.2.2. Notice that when we get to the end of the column we simply move over three digits to 028 and proceed up the column. We could have started at the top with the number 369.

Thus we have drawn a simple random sample of size 10 from a population of size 150. In future discussion, whenever the term simple random sample is used, it will be understood that the sample has been drawn in this or an equivalent manner.

Exercises

4.2.1. Using the table of random numbers, select a new random starting point, and draw another simple random sample of size 10 from the data in Table 4.2.1.

4.2.2. Draw a simple random sample of size 5 from the data in Table 1.6.1.

4.3 SAMPLING DISTRIBUTIONS

We come now to the main topic of this chapter, *sampling distributions*. The importance of a clear understanding of sampling distributions cannot be overemphasized, as this concept is the very key to the understanding of statistical inference. Let us begin with the following definition.

Definition

The distribution of all possible values which can be assumed by some statistic, computed from samples of the same size randomly drawn from the same population, is called the **sampling distribution** *of that statistic.*

Sampling distributions may be constructed empirically when sampling from a discrete, finite population. To construct a sampling distribution we proceed as follows.

1. From a discrete, finite population of size N, randomly draw all possible samples of size n.
2. Compute the statistic of interest for each sample.
3. List in one column the different distinct observed values of the statistic and, in another column, list the corresponding frequency of occurrence of each distinct observed value of the statistic.

The actual construction of a sampling distribution is a formidable undertaking if the population is of any appreciable size and is an impossible task if the population is infinite. In such cases, sampling distributions may be approximated by taking a large number of samples of a given size.

We usually are interested in knowing three things about a given sampling distribution: its mean, its variance, and its functional form (how it looks when graphed).

We can recognize the difficulty of constructing a sampling distribution according to the steps given above when the population is of any appreciable size. We also run into a problem when considering the construction of a sampling distribution for a continuous variable. The best we can do experimentally in this case is to approximate the sampling distribution of a statistic.

Both of these problems may be obviated by means of mathematics. Although the procedures involved are not compatible with the mathematical level of this text, sampling distributions can be derived mathematically. The interested reader can consult one of many mathematical statistics textbooks, for example, Hoel (1), and Anderson and Bancroft (2).

In the sections that follow some of the more frequently encountered sampling distributions are discussed.

4.4 DISTRIBUTION OF THE SAMPLE MEAN

An important sampling distribution is the distribution of the sample mean. Let us see how we might construct this sampling distribution by following the steps outlined in the previous section.

Example 4.4.1

Suppose we have a population of size $N = 5$, consisting of the ages of five children who are outpatients in a community mental health center. The

Table 4.4.1

All Possible Samples of Size $n = 2$ from a Population of Size $N = 5$. Samples Above or Below the Principal Diagonal Result When Sampling Is Without Replacement. Sample Means are in Parentheses.

		Second Draw				
		6	8	10	12	14
First Draw	6	6, 6 (6)	6, 8 (7)	6, 10 (8)	6, 12 (9)	6, 14 (10)
	8	8, 6 (7)	8, 8 (8)	8, 10 (9)	8, 12 (10)	8, 14 (11)
	10	10, 6 (8)	10, 8 (9)	10, 10 (10)	10, 12 (11)	10, 14 (12)
	12	12, 6 (9)	12, 8 (10)	12, 10 (11)	12, 12 (12)	12, 14 (13)
	14	14, 6 (10)	14, 8 (11)	14, 10 (12)	14, 12 (13)	14, 14 (14)

ages are as follows: $x_1 = 6$, $x_2 = 8$, $x_3 = 10$, $x_4 = 12$, and $x_5 = 14$. The mean, μ, of this population is equal to $\sum x_i/N = 10$ and the variance

$$\sigma^2 = \frac{\sum(x_i - \mu)^2}{N} = \frac{40}{5} = 8$$

Let us compute another measure of dispersion as follows:

$$S^2 = \frac{\sum(x_i - \mu)^2}{N - 1} = \frac{40}{4} = 10$$

We will refer to this quantity again in the next chapter. Let us draw all possible samples of size $n = 2$ from this population. These samples, along with their means, are shown in Table 4.4.1.

We see in this example that when sampling is with replacement, there are 25 possible samples. In general, when sampling with replacement, the number of possible samples is equal to N^n.

We may construct the sampling distribution of $\bar{x}$ by listing the different values of $\bar{x}$ in one column and their frequency of occurrence in another, as in Table 4.4.2.

We see that the data of Table 4.4.2 satisfy the requirements for a probability distribution. The individual probabilities are all greater than zero, and their sum is equal to 1.

It was stated earlier that we are usually interested in the functional form of a sampling distribution, its mean, and its variance.

Table 4.4.2

Sampling Distribution of $\bar{x}$ Computed from Samples in Table 4.4.1

$\bar{x}$	**Frequency**	**Relative Frequency**
6	1	1/25
7	2	2/25
8	3	3/25
9	4	4/25
10	5	5/25
11	4	4/25
12	3	3/25
13	2	2/25
14	1	1/25
Total	25	25/25

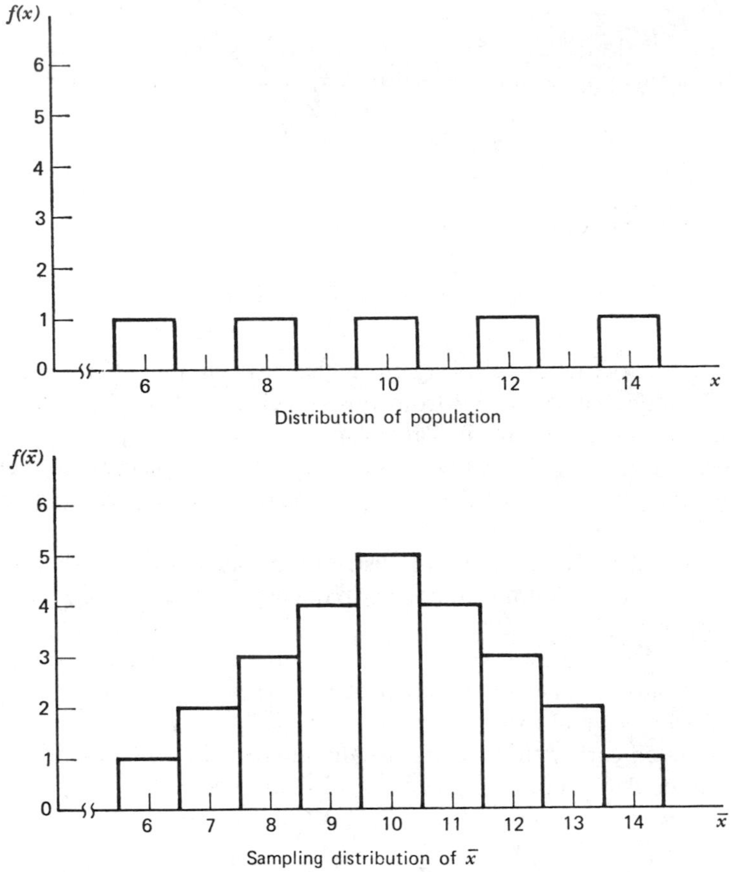

Figure 4.4.1. Distribution of population and sampling distribution of $\bar{x}$.

Let us look at the distribution of $\bar{x}$ plotted as a histogram, along with the distribution of the population, both of which are shown in Figure 4.4.1. The reader is no doubt impressed with the radical difference in appearance between the histogram of the population and the histogram of the sampling distribution of $\bar{x}$. Whereas the former is uniformly distributed, the latter gradually rises to a peak and then drops off with perfect symmetry. Now let us compute the mean, which we will call $\mu_{\bar{x}}$, of our sampling distribution. To do this we add the 25 sample means and divide by 25. Thus

$$\mu_{\bar{x}} = \frac{\sum \bar{x}_i}{N^n} = \frac{6 + 7 + 7 + 8 + \cdots + 14}{25} = \frac{250}{25} = 10$$

We note with interest that the mean of the sampling distribution of $\bar{x}$ has the same value as the mean of the original population.

Finally, we may compute the variance of $\bar{x}$, which we call $\sigma_{\bar{x}}^2$, as follows:

$$\sigma_{\bar{x}}^2 = \frac{\sum(\bar{x}_i - \mu_{\bar{x}})^2}{N^n}$$

$$= \frac{(6-10)^2 + (7-10)^2 + (7-10)^2 + \cdots + (14-10)^2}{25}$$

$$= \frac{100}{25} = 4$$

We note that the variance of the sampling distribution is not equal to the population variance. It is of interest to observe, however, that the variance of the sampling distribution is equal to the population variance divided by the size of the sample used to obtain the sampling distribution. That is,

$$\sigma_{\bar{x}}^2 = \frac{\sigma^2}{n} = \frac{8}{2} = 4$$

The square root of the variance of the sampling distribution, $\sqrt{\sigma_{\bar{x}}^2} = \sigma/\sqrt{n}$, is called the *standard error of the mean* or, simply, the *standard error.*

These results are not coincidences but are examples of the characteristics of sampling distributions in general, when sampling is with replacement or when sampling is from an infinite population. To generalize, we distinguish between two situations: sampling from a normally distributed population and sampling from a nonnormally distributed population.

When sampling is from a normally distributed population, the distribution of the sample mean will possess the following properties:

1. *The distribution of* $\bar{x}$ *will be normal.*
2. *The mean,* $\mu_{\bar{x}}$, *of the distribution of* $\bar{x}$ *will be equal to the mean of the population from which the samples were drawn.*
3. *The variance,* $\sigma_{\bar{x}}^2$, *of the distribution of* $\bar{x}$ *will be equal to the variance of the population divided by the sample size.*

For the case where sampling is from a nonnormally distributed population, we refer to an important mathematical theorem known as the *central limit theorem.* The importance of this theorem in statistical inference may be summarized in the following statement.

CENTRAL LIMIT THEOREM

Given a population of any functional form with a mean, μ, *and finite variance,* σ^2, *the sampling distribution of* $\bar{x}$, *computed from samples of size* n *from this population, will be approximately normally distributed with mean,* μ, *and variance,* $\sigma^2/$n, *when the sample size is large.*

Note that the central limit theorem allows us to sample from nonnormally distributed populations with a guarantee of approximately the same results as would be obtained if the populations were normally distributed provided that we take a large sample.

The importance of this will become evident later when we learn that a normally distributed sampling distribution is a powerful tool in statistical inference. In the case of the sample mean, we are assured of at least an approximately normally distributed sampling distribution under three conditions: (1) when sampling from a normally distributed population; (2) when sampling from a nonnormally distributed population and our sample is large; (3) when sampling from a population whose functional form is unknown to us so long as our sample size is large.

The logical question that arises at this point is: How large does the sample have to be in order for the central limit theorem to apply? There is no one answer, since the size of the sample needed depends on the extent of nonnormality present in the population. One rule of thumb states that, in most practical situations, a sample of size 30 is satisfactory. Let us add that, in general, the approximation to normality of the sampling distribution of $\bar{x}$ becomes better and better as the sample size increases.

The above results have been given on the assumption that sampling is either with replacement or that the samples are drawn from infinite populations. In general, we do not sample with replacement, and in many practical situations it may be necessary to sample from a finite population; hence, we need to become familiar with the behavior of the sampling distribution of the sample mean under these conditions. Before making any general statements, let us again look at the data in Table 4.4.1. The sample means that result when sampling is without replacement are those above the principal diagonal, which are the same as those below the principal diagonal, if we ignore the order in which the observations were drawn. We see that there are 10 possible samples. In general, when drawing samples of size n from a finite population of size N without replacement, and ignoring the order in which the sample values are drawn, the number of possible samples is given by the combination of N things taken n at a time. In our present example we have

$$\binom{N}{n} = \frac{N!}{n!(N-n)!} = \frac{5!}{2!3!} = \frac{5 \cdot 4 \cdot 3!}{2!3!} = 10 \text{ possible samples}$$

The mean of the 10 sample means is

$$\mu_{\bar{x}} = \frac{\sum x_i}{\binom{N}{n}} = \frac{7 + 8 + 9 + \cdots + 13}{10} = \frac{100}{10} = 10$$

We see that once again the mean of the sampling distribution is equal to the population mean.

The variance of this sampling distribution is found to be

$$\sigma_{\bar{x}}^2 = \frac{\sum(\bar{x}_i - \mu_{\bar{x}})^2}{\binom{N}{n}} = \frac{30}{10} = 3$$

and we note that this time the variance of the sampling distribution is not equal to the population variance divided by the sample size, since $\sigma_{\bar{x}}^2 = 3 \neq 8/2 = 4$. There is, however, an interesting relationship which we discover by multiplying σ^2/n by $(N - n)/(N - 1)$. That is

$$\frac{\sigma^2}{n} \cdot \frac{N-n}{N-1} = \frac{8}{2} \cdot \frac{5-2}{4} = 3$$

This result tells us that if we multiply the variance of the sampling distribution that would be obtained if sampling were with replacement, by the factor $(N - n)/(N - 1)$, we obtain the value of the variance of the sampling distribution that results when sampling without replacement. We may generalize these results with the following statement.

When sampling is without replacement from a finite population the sampling distribution of $\bar{x}$ *will have mean* μ *and variance,*

$$\frac{\sigma^2}{n} \cdot \frac{N-n}{N-1}$$

If the sample size is large, the central limit theorem applies and the sampling distribution of $\bar{x}$ will be approximately normally distributed.

The factor $(N - n)/(N - 1)$ is called the finite population correction and can be ignored when the sample size is small in comparison with the population size. When the population is much larger than the sample, the difference between σ^2/n and $(\sigma^2/n)[(N - n)/(N - 1)]$ will be negligible. Suppose a population contains 10,000 observations and a sample from this population consists of 25 observations, the finite population correction would be equal to $(10{,}000 - 25)/(9999) = .9976$. To multiply .9976 times σ^2/n is almost equivalent to multiplying by 1. Most practicing statisticians do not use the finite population correction unless the sample contains more than 5 percent of the observations in the population. That is, the finite population correction is usually ignored when $n/N \leq .05$.

Applications. As we shall see in succeeding chapters, a knowledge and understanding of sampling distributions will be a necessary requirement for understanding the concepts of statistical inference. The simplest application of our knowledge of the sampling distribution of the sample mean is in computing the probability of obtaining a sample with a mean of some specified magnitude. Let us illustrate with some examples.

Example 4.4.2

Suppose it is known that in a certain large human population, cranial length is approximately normally distributed with a mean of 185.6 mm and a standard deviation of 12.7 mm. What is the probability that a random sample of size 10 from this population will have a mean greater than 190?

Solution. We know that the single sample under consideration is one of the all possible samples of size 10 which can be drawn from the population, so that the mean which it yields is one of the $\bar{x}$'s constituting the sampling distribution of $\bar{x}$ which, theoretically, could be derived from this population.

When we say that the population is approximately normally distributed, we assume that the sampling distribution of $\bar{x}$ will be, for all practical purposes, normally distributed. We also know that the mean and standard deviation of the sampling distribution are equal to 185.6 and $\sqrt{(12.7)^2/10} = 12.7/\sqrt{10} = 4.02$, respectively. We assume that the population is large relative to the sample so that the finite population correction can be ignored.

We learned in the preceding chapter that whenever we have a random variable that is normally distributed, we may very easily transform it to the unit normal distribution. Our random variable now is $\bar{x}$, the mean of its distribution is $\mu_{\bar{x}}$, and its standard deviation is $\sigma_{\bar{x}} = \sigma/\sqrt{n}$. By appropriately modifying the formula given previously, we arrive at the following formula for transforming the normal distribution of $\bar{x}$ to the unit normal distribution.

$$z = \frac{\bar{x} - \mu_{\bar{x}}}{\sigma/\sqrt{n}} \tag{4.4.1}$$

The probability that answers our question is represented by the area to the right of $\bar{x} = 190$ under the curve of the sampling distribution. This area is equal to the area to the right of

$$z = \frac{190 - 185.6}{4.02} = \frac{4.4}{4.02} = 1.09$$

By consulting the unit normal table we find that the area to the right of 1.09 is .1379; hence, we say that the probability is .1379 that a sample of size 10 will have a mean greater than 190.

Figure 4.4.2 shows the relationship between the original population, the sampling distribution of $\bar{x}$, and the unit normal distribution.

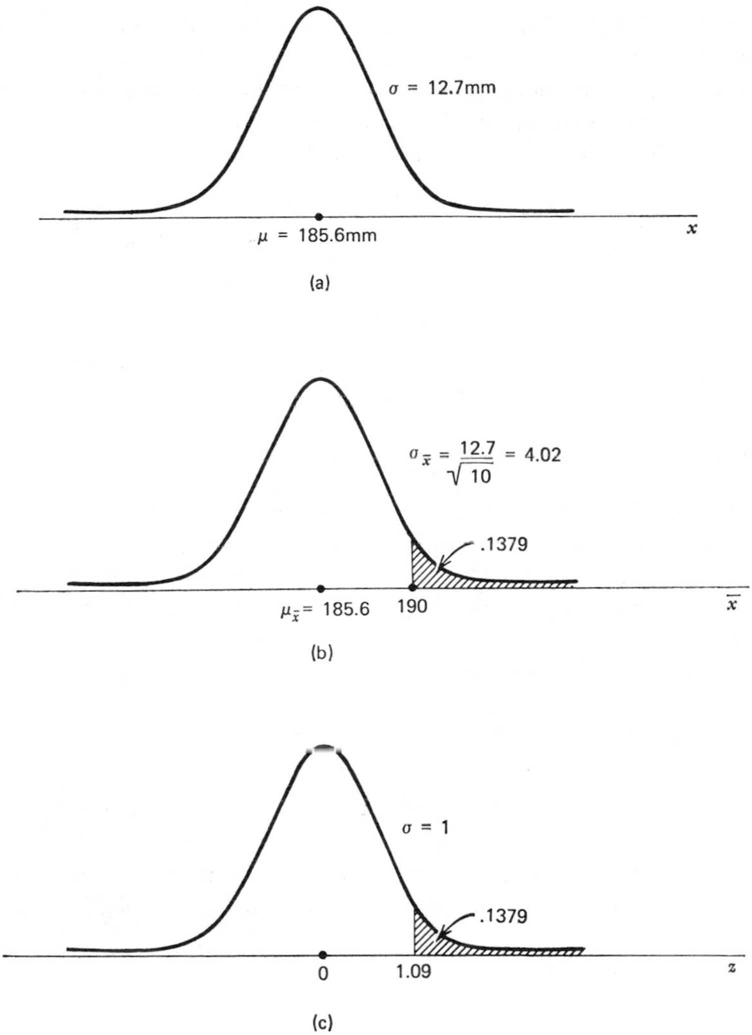

Figure 4.4.2. Population distribution, sampling distribution and unit normal distribution, Example 4.4.3. (a) Population distribution. (b) Sampling distribution of $\bar{x}$ for samples of size 10. (c) Unit normal distribution.

Example 4.4.3

If the mean and standard deviation of serum iron values for healthy men are 120 and 15 micrograms per 100 ml, respectively, what is the probability that a random sample of 50 normal men will yield a mean between 115 and 125 micrograms per 100 ml?

Solution. The functional form of the population of serum iron values is not specified, but since we have a sample size greater than 30, we make use of the central limit theorem and transform the resulting approximately normal sampling distribution of $\bar{x}$ (which has a mean of 120 and a standard deviation of $15/\sqrt{50} = 2.12$) to the unit normal. The probability we seek is

$$
\begin{aligned}
P(115 \leq \bar{x} \leq 125) &= P\left(\frac{115 - 120}{2.12} \leq z \leq \frac{125 - 120}{2.12}\right) \\
&= P(-2.36 \leq z \leq 2.36) \\
&= 2(.4909) \\
&= .9818
\end{aligned}
$$

Exercises

4.4.1. Suppose it is known that the hourly wages of a certain type of hospital employee are approximately normally distributed with a mean and standard deviation of \$4.50 and \$.50, respectively. If a random sample of size 16 is selected from this population, find the probability that the mean hourly wage for the sample will be:

(a) Greater than \$4.25.
(b) Between \$4.25 and \$4.75.
(c) Greater than \$4.80.
(d) Less than \$4.20.

4.4.2. It has been found that, following a period of training, the mean time required for certain handicapped persons to perform a particular task is 25 seconds with a standard deviation of 5 seconds. Assuming a normal distribution of times, find the probability that a sample of 25 individuals will yield a mean:

(a) Of 26 seconds or more.
(b) Between 24 and 27 seconds.
(c) 26 seconds or less.
(d) Greater than 22 seconds.

4.4.3. If the uric acid values in normal adult males are approximately normally distributed with a mean and standard deviation of 5.7 and 1 mgs percent respectively, find the probability that a sample of size 9 will yield a mean:

(a) Greater than 6.
(b) Between 5 and 6.
(c) Less than 5.2.

4.4.4. For a certain large segment of the population, for a particular year, suppose the mean number of days of disability is 5.4 with a standard deviation of 2.8 days. Find the probability that a random sample of size 49 from this population will have a mean:

(a) Greater than 6 days.
(b) Between 4 and 6 days.
(c) Between $4\frac{1}{2}$ and $5\frac{1}{2}$ days.

4.4.5. Given a normally distributed population with a mean of 100 and a standard deviation of 20, find the following probabilities based on a sample of size 16:

(a) $P(\bar{x} \geq 100)$.
(b) $P(96 \leq \bar{x} \leq 108)$.
(c) $P(\bar{x} \leq 110)$.

4.4.6. Given: $\mu = 50$, $\sigma = 16$, $n = 64$, find:

(a) $P(45 \leq \bar{x} \leq 55)$.
(b) $P(\bar{x} > 53)$.
(c) $P(\bar{x} < 47)$.
(d) $P(49 \leq \bar{x} \leq 56)$.

4.5 DISTRIBUTION OF THE DIFFERENCE BETWEEN TWO SAMPLE MEANS

Frequently the interest in an investigation is focused on two populations. Specifically, an investigator may wish to know something about the difference between two population means. In one investigation, for example, a researcher may wish to know if it is reasonable to conclude that two population means are different. In another situation, the researcher may desire knowledge about the magnitude of the difference between two population means. A medical research team, for example, may want to know whether or not the mean serum cholesterol level is higher in a population of sedentary office workers than in a population of laborers. If the researchers are able to conclude that the population means are different they may wish to know by how much they differ. A knowledge of the sampling distribution of the difference between two means is useful in investigations of this type.

Example 4.5.1

Suppose we have two groups of individuals—one group (Group 1) has experienced some condition felt to be associated with mental retardation, and the other group (Group 2) has not experienced the condition. The distribution of intelligence scores in each of the two groups is believed to be approximately normally distributed with a standard deviation of 20.

Suppose, further, that we take a sample of 15 individuals from each group and compute for each sample the mean intelligence score with the following results: $\bar{x}_1 = 92$ and $\bar{x}_2 = 105$. If there is no difference between the two groups, with respect to their true mean intelligence scores, what is the probability of observing this large a difference between sample means?

To answer this question we need to know the nature of the sampling distribution of the relevant statistic, the *difference between two sample means*, $\bar{x}_1 - \bar{x}_2$. Notice that we seek a probability associated with the difference between two sample means rather than a single mean.

Although, in practice, we would not attempt to construct the desired sampling distribution, we can conceptualize the manner in which it could be done when sampling is from finite populations. We would begin by selecting from Group 1 all possible samples of size 15 and computing the mean for each sample. We know that there would be $\binom{N_1}{n_1}$ such samples where N_1 is the group size and $n_1 = 15$. Similarly, we would select all possible samples of size 15 from Group 2 and compute the mean for each of these samples. We would then take all possible pairs of sample means, one from Group 1 and one from Group 2, and take the difference. Table 4.5.1 shows the results of following this procedure.

It is the distribution of the differences between sample means that we seek. If we plotted the sample differences against their frequency of occurrence, we would obtain a normal distribution with a mean equal to $\mu_1 - \mu_2$, the difference between the true group, or population, means, and a variance equal to $(\sigma_1^2/n_1) + (\sigma_2^2/n_2)$.

For our present example we would have a normal distribution with a mean of 0 (if there is no difference between the true population means) and a variance of $[(20)^2/15] + [(20)^2/15] = 53.3$. The graph of the sampling distribution is shown in Figure 4.5.1.

Table 4.5.1

Working Table for Constructing the Distribution of the Difference Between Two Sample Means

Samples from Group 1	**Samples from Group 2**	**Sample Means Group 1**	**Sample Means Group 2**	**All Possible Differences Between Means**
n_{11}	n_{12}	$\bar{x}_{11}$	$\bar{x}_{12}$	$\bar{x}_{11} - \bar{x}_{12}$
n_{21}	n_{22}	$\bar{x}_{21}$	$\bar{x}_{22}$	$\bar{x}_{11} - \bar{x}_{22}$
n_{31}	n_{32}	$\bar{x}_{31}$	$\bar{x}_{32}$	$\bar{x}_{11} - \bar{x}_{32}$
$\vdots$	$\vdots$	$\vdots$	$\vdots$	$\vdots$
$n_{\binom{N_1}{n_1}1}$	$n_{\binom{N_2}{n_2}2}$	$\bar{x}_{\binom{N_1}{n_1}1}$	$\bar{x}_{\binom{N_2}{n_2}2}$	$\bar{x}_{\binom{N_1}{n_1}1} - \bar{x}_{\binom{N_2}{n_2}2}$

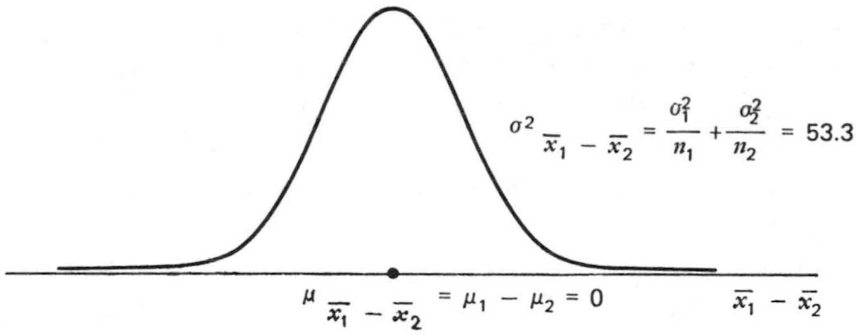

Figure 4.5.1. Graph of the sampling distribution of $\bar{x}_1 - \bar{x}_2$ when there is no difference between population means, Example 4.5.1.

We know that this normal distribution can be transformed to the unit normal distribution by means of a modification of a previously learned formula. The new formula is as follows:

$$z = \frac{(\bar{x}_1 - \bar{x}_2) - (\mu_1 - \mu_2)}{\sqrt{\dfrac{\sigma_1^{\,2}}{n_1} + \dfrac{\sigma_2^{\,2}}{n_2}}} \tag{4.5.1}$$

The area under the curve of $\bar{x}_1 - \bar{x}_2$ corresponding to the probability we seek is the area to the left of $\bar{x}_1 - \bar{x}_2 = 92 - 105 = -13$. The z value corresponding to -13, assuming there is no difference between population means, is

$$z = \frac{-13 - 0}{\sqrt{\dfrac{(20)^2}{15} + \dfrac{(20)^2}{15}}} = \frac{-13}{\sqrt{53.3}} = \frac{-13}{7.3} = -1.78$$

By consulting Table F, we find that the area under the unit normal curve to the left of -1.78 is equal to $.5 - .4625 = .0375$. In answer to our original question, we say that if there is no difference between population means, the probability of obtaining a difference between sample means as large as or larger than 13 is .0375.

The procedure we have just followed is valid even when the sample sizes, n_1 and n_2, are different and when the population variances, $\sigma_1^{\,2}$ and $\sigma_2^{\,2}$ have different values. The theoretical results on which this procedure is based may be summarized as follows.

Given two normally distributed populations with means, μ_1 and μ_2, and variances, $\sigma_1^{\,2}$ and $\sigma_2^{\,2}$, respectively, the sampling distribution of the difference, $\bar{x}_1 - \bar{x}_2$, between the means of independent samples of size n_1 and n_2 drawn from these populations is normally distributed with mean, $\mu_1 - \mu_2$, and variance, $(\sigma_1^{\,2}/n_1) + (\sigma_2^{\,2}/n_2)$.

Sampling from Nonnormal Populations. Many times a researcher is faced with one or the other of the following problems: the necessity of (1) sampling from nonnormally distributed populations, or (2) sampling from populations whose functional forms are not known. A solution to these problems is to take large samples, since when the sample sizes are large the central limit theorem applies and the distribution of the difference between two sample means is approximately normally distributed with a mean equal to $\mu_1 - \mu_2$ and a variance of $(\sigma_1{}^2/n_1) + (\sigma_2{}^2/n_2)$. To find probabilities associated with specific values of the statistic, then, our procedure would be the same as that given above when sampling from normally distributed populations.

Example 4.5.2

Suppose it has been established that for a certain type client the average length of a home visit by a public health nurse is 45 minutes with a standard deviation of 15 minutes, and that for a second type client the average home visit is 30 minutes long with a standard deviation of 20 minutes. If a nurse randomly visits 35 clients from the first and 40 from the second group, what is the probability that the average length of home visit will differ between the two groups by as much as 20 minutes?

Solution. No mention is made of the functional form of the two populations, so let us assume that this characteristic is either unknown, or that the populations are not normally distributed. Since the sample sizes are large (greater than 30) in both cases, we draw on the results of the central limit theorem to answer the question posed. We know that the difference between sample means is approximately normally distributed with the following mean and variance:

$$\mu_{\bar{x}_1 - \bar{x}_2} = \mu_1 - \mu_2 = 45 - 30 = 15$$

$$\sigma^2_{\bar{x}_1 - \bar{x}_2} = \frac{\sigma_1{}^2}{n_1} + \frac{\sigma_2{}^2}{n_2} = \frac{(15)^2}{35} + \frac{(20)^2}{40} = 16.4286$$

The area under the curve of $\bar{x}_1 - \bar{x}_2$ which we seek is that area to the right of 20. The corresponding value of z in the unit normal is

$$z = \frac{(\bar{x}_1 - \bar{x}_2) - (\mu_1 - \mu_2)}{\sqrt{\dfrac{\sigma_1{}^2}{n_1} + \dfrac{\sigma_2{}^2}{n_2}}} = \frac{20 - 15}{\sqrt{16.4286}} = \frac{5}{4.05} = 1.23$$

In Table F we find the area to the right of $z = 1.23$ is $.5 - .3907 = .1093$. We say, then, that the probability of the nurse's random visits resulting in a difference between the two groups as great or greater than 20 minutes is .1093. The curve of $\bar{x}_1 - \bar{x}_2$ and the corresponding unit normal curve are shown in Figure 4.5.2.

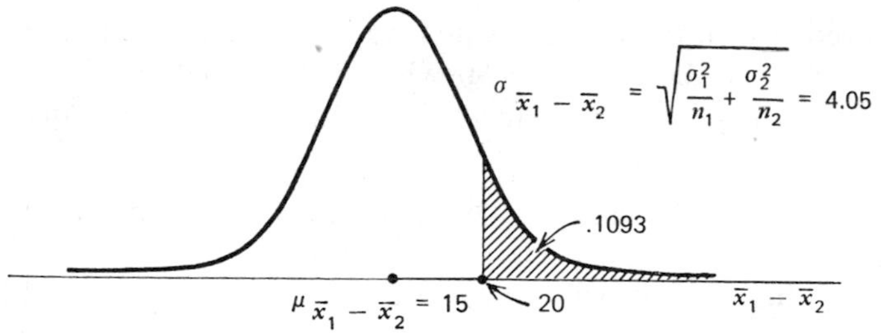

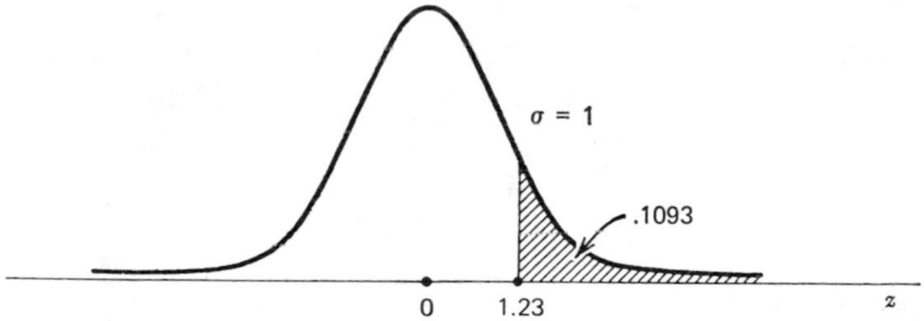

Figure 4.5.2. Sampling distribution of $\bar{x}_1 - \bar{x}_2$ *and the corresponding unit normal distribution, home visit example.*

Exercises

4.5.1. A researcher is willing to assume that levels of vitamin A in the livers of two human populations are each normally distributed. The variances for the two populations are assumed to be as follows:

Population 1: $\sigma_1{}^2 = 19{,}600$

Population 2: $\sigma_2{}^2 = 8100$

What is the probability that a random sample of size 15 from the first population and 10 from the second population will yield a value of $\bar{x}_1 - \bar{x}_2$ greater than or equal to 50 if there is no difference in the population means?

4.5.2. In a study of annual family expenditures for general health care, two populations were surveyed with the following results:

Population 1: $n_1 = 40$, $\bar{x}_1 = \$346$

Population 2: $n_2 = 35$, $\bar{x}_2 = 300$

If it is known that the population variances are $\sigma_1{}^2 = 2800$ and $\sigma_2{}^2 = 3250$, what is the probability of obtaining sample results as extreme as those shown above if there is no difference in the means of the two populations?

4.5.3. Given two normally distributed populations with equal means and variances of $\sigma_1^2 = 100$ and $\sigma_2^2 = 80$, what is the probability that samples of size $n_1 = 25$ and $n_2 = 16$ will yield a value of $\bar{x}_1 - \bar{x}_2$ greater than or equal to 8?

4.5.4. Given two nonnormally distributed populations with equal means and variances of $\sigma_1^2 = 240$ and $\sigma_2^2 = 350$, what is the probability that samples of size $n_1 = 40$ and $n_2 = 35$ will yield a value of $\bar{x}_1 - \bar{x}_2$ as large as 12?

4.6 DISTRIBUTION OF THE SAMPLE PROPORTION

In the previous sections we have dealt with the sampling distributions of statistics computed from measured variables. We are frequently interested, however, in the sampling distribution of statistics, such as a sample proportion, that result from counts or frequency data.

Example 4.6.1

Suppose we know that in a certain human population .08 are colorblind. If we designate a population proportion by p, we can say that in this example $p = .08$. If we randomly select 150 individuals from this population, what is the probability that the proportion who are colorblind will be as great as .15?

To answer this question we need to know the properties of the sampling distribution of the sample proportion. We will designate the sample proportion by the symbol $\tilde{p}$.

The reader will recognize the similarity between the present example and those presented in Section 3.3, which dealt with the binomial distribution. Indeed, the variable colorblindness is a binomial variable, since an individual can be classified into one or the other of two mutually exclusive categories, colorblind or not colorblind. In Section 3.3, we were given the same information and were asked to find the number with the characteristic of interest, whereas here we are seeking the proportion in the sample possessing the characteristic of interest. We could with a sufficiently large table of binomial probabilities, such as Table C, determine the probability associated with the number corresponding to the proportion of interest. As we shall see, this will not be necessary, since there is available an alternative procedure, when sample sizes are large, that is generally more convenient.

The sampling distribution of a sample proportion would be constructed experimentally in exactly the same manner as was suggested in the case of the arithmetic mean and the difference between two means. From the population, which we assume to be finite, we would take all possible samples of a given size and for each sample compute the sample proportion, $\tilde{p}$. We would then prepare a frequency distribution of $\tilde{p}$ by listing the different distinct values of $\tilde{p}$ along with their frequencies of occurrence. This frequency distribution (as well as the corresponding relative frequency distribution) would constitute the sampling distribution of $\tilde{p}$.

When the sample size is large, the distribution of sample proportions is approximately normally distributed by virtue of the central limit theorem. The mean of the distribution, $\mu_{\tilde{p}}$, that is, the average of the all possible sample proportions, will be equal to the true population proportion, p, and the variance of the distribution $\sigma_{\tilde{p}}^2$ will be equal to $p(1 - p)/n$.

The question that now arises is: How large does the sample size have to be for the use of the normal approximation to be valid? A widely used criterion is that both np and $n(1 - p)$ must be greater than 5, and we will abide by that rule in this text.

We are now in a position to answer the question regarding colorblindness in the sample of 150 individuals from a population in which .08 are colorblind. Since both np and $n(1 - p)$ are greater than 5 ($150 \times .08 = 12$ and $150 \times .92 = 138$), we can say that, in this case, $\tilde{p}$ is approximately normally distributed with a mean, $\mu_{\tilde{p}} = p = .08$ and $\sigma_{\tilde{p}}^2 = p(1 - p)/n = (.08)(.92)/150 = .00049$. The probability we seek is the area under the curve of $\tilde{p}$ that is to the right of .15. This area is equal to the area under the unit normal curve to the right of

$$z = \frac{\tilde{p} - p}{\sqrt{\dfrac{p(1 - p)}{n}}} = \frac{.15 - .08}{\sqrt{.00049}} = \frac{.07}{.022} = 3.18$$

standard deviation

The transformation to the unit normal distribution has been accomplished in the usual manner: z is found by dividing the difference between a value of the statistic and the mean by the standard error. From Table F we find that the area to the right of $z = 3.18$ is less than $.5 - .4990 = .0010$. We may say, then, that the probability of observing $\tilde{p} \geq .15$ in a random sample of size $n = 150$ from a population in which $p = .08$ is less than .0010. If we should, in fact, draw such a sample most people would consider it a rather rare event.

The normal approximation may be improved by the *correction for continuity*, a device that makes an adjustment for the fact that a discrete distribution is being approximated by a continuous distribution. To employ the correction for continuity $1/2n$ is subtracted from the absolute value of $\tilde{p} - p$ in computing z to give

$$z_c = \frac{|\tilde{p} - p| - 1/2n}{\sqrt{pq/n}} \tag{4.6.1}$$

where $q = 1 - p$. The correction for continuity will not make a great deal of difference when n is large. In the above example

$$z_c = \frac{|.15 - .08| - 1/300}{\sqrt{.00049}} = 3.01$$

and $P(\tilde{p} \geq .15) = .5 - .4987 = .0013$, a result not greatly different from that obtained without the correction for continuity.

Example 4.6.2

Suppose it is known that in a certain population of women, 90 percent entering their third trimester of pregnancy have had some prenatal care. If a random sample of size 200 is drawn from this population, what is the probability that the sample proportion who have had some prenatal care will be less than .85?

Solution. We can assume that the sampling distribution of p is approximately normally distributed with $\mu_{\tilde{p}} = .90$ and $\sigma_{\tilde{p}}^2 = (.1)(.9)/200 = .00045$. We compute

$$z = \frac{.85 - .90}{\sqrt{.00045}} = \frac{-.05}{.021} = -2.38$$

The area to the left of -2.38 under the unit normal curve is $.5 - .4913 = .0087$. Therefore, $P(\tilde{p} \leq .85) = P(z \leq -2.38) = .0087$.

Exercises

4.6.1. If, in a population of adults, .15 are on some sort of diet, what is the probability that a random sample of size 100 will yield a proportion who are on a diet:

(a) Greater than or equal to .20?
(b) Between .10 and .20?
(c) No greater than .12?

4.6.2. In a certain city it is felt that 20 percent of the households have at least one member who is suffering from some ill effect due to air pollution. A random sample of 150 households yielded $\tilde{p} = .27$. If the 20 percent figure is correct, what is the probability of obtaining a sample proportion this large or larger?

4.6.3. In a random sample of 75 adults, 35 said they felt that cancer of the breast is curable. If, in the population from which the sample was drawn, the true proportion who feel cancer of the breast can be cured is .55, what is the probability of obtaining a sample proportion as small or smaller than was obtained in this sample?

4.6.4. The standard drug used to treat a certain disease is known to prove effective within three days in 75 percent of the cases in which it is used. In evaluating the effectiveness of a new drug in treating the same disease, it was given to 150 persons suffering from the disease. At the end of three days 97 persons had recovered. If the new drug is equally as effective as the standard, what is the probability of observing this small a proportion recovering?

4.6.5. Given a population in which $p = .6$ and a random sample from this population of size 100 find:

(a) $P(\tilde{p} \geq .65)$
(b) $P(\tilde{p} \leq .58)$
(c) $P(.56 \leq \tilde{p} \leq .63)$

4.7 DISTRIBUTION OF THE DIFFERENCE BETWEEN TWO SAMPLE PROPORTIONS

Often there are two population proportions in which we are interested and we desire to assess the probability associated with a difference in proportions computed from samples drawn from each of these populations. The relevant sampling distribution is the distribution of the difference between two sample proportions. The characteristics of this sampling distribution may be summarized as follows:

If independent random samples of size n_1 and n_2 are drawn from two populations of binomial variables where the proportion of observations with the characteristic of interest in the two populations are p_1 and p_2, respectively, the distribution of the difference between sample proportions, $\tilde{p}_1 - \tilde{p}_2$, is approximately normal with mean

$$\mu_{\tilde{p}_1 - \tilde{p}_2} = p_1 - p_2$$

and variance

$$\sigma^2_{\tilde{p}_1 - \tilde{p}_2} = \frac{p_1(1 - p_1)}{n_1} + \frac{p_2(1 - p_2)}{n_2}$$

when n_1 and n_2 are large.

To physically construct the sampling distribution of the difference between two sample proportions, we would proceed in the manner described in Section 4.5 for constructing the sampling distribution of the difference between two means.

Given two sufficiently small populations, one would draw, from population 1, all possible simple random samples of size n_1 and compute, from each set of sample data, the sample proportion $\tilde{p}_1$. From population 2, one would draw independently all possible simple random samples of size n_2 and compute, for each set of sample data, the sample proportion $\tilde{p}_2$. One would compute the differences between all possible pairs of sample proportions, where one member of each pair was a value of $\tilde{p}_1$ and the other a value of $\tilde{p}_2$. The sampling distribution of the difference between sample proportions, then, would consist of all such distinct differences, accompanied by their frequencies (or relative frequencies) of occurrence. For large finite or infinite populations one could approximate the sampling distribution of the difference between sample proportions by drawing a large number of independent simple random samples and proceeding in the manner just described.

Example 4.7.1

Suppose that the proportion of moderate to heavy users of illegal drugs in one population, Group 1, is .50 while in another population, Group 2, the proportion is .33. What is the probability that samples of size 100 drawn from each of the populations will yield a value of $\tilde{p}_1 - \tilde{p}_2$ as large as .30?

We assume that the sampling distribution of $\tilde{p}_1 - \tilde{p}_2$ is approximately normal with mean

$$\mu_{\tilde{p}_1 - \tilde{p}_2} = .50 - .33 = .17$$

and variance

$$\sigma^2_{\tilde{p}_1 - \tilde{p}_2} = \frac{(.33)(.67)}{100} + \frac{(.5)(.5)}{100}$$
$$= .004711$$

The area corresponding to the probability we seek is the area under the curve of $\tilde{p}_1 - \tilde{p}_2$ to the right of .30. Transforming to the unit normal distribution gives

$$z = \frac{(\tilde{p}_1 - \tilde{p}_2) - (p_1 - p_2)}{\sqrt{\dfrac{p_1(1 - p_1)}{n_1} + \dfrac{p_2(1 - p_2)}{n_2}}} = \frac{.30 - .17}{\sqrt{.004711}} = 1.89$$

Consulting Table F, we find that the area under the unit normal curve that lies to the right of $z = 1.89$ is $.5 - .4706 = .0294$. The probability of observing a difference as large as .30 is, then, .0294.

Example 4.7.2

In a certain population of teenagers it is known that 10 percent of the boys are obese. If the same proportion of girls in the population are obese, what is the probability that a random sample of 250 boys and 200 girls will yield a value of $\tilde{p}_1 - \tilde{p}_2 \geq .06$?

We assume that the sampling distribution of $\tilde{p}_1 - \tilde{p}_2$ is approximately normal. If the proportion of obese individuals is the same in the two groups, the mean of the distribution will be 0 and the variance will be

$$\sigma^2_{\tilde{p}_1-\tilde{p}_2} = \frac{p_1(1-p_1)}{n_1} + \frac{p_2(1-p_2)}{n_2} = \frac{(.1)(.9)}{250} + \frac{(.1)(.9)}{200}$$

$$= .00081$$

The area of interest under the curve of $\tilde{p}_1 - \tilde{p}_2$ is that to the right of .06. The corresponding z value is

$$z = \frac{.06 - 0}{\sqrt{.00081}} = 2.11$$

Consulting Table F, we find that the area to the right of $z = 2.11$ is $.5 - .4826 = .0174$.

Exercises

4.7.1. In a certain population of retarded children it is known that the proportion who are hyperactive is .40. A random sample of size 120 was drawn from this population, and a random sample of size 100 was drawn from another population of retarded children. If the proportion of hyperactive children is the same in both populations, what is the probability that the sample would yield a difference, $\tilde{p}_1 - \tilde{p}_2$, of .16 or more?

4.7.2. In a certain area of a large city it is hypothesized that 40 percent of the houses are in a dilapidated condition. A random sample of 75 houses from this section and 90 houses from another section yielded a difference, $\tilde{p}_1 - \tilde{p}_2$ of .09. If there is no difference between the two areas in the proportion of dilapidated houses, what is the probability of observing a difference this large or larger?

4.8 SUMMARY

This chapter is concerned with sampling and sampling distributions. Simple random sampling, the type of sampling that is basic to statistical inference, is defined, and a procedure for drawing this type of sample is explained. The concept of a sampling distribution is introduced and the following important sampling distributions are covered:

1. The distribution of a single sample mean.
2. The distribution of the difference between two sample means.
3. The distribution of a sample proportion.
4. The distribution of the difference between two sample proportions.

We emphasize the importance of this material and urge readers to make sure that they understand it before proceeding to the next chapter.

Review Questions and Exercises

1. What are the two types of sampling?
2. Why is nonprobability sampling not covered in this text?
3. Define or explain the following terms:
   (a) Probability sample
   (b) Simple random sample
   (c) Sampling with replacement
   (d) Sampling without replacement
   (e) Sampling distribution
4. Explain how a sampling distribution may be constructed from a finite population.
5. Describe the sampling distribution of the sample mean when sampling is with replacement from a normally distributed population.
6. Explain the central limit theorem.
7. How does the sampling distribution of the sample mean, when sampling without replacement, differ from the sampling distribution obtained when sampling is with replacement?
8. Describe the sampling distribution of the difference between two sample means.
9. Describe the sampling distribution of the sample proportion when large samples are drawn.
10. Describe the sampling distribution of the difference between two sample means when large samples are drawn.
11. Explain the procedure you would follow in constructing the sampling distribution of the difference between sample proportions based on large samples from a finite population.
12. Suppose it is known that the response time of healthy subjects to a particular stimulus is a normally distributed random variable with a mean of 15 seconds and a variance of 16. What is the probability that a random sample of 16 subjects will have a mean response time of 12 seconds or more?
13. A certain firm has 2000 employees. During a recent year, the mean amount per employee spent on personal medical expenses was \$31.50, and the standard deviation was \$6.00. What is the probability that a

simple random sample of 36 employees will yield a mean between \$30 and \$33?

14. Suppose it is known that in a certain population of drug addicts the mean duration of abuse is 5 years and the standard deviation is 3 years. What is the probability that a random sample of 36 subjects from this population will yield a mean duration of abuse between 4 and 6 years?

15. Suppose the mean daily protein intake for a certain population is 125 grams, while for another population the mean is 100 grams. If daily protein intake values in the two populations are normally distributed with a standard deviation of 15 grams, what is the probability that random and independent samples of size 25 from each population will yield a difference between sample means of 12 or less?

16. Suppose that two drugs, purported to reduce the response time to a certain stimulus, are under study by a drug manufacturer. The researcher is willing to assume that response times, following administration of the two drugs, are normally distributed with equal variances of 60. As part of the evaluation of the two drugs Drug A is to be administered to 15 subjects, and Drug B is to be administered to 12 subjects. The researcher would like to know between what two values the central 95 percent of all differences between sample means would lie if the drugs are equally effective and the experiment were repeated a large number of times using these sample sizes.

17. Suppose it is known that the serum albumin concentration in a certain population of individuals is normally distributed with a mean of 4.2 g/100 ml and a standard deviation of .5. A random sample of nine of these individuals placed on a daily dosage of a certain oral steroid yielded a mean serum albumin concentration value of 3.8 g/100 ml. Does it appear likely from these results that the oral steroid reduces the level of serum albumin?

18. A survey conducted in a large metropolitan area revealed that among high school students, 35 percent have, at one time or another, smoked marijuana. If, in a random sample of 150 of these students, only 40 admit to having ever smoked marijuana, what would you conclude?

19. Sixty percent of the employees of a large firm were absent due to sickness three or more days last year. If a simple random sample of 150 of these employees is selected, what is the probability that the proportion in the sample who were absent three or more days due to sickness will be between .50 and .65?

20. A psychiatric social worker believes that in both Community A and Community B, the proportion of adolescents suffering from some emotional or mental problem is .20. In a sample of 150 adolescents from Community A 15 had an emotional or mental problem. In a sample of

100 from Community B, the number was 16. If the social worker's belief is correct, what is the probability of observing a difference as great as was observed between these two samples?

21. Two drugs, A and B, are purported to be equally effective in reducing the level of anxiety in a certain type of emotionally disturbed person. The proportion of persons with whom the drugs are effective is believed to be .80. A random sample of 100 emotionally disturbed persons were given Drug A and 85 experienced a reduction in anxiety level. Drug B was effective with 105 of an independent random sample of 150 emotionally disturbed subjects. If the two drugs are, in fact, equally effective as believed, what is the probability of observing a difference in sample proportions as large as or larger than that observed?

References

References cited

1. Paul G. Hoel, *Introduction to Mathematical Statistics*, Third Edition, Wiley, New York, 1962.
2. R. L. Anderson and T. A. Bancroft, *Statistical Theory in Research*, McGraw-Hill, New York, 1952.

5

ESTIMATION

5.1 INTRODUCTION

We come now to a consideration of *estimation*, the first of the two general areas of statistical inference. The second general area, *hypothesis testing*, is examined in the next chapter.

In Chapter 1 inferential statistics is defined as the procedure whereby one reaches decisions about a large body of data by examining only a small portion of that data. More specifically, the large body of data, and the small portion thereof, that are referred to in that definition are, respectively, a population, and a sample drawn from that population. This leads to the following restatement of the definition of statistical inference.

Definition

Statistical inference is the procedure whereby inferences about a population are made on the basis of the results obtained from a sample drawn from that population.

The process of estimation entails calculating, from the data of a sample, some statistic that is offered as an approximation of the corresponding parameter of the population from which the sample was drawn.

The rationale behind estimation in the health sciences field rests on the assumption that workers in this field have an interest in the parameters of various populations. If this be the case, there are two good reasons why one must rely on estimating procedures to obtain information regarding these parameters. First, many populations of interest, although finite, are so large that a 100 percent examination would be prohibitive from the standpoint of cost. Second, populations that are infinite are incapable of complete examination.

Suppose the administrator of a large hospital is interested in the average age of patients admitted to his hospital during a given year. He may consider it too expensive to go through the records of all patients admitted during that particular year and, consequently, elects to examine a sample of the records from which he can compute an estimate of the average age of patients admitted that year.

A physician in general practice may be interested in knowing what proportion of a certain type of individual, treated with a particular drug, suffers undesirable side effects. No doubt, her concept of the population consists of all those persons who ever have been or ever will be treated with this drug. Deferring a conclusion until the entire population has been observed could have an adverse effect on her practice.

These two examples have implied an interest in estimating, respectively, a population mean and a population proportion. Other parameters, the estimation of which we shall cover in this chapter, are the difference between two means, the difference between two proportions, the population variance, and the ratio of two variances.

We shall find that for each of these parameters we can compute two types of estimate: a point estimate and an interval estimate. A *point estimate* is a single numerical value used to estimate the corresponding population parameter. An *interval estimate* consists of two numerical values defining an interval which, with varying degrees of confidence, we feel includes the parameter being estimated. These concepts will be elaborated on in the succeeding sections.

Note that a single computed value has been referred to as an *estimate.* The rule that tells us how to compute this value, or estimate, is referred to as an *estimator*. Estimators are usually presented as formulas. For example,

$$\bar{x} = \frac{\sum x_i}{n}$$

is an estimator of the population mean, μ. The single numerical value that results from evaluating this formula is called an estimate of the parameter, μ.

In many cases, a parameter may be estimated by more than one estimator. For example we could use the sample median to estimate the population mean. How then do we decide which estimator to use for estimating a given parameter? The decision is based on criteria that reflect the "goodness" of particular estimators. When measured against these criteria, some estimators are better than others. One of these criteria is the property of *unbiasedness.*

An estimator, say t, of the parameter θ is said to be an unbiased estimator of θ if $E(t) = \theta$. $E(t)$ is read, "the expected value of t." For a finite population, $E(t)$ is obtained by taking the average value of t computed from all possible samples of a given size that may be drawn from the population. For an infinite population, $E(t)$ is defined in terms of calculus.

In the previous chapter we have seen that the sample mean, the sample proportion, the difference between two sample means, and the difference between two sample proportions are each unbiased estimates of their corresponding parameters. This property was implied when the parameters were said to be the means of the respective sampling distributions. For example, since the mean of the sampling distribution of $\bar{x}$ is equal to μ, we know that $\bar{x}$ is an unbiased estimator of μ. The other criteria of good estimators will not be discussed in this book. The interested reader will find them covered in detail by Freund (1) and Mood and Graybill (2), among others. A much less mathematically rigorous treatment may be found in Yamane (3).

Sampled Populations and Target Populations. The health researcher who uses statistical inference procedures must be aware of the difference between two kinds of population—the *sampled population* and the *target population.* The sampled population is the population from which one actually draws a sample. The target population is the population about which one wishes to make an inference. These two populations may or may not be the same. Statistical inference procedures allow one to make inferences about sampled populations (provided proper sampling methods have been employed). Only when the target population and the sampled population are the same is it possible for one to use statistical inference procedures to reach conclusions about the target population. If the sampled population and the target population are different, the researcher can reach conclusions about the target population only on the basis of nonstatistical considerations.

Suppose, for example, that a researcher wishes to assess the effectiveness of some method for treating rheumatoid arthritis. The target population consists of all patients sufferering from the disease. It is not practical to draw a sample from this population. The researcher may, however, select a sample from all rheumatoid arthritis patients seen in some specific clinic. These patients constitute the sampled population, and if proper sampling methods are used, inferences about this sampled population may be drawn on the basis of the information in the sample. If the researcher wishes to make inferences about all rheumatoid arthritis sufferers, he or she must rely on nonstatistical means to do so. Perhaps the researcher knows that the sampled population is similar, with respect to all important characteristics, to the target population. That is, the researcher may know that the age, sex, severity of illness, duration of illness compositions, and so on, are similar. And on the strength of this knowledge, the researcher may be willing to extrapolate his or her findings to the target population.

In many situations the sampled population and the target population are identical, and, when this is the case, inferences about the target population are straightforward. The researcher should however, be aware that this is not always the case and not fall into the trap of drawing unwarranted inferences about a population that is different from the one that is sampled.

Random and Nonrandom Samples. In the examples and exercises of this book, we assume that the data available for analysis have come from random samples. The strict validity of the statistical procedures discussed depend on this assumption. In many instances in real-world applications it is impossible or impractical to use truly random samples. In animal experiments, for example, researchers usually use whatever animals are available from suppliers or their own breeding stock. If the researchers had to depend on randomly selected material, very little research of this type would be conducted. Again, nonstatistical considerations must play a part in the generalization process. Researchers may contend that the samples actually used are equivalent to simple random samples, since there is no reason to believe that the material actually used is not representative of the population about which inferences are desired.

In many health research projects, samples of convenience, rather than random samples, are employed. Researchers may have to rely on volunteer subjects or on readily available subjects such as students in their classes. Again, generalizations must be made on the basis of nonstatistical considerations. The consequences of such generalizations, however, may be useful or they may range from misleading to disastrous.

In some situations it is possible to introduce randomization into an experiment even though available subjects are not randomly selected from some well-defined population. In comparing two treatments, for example, each subject may be randomly assigned to one or the other of the treatments. Inferences in such cases apply to the treatments and not the subjects, and hence the inferences are valid.

5.2 CONFIDENCE INTERVAL FOR A POPULATION MEAN

Suppose researchers wish to estimate the mean of some normally distributed population. They draw a random sample of size n from the population, and compute $\bar{x}$, which they use as a point estimate of μ. Although this estimate of μ possesses all the qualities of a good estimator, we know that because of the vagaries of sampling, $\bar{x}$ cannot be expected to be equal to μ.

It would be much more meaningful, therefore, to estimate μ by an interval that somehow communicates the probable magnitude of μ.

To obtain such an interval estimate, we must draw on our knowledge of sampling distributions. In the present case, since we are concerned with the sample mean as an estimator of a population mean, we must recall what we know about the sampling distribution of the sample mean.

In the previous chapter we learned that if sampling is from a normally distributed population, the sampling distribution of the sample mean will be normally distributed with a mean, $\mu_{\bar{x}}$, equal to the population mean, μ, and a variance, $\sigma_{\bar{x}}^2$, equal to σ^2/n. We could plot the sampling distribution if we only knew where to locate it on the x-axis. From our knowledge of normal distributions, in general, we know even more about the distribution of $\bar{x}$ in this case. We know, for example, that regardless of where it is located, approximately 95 percent of the possible values of $\bar{x}$ constituting the distribution are within two standard deviations of the mean. The two points that are two standard deviations from the mean are: $\mu - 2\sigma_{\bar{x}}$ and $\mu + 2\sigma_{\bar{x}}$, so that the interval, $\mu \pm 2\sigma_{\bar{x}}$, will contain approximately 95 percent of the possible values of $\bar{x}$. We know that μ and, hence, $\mu_{\bar{x}}$ are unknown, but we may arbitrarily place the sampling distribution of $\bar{x}$ on the $\bar{x}$-axis.

Since we do not know the value of μ, not a great deal is accomplished by the expression $\mu \pm 2\sigma_{\bar{x}}$. We do, however, have a point estimate of μ which is $\bar{x}$. Would it be useful to construct an interval about this point estimate of μ? The answer is, yes. Suppose we constructed intervals about every possible value of $\bar{x}$ computed from all possible samples of size n from the population of interest. We would have a large number of intervals of the form $\bar{x} \pm 2\sigma_{\bar{x}}$ with widths all equal to the width of the interval about the unknown μ. Approximately 95 percent of these intervals would have centers falling within the $\pm 2\sigma_{\bar{x}}$ interval about μ. Each of the intervals whose centers fall within $2\sigma_{\bar{x}}$ of μ would contain μ. These concepts are illustrated in Figure 5.2.1. In Figure 5.2.1 we see that $\bar{x}_1$, $\bar{x}_3$, and $\bar{x}_4$ all fall within the $2\sigma_{\bar{x}}$ interval about μ and, consequently, the $2\sigma_x$ intervals about these sample means include the value

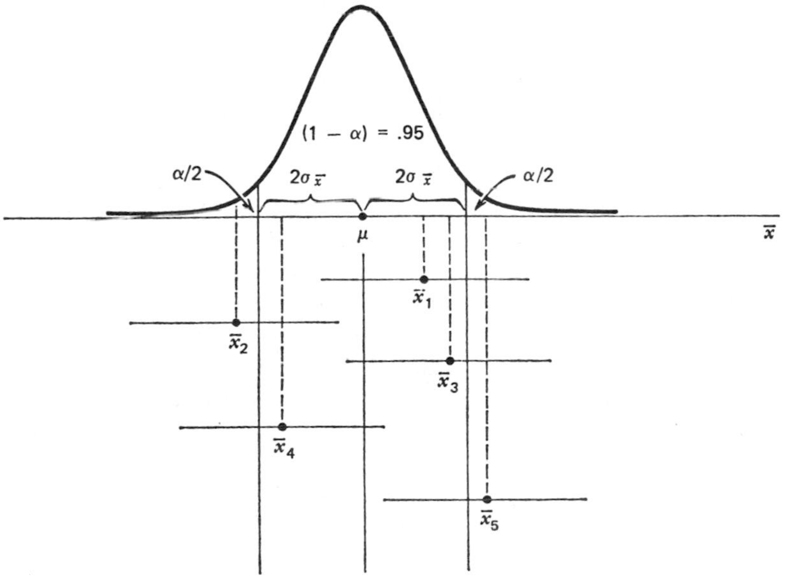

Figure 5.2.1. The 95 percent confidence intervals for μ.

of μ. The sample means $\bar{x}_2$ and $\bar{x}_5$ do not fall within the $2\sigma_{\bar{x}}$ interval about μ, and the $2\sigma_{\bar{x}}$ intervals about them do not include μ.

Example 5.2.1

Suppose a researcher, interested in obtaining an estimate of the average level of some enzyme in a certain human population, takes a sample of 10 individuals, determines the level of the enzyme in each, and computes a sample mean of $\bar{x} = 22$. Suppose further it is known that the variable of interest is approximately normally distributed with a variance of 45. An approximate 95 percent confidence interval for μ is given by

$$\bar{x} \pm 2\sigma_{\bar{x}}$$
$$22 \pm 2\sqrt{\tfrac{45}{10}}$$
$$22 \pm 2(2.12)$$
$$17.76,\ 26.24$$

Let us examine the composition of this interval estimate. It contains in its center the point estimate of μ. The 2 we recognize as a value from the unit normal distribution that tells us within how many standard errors lie approximately 95 percent of the possible values of $\bar{x}$. This value of z is referred to as the *reliability coefficient*. The last component, $\sigma_{\bar{x}}$, is the standard error, or standard deviation of the sampling distribution of $\bar{x}$. In general, then, an interval estimate may be expressed as follows:

$$\text{estimator} \pm (\text{reliability coefficient}) \times (\text{standard error}) \qquad (5.2.1)$$

In particular, when sampling from a normal distribution with known variance an interval estimate for μ may be expressed as

$$\bar{x} \pm z_{(1-\alpha/2)}\sigma_{\bar{x}} \qquad (5.2.2)$$

How do we interpret the interval given by 5.2.2? In the present example, where the reliability coefficient is equal to 2, we say that in repeated sampling approximately 95 percent of the intervals constructed by 5.2.2 will include the population mean. This interpretation is based on the probability of occurrence of different values of $\bar{x}$. We may generalize this interpretation if we designate the total area, under the curve of $\bar{x}$, which is outside the interval $\mu \pm 2\sigma_{\bar{x}}$ as α and the area within the interval as $1 - \alpha$ and give the following *probabilistic interpretation* of 5.2.2.

In repeated sampling, from a normally distributed population, $100(1 - \alpha)$ *percent of all intervals of the form* $\bar{x} \pm z_{(1-\alpha/2)}\sigma_{\bar{x}}$ *will in the long run include the population mean,* μ.

The quantity $1 - \alpha$, in this case .95, is called the *confidence coefficient*, and the interval $\bar{x} \pm z_{(1-\alpha/2)}\sigma_{\bar{x}}$ is called a *confidence interval* for μ. When $(1 - \alpha) = .95$, the interval is called the 95 percent confidence interval for μ. In the present example we say that we are 95 percent confident that the population mean is between 17.76 and 26.24. This is called the *practical interpretation* of 5.2.2. In general, it may be expressed as follows.

We are $100(1 - \alpha)$ *percent confident that the single computed interval,* $\bar{x} \pm z_{(1-\alpha/2)}\sigma_{\bar{x}}$, *contains the population mean,* μ.

In the example given here we might prefer, rather than 2, the more exact value of z, 1.96, corresponding to a confidence coefficient of .95. The researcher may use any confidence coefficient he wishes, the most frequently used values are .90, .95, and .99.

Example 5.2.2

A physical therapist wished to estimate, with 99 percent confidence, the mean maximal strength of a particular muscle in a certain group of individuals. He is willing to assume that strength scores are approximately normally distributed with a variance of 144. A sample of 15 subjects who participated in the experiment yielded a mean of 84.3. The z value corresponding to a confidence coefficient of .99 is found in Table F to be 2.58. This is our reliability coefficient. The standard error is $\sigma_{\bar{x}} = 12/\sqrt{15} = 3.10$. Our 99 percent confidence interval for μ, then, is

$$84.3 \pm 2.58(3.10)$$

$$84.3 \pm 8.0$$

$$76.3, 92.3$$

We say we are 99 percent confident that the population mean is between 76.3 and 92.3 since, in repeated sampling, 99 percent of all intervals that could be constructed in the manner just described would include the population mean.

Sampling from Nonnormal Populations. It will not always be possible or prudent to assume that the population of interest is normally distributed. Thanks to the central limit theorem, this will not deter us if we are able to select a large enough sample. We have learned that for large samples, the sampling distribution of $\bar{x}$ is approximately normally distributed regardless of how the parent population is distributed.

Example 5.2.3

In a study of patient flow through the offices of general practitioners, it was found that a sample of 35 patients arriving late for appointments were 17.2 minutes late for appointments, on the average. Previous research had shown the standard deviation to be about 8 minutes. The population distribution was felt to be nonnormal. What is the 90 percent confidence interval for μ, the true average amount of time late for appointments?

Since the sample size is fairly large (greater than 30), and since the population standard deviation is known, we draw on the central limit theorem and assume the sampling distribution of $\bar{x}$ to be approximately normally distributed. From Table F we find the reliability coefficient, corresponding to a confidence coefficient of .90, to be about 1.645, if we interpolate. The standard error is $\sigma_{\bar{x}} = 8/\sqrt{35} = 1.35$, so that our 90 percent confidence interval for μ is

$$17.2 \pm 1.645(1.35)$$

$$17.2 \pm 2.2$$

$$15.0, 19.4$$

Exercises

5.2.1. In an experiment designed to estimate the average number of heartbeats per minute for a certain population, under the conditions of the experiment, the average number of heartbeats per minute for 49 subjects was found to be 90. If it is reasonable to assume that these 49 patients constitute a random sample, and that the population is normally distributed with a standard deviation of 10, find:

(a) The 90 percent confidence interval for μ.
(b) The 95 percent confidence interval for μ.
(c) The 99 percent confidence interval for μ.

5.2.2. The mean serum indirect bilirubin level of 16 four-day-old infants was found to be 5.98 mg/100 cc. Assuming bilirubin levels in four-day-old infants are approximately normally distributed with a standard deviation of 3.5 mg/100 cc., find:

(a) The 90 percent confidence interval for μ.
(b) The 95 percent confidence interval for μ.
(c) The 99 percent confidence interval for μ.

5.2.3. In a length of hospitalization study conducted by several cooperating hospitals, a random sample of 64 peptic ulcer patients was drawn from a list of all peptic ulcer patients ever admitted to the participating hospitals and the length of hospitalization per admission was determined for each. The mean length of hospitalization was found to be 8.25 days. If the population standard deviation is known to be 3 days, find:

(a) The 90 percent confidence interval for μ.
(b) The 95 percent confidence interval for μ.
(c) The 99 percent confidence interval for μ.

5.2.4. A sample of 100 apparently normal adult males, 25 years old, had a mean systolic blood pressure of 125. If it is felt that the population standard deviation is 15, find:

(a) The 90 percent confidence interval for μ.
(b) The 95 percent confidence interval for μ.

5.3 CONFIDENCE INTERVAL FOR THE DIFFERENCE BETWEEN TWO POPULATION MEANS

Sometimes there arise instances in which we are interested in estimating the difference between two population means. From each of the populations a sample is drawn, and from the data of each, the sample means $\bar{x}_1$ and $\bar{x}_2$, respectively, are computed. We learned in the previous chapter that the estimator $\bar{x}_1 - \bar{x}_2$ yields an unbiased estimate of $\mu_1 - \mu_2$, the difference between the population means. We also know from Chapter 4 that, depending on the conditions, the sampling distribution of $\bar{x}_1 - \bar{x}_2$ may be, at least, approximately normally distributed, so that in many cases we make use of the theory relevant to normal distributions to compute a confidence interval for $\mu_1 - \mu_2$. Let us illustrate, first for the case where sampling is from a normal distribution, and then for the case where the assumption of normally distributed populations cannot be made.

Example 5.3.1

In a large hospital for the treatment of the mentally retarded, a sample of 12 individuals with mongolism yielded a mean serum uric acid value of $\bar{x}_1 = 4.5$ mg/100 ml. In a general hospital a sample of 15 normal individuals of the same age and sex were found to have a mean value of $\bar{x}_2 = 3.4$. If it is reasonable to assume that the two populations of values are normally distributed with variances equal to 1, find the 95 percent confidence interval for $\mu_1 - \mu_2$.

For a point estimate of $\mu_1 - \mu_2$, we use $\bar{x}_1 - \bar{x}_2 = 4.5 - 3.4 = 1.1$. The reliability coefficient corresponding to .95 is found in Table F to be 1.96. The standard error is

$$\sigma_{\bar{x}_1 - \bar{x}_2} = \sqrt{\frac{{\sigma_1}^2}{n_1} + \frac{{\sigma_2}^2}{n_2}} = \sqrt{\frac{1}{12} + \frac{1}{15}} = .39$$

The 95 percent confidence interval, then, is

$$1.1 \pm 1.96(.39)$$
$$1.1 \pm .8$$
$$.3, 1.9$$

We say that we are 95 percent confident that the true difference, $\mu_1 - \mu_2$, is between .3 and 1.9, because, in repeated sampling, 95 percent of the intervals constructed in this same manner would include the difference between the true means.

Sampling from Nonnormal Populations. The construction of a confidence interval for the difference between two population means when sampling is from nonnormal populations proceeds in the same manner as above if the sample sizes, n_1 and n_2, are large. Again, this is a result of the central limit theorem.

Example 5.3.2

The average family income of a sample of 75 patients admitted to hospital A was $\bar{x}_1 = \$6800$, while the average based on a sample of 80 patients from hospital B was found to be $\bar{x}_2 = \$4450$. If the population standard deviations are $\sigma_1 = \$600$ and $\sigma_2 = \$500$, find the 99 percent confidence interval for $\mu_1 - \mu_2$, the difference between population means.

The point estimate of $\mu_1 - \mu_2$ is $\bar{x}_1 - \bar{x}_2 = \$6800 - \$4450 = \$2350$. From Table F we find the reliability coefficient to be 2.58. The standard error is

$$\sigma_{\bar{x}_1 - \bar{x}_2} = \sqrt{\frac{(600)^2}{75} + \frac{(500)^2}{80}} = 89$$

Our 99 percent confidence interval is

$$\$2350 \pm 2.58(89)$$
$$\$2350 \pm 230$$
$$\$2120, \$2580$$

We interpret this interval in the usual ways.

Exercises

5.3.1. In a study using educable mentally retarded children, 11 boys and 10 girls, after a year of academic schooling combined with therapy, were given achievement tests. The mean score for boys was $\bar{x}_1 = 67.0$ and for girls $\bar{x}_2 = 61.5$. If it is reasonable to assume that scores for similar children under similar circumstances are normally distributed with standard deviations, $\sigma_1 = 11$ and $\sigma_2 = 10$, find:

(a) The 90 percent confidence interval for $\mu_1 - \mu_2$.
(b) The 95 percent confidence interval for $\mu_1 - \mu_2$.
(c) The 99 percent confidence interval for $\mu_1 - \mu_2$.

5.3.2. A sample of 10 twelve-year-old girls and a sample of 10 twelve-year-old boys yielded mean heights, respectively, of $\bar{x}_1 = 59.8$ inches and $\bar{x}_2 = 58.5$ inches. Assuming normal distributions of heights with $\sigma_1 = 2$ inches and $\sigma_2 = 3$ inches, find:

(a) The 90 percent confidence interval for $\mu_1 - \mu_2$.
(b) The 95 percent confidence interval for $\mu_1 - \mu_2$.
(c) The 99 percent confidence interval for $\mu_1 - \mu_2$.

5.3.3. A sample of 100 patients with disease A, admitted to a chronic disease hospital, remained in the hospital, on the average, 35 days. Another sample of 100 patients with disease B stayed, on the average, 28 days. If the population variances are 100 and 225, respectively, find:

(a) The 90 percent confidence interval for $\mu_A - \mu_B$.
(b) The 95 percent confidence interval for $\mu_A - \mu_B$.
(c) The 99 percent confidence interval for $\mu_A - \mu_B$.

5.4 CONFIDENCE INTERVAL FOR A POPULATION PROPORTION

Many questions of interest to the health worker relate to population proportions. What proportion of patients who receive a particular type of treatment recover? What proportion of some population has a certain disease? What proportion of a population are immune to a certain disease?

To estimate a population proportion we proceed in the same manner as when estimating a population mean. A sample is drawn from the population of interest, and the sample proportion, $\hat{p}$, is computed. This sample proportion is used as the point estimator of the population proportion. A confidence interval is obtained by the general formula:

$$\text{estimator} \pm (\text{reliability coefficient}) \times (\text{standard error})$$

In the previous chapter we have seen that when both np and $n(1 - p)$ are greater than 5, we may consider the sampling distribution of $\hat{p}$ to be quite close to the normal distribution. When this condition is met, our reliability coefficient is some value of z from the unit normal distribution. The standard error, we have seen, is equal to $\sigma_{\hat{p}} = \sqrt{p(1 - p)/n}$. Since p, the parameter we are trying to estimate, is unknown, we must use $\tilde{p}$ as an estimate. Thus we estimate $\sigma_{\tilde{p}}$ by $\sqrt{\tilde{p}(1-\tilde{p})/n}$, and our $100(1-\alpha)$ percent confidence interval for p is given by

$$\tilde{p} \pm z_{(1-\alpha/2)}\sqrt{\tilde{p}(1-\tilde{p})/n} \tag{5.4.1}$$

We give this interval both the probabilistic and practical interpretations.

Example 5.4.1

A survey was conducted to study the dental health practices, and attitudes of a certain urban adult population. Of 300 adults interviewed, 123 said that they regularly had a dental checkup twice a year.

The best point estimate of the population proportion is $\tilde{p} = 123/300 = .41$. The size of the sample and our estimate of p are of sufficient magnitude to justify use of the unit normal distribution in constructing a confidence interval. The reliability coefficient corresponding to a confidence level of .95, for example, is 1.96 and our estimate of the standard error, $\sigma_{\tilde{p}}$, is $\sqrt{\tilde{p}(1-\tilde{p})/n} = \sqrt{.41(.59)/300} = .028$. The 95 percent confidence interval for p, based on these data, is

$$.41 \pm 1.96(.028)$$
$$.41 \pm .05$$
$$.36, .46$$

We say we are 95 percent confident that the true proportion, p, is between .36 and .46 since, in repeated sampling, 95 percent of the intervals constructed in the manner of the present single interval would include the true p.

Exercises

5.4.1. A medical record librarian drew a random sample of 100 patients' charts and found that in 8 percent of them, the face sheet had at least one item of information contradictory to other information in the record. Construct the 90, 95, and 99 percent confidence intervals for the true proportion of charts containing such discrepancies.

5.4.2. A survey, resulting in a random sample of 150 households in a certain urban community, revealed that in 87 percent of the cases, at least one member of the household had some form of health insurance. Construct the 90, 95, and 99 percent confidence intervals for p, the true proportion of households in the community with the characteristic of interest.

5.4.3. In a study designed to assess the relationship between a certain drug and a certain anomaly in chick embryos, 50 fertilized eggs were injected with the drug on the fourth day of incubation. On the twentieth day of incubation the embryos were examined and in 12 the presence of the abnormality was observed. Find the 90, 95, and 99 percent confidence intervals for p.

5.5 CONFIDENCE INTERVAL FOR THE DIFFERENCE BETWEEN TWO POPULATION PROPORTIONS

The magnitude of the difference between two population proportions is often of interest. We may want to compare, for example, men and women, two age groups, two socioeconomic groups, or two diagnostic groups with respect to the proportion possessing some characteristic of interest. An unbiased point estimator of the difference in two population proportions is provided by the difference in sample proportions, $\tilde{p}_1 - \tilde{p}_2$. Since, as we have seen, when n_1 and n_2 are large and the population proportions are not too close to 0 or 1, the central limit theorem applies, normal distribution theory may be employed to obtain confidence intervals. The standard error of the estimate must be estimated by

$$\sqrt{\frac{\tilde{p}_1(1-\tilde{p}_1)}{n_1}+\frac{\tilde{p}_2(1-\tilde{p}_2)}{n_2}}$$

since the population proportions are unknown. A $100(1-\alpha)$ percent confidence interval for $p_1 - p_2$ is given by

$$(\tilde{p}_1 - \tilde{p}_2) \pm z_{(1-\alpha/2)}\sqrt{\frac{\tilde{p}_1(1-\tilde{p}_1)}{n_1}+\frac{\tilde{p}_2(1-\tilde{p}_2)}{n_2}} \qquad (5.5.1)$$

We may interpret this interval from both the probabilistic and practical points of view.

Example 5.5.1

Two hundred patients suffering from a certain disease were randomly divided into two equal groups. Of the first group, who received the standard treatment, 78 recovered within three days. Out of the other 100, who were treated by a new method, 90 recovered within three days. The physician wished to estimate the true difference in the proportions who would recover within three days.

Our best point estimate of the difference in the population proportions is $\tilde{p}_1 - \tilde{p}_2 = .78 - .90 = -.12$. The 95 percent confidence interval for $p_1 - p_2$ is

$$(.78 - .90) \pm 1.96 \sqrt{\frac{(.78)(.22)}{100} + \frac{(.90)(.10)}{100}}$$

$$-.12 \pm 1.96(.05)$$

$$-.12 \pm .10$$

$$-.22, -.02$$

We say we are 95 percent confident that the true difference is between .02 and .22, because we know that, in repeated sampling, about 95 percent of the intervals that may be constructed in the manner just described will include the true difference.

Note that the negative signs merely reflect the fact that better results were obtained by using the new treatment. The interval could just as well have been constructed around $\tilde{p}_2 - \tilde{p}_1$, in which case the end points of the interval would have been positive.

Exercises

5.5.1. Out of a sample of 150, selected from patients admitted over a two-year period to a large hospital, 129 had some type of hospitalization insurance. In a sample of 160 similarly selected patients, from a second hospital, 144 had some type of hospitalization insurance. Find the 90, 95, and 99 percent confidence intervals for the true difference in population proportions.

5.5.2. In a survey conducted in two sections of a large metropolitan area, the following results were obtained with respect to abnormal blood pressure.

Area	Number of Persons Screened	Number Abnormal on Screening
1	200	20
2	250	38

Construct the 90, 95, and 99 percent confidence intervals for the difference between the two population proportions.

5.5.3. In a study designed to assess the side effects of two drugs, 50 animals were given Drug A, and 50 animals were given Drug B. Of the 50 receiving Drug A, 11 showed undersirable side effects, while 8 of those receiving Drug B reacted similarly. Find the 90, 95, and 99 percent confidence intervals for $p_A - p_B$.

5.6 THE *t* DISTRIBUTION

In Sections 5.2 and 5.3, procedures were outlined for constructing confidence intervals for a population mean and the difference between two population means. These procedures, we recall, require a knowledge of the variances of the populations from which the samples are drawn. It may seem somewhat strange that one can have knowledge of the population variance and not know the value of the population mean. Indeed, it is the usual case, in situations such as have been presented, that the population variance, as well as the population mean, is unknown. This condition presents a problem with respect to constructing confidence intervals. Although, for example, the statistic

$$z = \frac{\bar{x} - \mu}{\sigma/\sqrt{n}}$$

is normally distributed, when the population is normally distributed, and is approximately normally distributed when n is large, regardless of the functional form of the population, we cannot make use of this fact because σ is unknown. However, all is not lost, and the most logical solution to the problem is the one followed. We use the sample standard deviation, $s = \sqrt{\sum(x_i - \bar{x})^2/(n-1)}$, to replace σ. When the sample size is large, say greater than 30, our faith in s as an approximation of σ is usually substantial, and we may feel justified in using normal distribution theory to construct confidence intervals for population means or differences between population means. In that event, we proceed as instructed in Sections 5.2 and 5.3.

It is when we have small samples that it becomes mandatory for us to find an alternative procedure for constructing confidence intervals.

As a result of the work of W. S. Gosset (4), writing under the pseudonym of "Student," an alternative, known as *Student's t distribution*, usually shortened to *t distribution*, is available to us.

The quantity

$$t = \frac{\bar{x} - \mu}{s/\sqrt{n}}$$

follows this distribution. The t distribution has the following properties.

1. It has a mean of 0.
2. It is symmetrical about the mean.
3. In general, it has a variance greater than 1, but the variance approaches 1 as the sample size becomes large.
4. The variable t ranges from $-\infty$ to $+\infty$.
5. The t distribution is really a family of distributions, since there is a different distribution for each sample value of $n - 1$, the divisor used in computing s^2. Figure 5.6.1 shows t distributions corresponding to several degrees-of-freedom values.

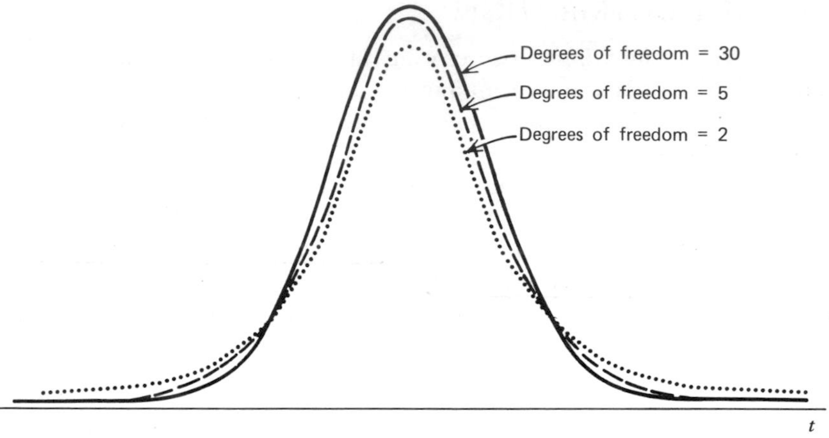

Figure 5.6.1. The t*-distribution for different degrees-of-freedom values.*

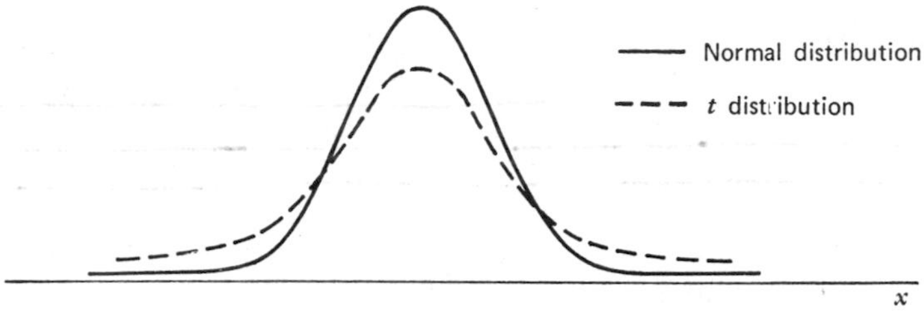

Figure 5.6.2. Comparison of normal distribution and t*-distribution.*

6. Compared to the normal distribution the t distribution is less peaked in the center and has higher tails. Figure 5.6.2 compares the t distribution with the normal.
7. The t distribution approaches the normal distribution as $n - 1$ approaches infinity.

The t distribution, like the unit normal, has been extensively tabulated. One such table is given as Table H in the Appendix.

The quantity $n - 1$ used in computing the sample variance, it will be recalled, is referred to as the degrees of freedom; hence, we say there is a diffferent t distribution for each degrees of freedom value and, as we shall see, we must take degrees of freedom into account when using the table of the t distribution.

The general procedure for constructing confidence intervals is not affected by our having to use the t distribution rather than the unit normal distribution. We still make use of the relationship expressed by

$$\text{estimator} \pm (\text{reliability coefficient}) \times (\text{standard error})$$

What is different is the source of the reliability coefficient. It is now obtained from the table of the t distribution rather than from the table of the unit normal distribution. To be more specific, *when sampling from a normal distribution whose standard deviation, σ, is unknown, the $100(1-\alpha)$ percent confidence interval for the population mean, μ, is given by*

$$\bar{x} \pm t_{(1-\alpha/2)} \frac{s}{\sqrt{n}} \tag{5.6.1}$$

Notice that a requirement for the valid use of the t distribution is that the sample must be drawn from a normal distribution. Experience has shown, however, that moderate departures from this requirement can be tolerated. As a consequence the t distribution is used even when it is known that the parent population deviates from normality. Most researchers require that an assumption of, at least, a mound-shaped population distribution be tenable.

Example 5.6.1

Serum amylase determinations were made on a sample of 15 apparently healthy subjects. The sample yielded a mean of 96 units/100 ml and a standard deviation of 35 units/100 ml. The population variance was unknown. We may use the sample mean, 96, as a point estimate of the population mean but, since the population standard deviation is unknown, we must assume the population of values to be at least approximately normally distributed before constructing a confidence interval for μ. Let us assume that such an assumption is reasonable and that a 95 percent confidence interval is desired. We have our estimator, $\bar{x}$, and our standard error is $s/\sqrt{n} = 35/\sqrt{15} = 9.04$. We need now to find the reliability coefficient, the value of t associated with a confidence coefficient of .95 and $n - 1 = 14$ degrees of freedom. Since a 95 percent confidence interval leaves .05 of the area under the curve of t to be equally divided between the two tails, we need the value of t to the right of which lies .025 of the area. We locate in Table H the column headed $t_{.975}$. This is the value of t to the left of which lies .975 of the area under the curve. The area to the right of this value is equal to the desired .025. We now locate the number 14 in the degrees of freedom column. The value at the intersection of the row labeled 14 and the column labeled $t_{.975}$ is the t we seek. This value of t, which is our reliability coefficient, is found to be 2.1448. We now construct our 95 percent confidence interval as follows:

$$96 \pm 2.1448(9.04)$$

$$96 \pm 19$$

$$77, 115$$

This interval may be interpreted from both the probabilistic and practical points of view. We say we are 95 percent confident that the true population mean, μ, is between 77 and 115 because, in repeated sampling, 95 percent of intervals constructed in like manner will include μ.

The t Distribution and the Difference Between Means. When population standard deviations are unknown, and it is desired to estimate the difference between two population means with a confidence interval, an additional assumption must be made before we can use the t distribution in the manner just described. The assumption that must be made is that the population variances, although unknown, are equal, that is, we must assume $\sigma_1^2 = \sigma_2^2$. The reasonableness of this assumption may be tested by an appropriate test to be discussed in a later section.

If the assumption of equal population variances is justified, the two sample variances which we compute from our two samples may be construed as estimates of the same thing, the common variance. It seems logical then that we should somehow capitalize on this in our analysis. We do just that and obtain a *pooled estimate* of the common variance. This pooled estimate is obtained by computing the weighted average of the two sample variances. Each sample variance is weighted by its degrees of freedom. If the sample sizes are equal, this weighted average turns out to be the arithmetic mean of the two sample variances. If the two sample sizes are unequal, the weighted average takes advantage of the additional information provided by the larger sample. The pooled estimate is given by the formula:

pooled estimate of the common variance

$$s_p^2 = \frac{(n_1 - 1)s_1^2 + (n_2 - 1)s_2^2}{n_1 + n_2 - 2} \tag{5.6.2}$$

The standard error of the estimate, then, is given by

$$\sqrt{\frac{s_p^2}{n_1} + \frac{s_p^2}{n_2}} = s_p \sqrt{\frac{1}{n_1} + \frac{1}{n_2}}$$

and the $100(1 - \alpha)$ percent confidence interval for $\mu_1 - \mu_2$ is given by

$$(\bar{x}_1 - \bar{x}_2) \pm t_{(1-\alpha/2)} s_p \sqrt{\frac{1}{n_1} + \frac{1}{n_2}} \tag{5.6.3}$$

The number of degrees of freedom used in determining the value of t to use in constructing the interval are $n_1 + n_2 - 2$, the denominator of Equation 5.6.2. We interpret this interval in the usual manner.

Example 5.6.2

To illustrate, let us refer to Example 5.6.1 and suppose that in addition to the apparently healthy normal subjects, serum amylase determinations were also made on 22 hospitalized subjects. Suppose the mean and standard deviation from this group are 120 and 40 units/ml, respectively. Let us designate the 15 normal subjects as group 2. Our point estimate of $\mu_1 - \mu_2$ is $120 - 96 = 24$.

To find a confidence interval, let us proceed under the assumption that the two populations under study are normally distributed and that the population variances are equal. Our first step is to obtain a pooled estimate of the common variance as follows:

$$s_p^{\,2} = \frac{14(35)^2 + 21(40)^2}{15 + 22 - 2} = 1450$$

The 95 percent confidence interval for $\mu_1 - \mu_2$ is as follows:

$$(120 - 96) \pm 2.0301 \sqrt{\frac{1450}{15} + \frac{1450}{22}}$$

$$24 \pm (2.0301)(38.08) \sqrt{\frac{1}{15} + \frac{1}{22}}$$

$$24 \pm 26$$

$$-2,\ 50$$

use $t_{.975}$ df = 35 (n_1+n_2-2)

Again, we say we are 95 percent confident that the true difference, $\mu_1 - \mu_2$, is between -2 and 50 because, in repeated sampling, 95 percent of intervals so constructed would include $\mu_1 - \mu_2$.

The Difference Between Two Means—Population Variances Not Equal. When one is reluctant to assume that the variances of two populations of interest are equal, even though the two populations may be assumed to be normal, it is not proper to use the t distribution as just outlined in constructing confidence intervals.

A solution to the problem of unequal variances was proposed by Behrens (5) and later was verified and generalized by Fisher (6, 7). Solutions have also been proposed by Neyman (8), Scheffé (9, 10), and Welch (11, 12). The problem is discussed in detail by Aspin (13), Trickett et al. (14), and Cochran (15). Cochran's approach is also found in Snedecor and Cochran (16).

The problem revolves around the fact that the quantity

$$t' = \frac{(\bar{x}_1 - \bar{x}_2) - (\mu_1 - \mu_2)}{\sqrt{\dfrac{s_1^{\,2}}{n_1} + \dfrac{s_2^{\,2}}{n_2}}}$$

does not follow a t distribution with $n_1 + n_2 - 2$ degrees of freedom when the population variances are not equal. One way of circumventing the problem is to use a modified value for the degrees of freedom. A convenient formula for doing this is given by Dixon and Massey (17) as follows:

difference between two means - variances not equal

$$df' = \frac{\left(\frac{s_1^2}{n_1} + \frac{s_2^2}{n_2}\right)^2}{\frac{(s_1^2/n_1)^2}{n_1} + \frac{(s_2^2/n_2)^2}{n_2}} \tag{5.6.4}$$

If the assumptions of normality hold true, t' is distributed approximately as t with degrees of freedom calculated by Equation 5.6.4. The $100(1 - \alpha)$ percent confidence interval for $\mu_1 - \mu_2$ then is given by

$$(\bar{x}_1 - \bar{x}_2) \pm t_{(1-\alpha/2)} \sqrt{\frac{s_1^2}{n_1} + \frac{s_2^2}{n_2}} \tag{5.6.5}$$

The numerical value of the degrees of freedom computed by Equation 5.6.4 may not be an integer. In this case, it is usually satisfactory to use the closest value of df' given in the table of the t distribution.

The interval obtained by this method is interpreted in the usual manner, but it must be kept in mind that the interval is only approximate.

Example 5.6.3

Total serum complement activity (C_{H50}) was assayed in 20 apparently healthy subjects and 10 subjects with disease. The following results were obtained:

Subjects	n	$\bar{x}$	s
With disease	10	62.6	33.8
Normal	20	47.2	10.1

The investigators had reason to believe that the sampled populations are approximately normally distributed, but they were unwilling to assume that the two unknown population variances are equal. Find the 95 percent confidence interval for $\mu_1 - \mu_2$.

The point estimate for $\mu_1 - \mu_2$ is $62.6 - 47.2 = 15.4$. The modified degrees of freedom value is

$$df' = \frac{\left(\frac{33.8^2}{10} + \frac{10.1^2}{20}\right)^2}{\frac{\left(\frac{33.8^2}{10}\right)^2}{10} + \frac{\left(\frac{10.1^2}{20}\right)^2}{20}} = \frac{(114.2440 + 5.1005)^2}{\frac{13051.6915}{10} + \frac{26.0151}{20}} = 10.9$$

The value of t corresponding to a confidence coefficient of .95 and 11 degrees of freedom is 2.2010, and our approximate 95 percent confidence interval for $\mu_1 - \mu_2$ is

$$15.4 \pm 2.2010 \sqrt{\frac{(33.8)^2}{10} + \frac{(10.1)^2}{20}}$$

$$15.4 \pm (2.2010)(10.92)$$

$$15.4 \pm 24.0$$

$$-8.6,\ 39.4$$

Exercises

5.6.1. Nine patients suffering from the same physical handicap, but otherwise comparable, were asked to perform a certain task as part of an experiment. The average time required to perform the task was seven minutes with a standard deviation of two minutes. Assuming normality, construct the 90, 95, and 99 percent confidence intervals for the true mean time required to perform the task by this type patient.

5.6.2. A hospital administrator took a sample of 25 overdue accounts from which were computed a mean of $250 and a standard deviation of $75. Assuming that the amounts of all overdue accounts are normally distributed, find the 90, 95, and 99 percent confidence intervals for μ.

5.6.3. A sample of 25 ten-year old boys yielded a mean weight and standard deviation of 73 and 10 pounds, respectively. Assuming a normally distributed population, find the 90, 95, and 99 percent confidence intervals for the mean of the population from which the sample came.

5.6.4. A sample of 16 ten-year-old girls gave a mean weight of 71.5 and a standard deviation of 12 pounds, respectively. Assuming normality, find the 90, 95, and 99 percent confidence intervals for μ.

5.6.5. Refer to Exercises 5.6.3 and 5.6.4. Assume the population variances are equal. Construct the 90, 95, and 99 percent confidence intervals for the difference in the two population means.

5.6.6. Transverse diameter measurements on the hearts of adult males and females gave the following results:

Group	Sample Size	$\bar{x}$ (Centimeters)	s (Centimeters)
Males	12	13.21	1.05
Females	9	11.00	1.01

Assuming normally distributed populations with equal variances, construct the 90, 95, and 99 percent confidence intervals for $\mu_1 - \mu_2$.

5.6.7. Twenty-four experimental animals with vitamin D deficiency were divided equally into two groups. Group 1 received treatment consisting of a diet that provided vitamin D. The second group was not treated. At the end of the experimental period, serum calcium determinations were made with the following results:

$$\text{Treated group: } \bar{x} = 11.1 \text{ mg/100 ml}, s = 1.5$$
$$\text{Untreated group: } \bar{x} = 7.8 \text{ mg/100 ml}, s = 2.0$$

Assuming normally distributed populations with equal variances construct the 90, 95, and 99 percent confidence intervals for the difference between population means.

5.6.8. Two groups of children were given visual acuity tests. Group 1 was composed of 11 children who receive their health care from private physicians. The mean score for this group was 26 with a standard deviation of 5. The second group, consisting of 14 children who receive their health care from the health department, had an average score of 21 with a standard deviation of 6. Assuming normally distributed populations with equal variances find the .90, .95, and .99 confidence intervals for $\mu_1 - \mu_2$.

5.6.9. The average length of stay of a sample of 20 patients discharged from a general hospital was seven days with a standard deviation of two days. A sample of 24 patients discharged from a chronic disease hospital has an average length of stay of 36 days with a standard deviation of 10 days. Assuming normally distributed populations with unequal variances, find the 95 percent confidence interval for the difference between population means.

5.7 DETERMINATION OF SAMPLE SIZE FOR ESTIMATING MEANS

The question of how large a sample to take arises early in the planning of any survey or experiment. This is an important question and should not be treated lightly. To take a larger sample than is needed to achieve the desired results is wasteful of resources, while very small samples often lead to results that are of no practical use. Let us consider, then, how one may go about determining the size sample that is needed in a given situation. In this section, we present a method for determining the sample size required for estimating a population mean, and in the next section we apply this method to the case of sample size determination when the parameter to be estimated is a population proportion. By straightforward extensions of these methods, sample sizes required for more complicated situations can be determined.

The objectives in interval estimation are to obtain narrow intervals with high reliability. If we look at the components of a confidence interval, we see that the width of the interval is determined by the magnitude of the quantity

$$\text{(reliability coefficient)} \times \text{(standard error)}$$

since the total width of the interval is twice this amount. For a given standard error, increasing reliability means a larger reliability coefficient. But a larger reliability coefficient for a fixed standard error makes for a wider interval.

On the other hand, if we fix the reliability coefficient, the only way to reduce the width of the interval is to reduce the standard error. Since the standard error is equal to $\sigma/\sqrt{n}$, and since σ is a constant, the only way to obtain a small standard error is to take a large sample. How large a sample? That depends on the size of σ, the population standard deviation, and the desired degree of reliability and desired interval width.

Let us suppose we want an interval that extends d units on either side of the estimator. We can write

$$d = \text{(reliability coefficient)} \times \text{(standard error)} \tag{5.7.1}$$

If sampling is to be with replacement, from an infinite population, or from a population that is sufficiently large to warrant our ignoring the finite population correction, Equation 5.7.1 becomes

$$d = z\frac{\sigma}{\sqrt{n}} \tag{5.7.2}$$

which, when solved for n, gives

$$\boxed{n = \frac{z^2\sigma^2}{d^2}} \tag{5.7.3}$$

When sampling is without replacement from a small finite population, the finite population correction is required and Equation 5.7.1 becomes

$$d = z\frac{\sigma}{\sqrt{n}}\sqrt{\frac{N-n}{N-1}} \tag{5.7.4}$$

which, when solved for n, gives

$$\boxed{n = \frac{Nz^2\sigma^2}{d^2(N-1) + z^2\sigma^2}} \tag{5.7.5}$$

If the finite population correction can be ignored, Equation 5.7.5 reduces to Equation 5.7.3.

The formulas for sample size require a knowledge of σ^2 but, as has been pointed out, the population variance is, as a rule, unknown. As a result, σ^2 has to be estimated. The most frequently used sources of estimates for σ^2 are the following.

1. A *pilot* or preliminary sample may be drawn from the population and the variance computed from this sample may be used as an estimate of σ^2. Observations used in the pilot sample may be counted as part of the final sample, so that n (the computed sample size) $-$ n_1 (the pilot sample size) $=$ n_2 (the number of observations needed to satisfy the total sample size requirement).
2. Estimates of σ^2 may be available from previous or similar studies.
3. If it is felt that the population from which the sample is to be drawn is approximately normally distributed, one may use the fact that the range is approximately equal to 6 standard deviations and compute $\sigma \approx R/6$. This method requires some knowledge of the smallest and largest value of the variable in the population.

Example 5.7.1

A health department nutritionist, wishing to conduct a survey among a population of teenage girls, to determine their average daily protein intake, is seeking the advice of a biostatistician relative to the size sample that should be taken.

What procedure does the biostatistician follow in providing assistance to the nutritionist? Before the statistician can be of help to the nutritionist, the latter must provide three items of information: the desired width of the confidence interval, the level of confidence desired, and the magnitude of the population variance.

Let us assume that the nutritionist would like an interval about 10 units wide, that is, the estimate should be within about 5 units of the true value in either direction. Let us also assume that a confidence coefficient of .95 is decided on, and that, from past experience, the nutritionist feels that the population standard deviation is probably about 20 grams. The statistician now has the necessary information to compute the sample size: $z = 1.96$, $\sigma = 20$, and $d = 5$. Let us assume that the population of interest is large so that the statistician may ignore the finite population correction and use Equation 5.7.3. On making proper substitutions, the value of n is found to be

$$n = \frac{(1.96)^2(20)^2}{(5)^2}$$

$$= 61.47$$

The nutritionist is advised to take a sample of size 62. When calculating a sample size by Equation 5.7.3 or Equation 5.7.5, we round up to the next largest whole number if the calculations yield a number that is not itself an integer.

Exercises

5.7.1. A hospital administrator wishes to estimate the mean weight of babies born in her hospital. How large a sample of birth records should be taken if she wants a 99 percent confidence interval that is one pound wide. Assume that a reasonable estimate of σ is one pound. What size sample is required if the confidence coefficient is lowered to .95?

5.7.2. The director of the rabies control section in a city health department wishes to draw a sample from the department's records of dog bites reported during the past year in order to estimate the mean age of persons bitten. He wants a 95 percent confidence interval, he will be satisfied to let $d = 2.5$, and from previous studies he estimates the population standard deviation to be about 15 years. How large a sample should be drawn?

5.7.3. A physician would like to know the mean fasting blood glucose value (mg/100 ml) of patients seen in a diabetes clinic over the past 10 years. Determine the number of records the physician should examine in order to obtain a 90 percent confidence interval for μ if the desired width of the interval is 6 units and a pilot sample yields a variance of 60.

5.8 DETERMINATION OF SAMPLE SIZE FOR ESTIMATING PROPORTIONS

The method of sample size determination when a population proportion is to be estimated is essentially the same as that described above for estimating a population mean. We make use of the fact that one-half the desired interval, d, may be set equal to the product of the reliability coefficient and the standard error.

Assuming random sampling and conditions warranting approximate normality of the distribution of $\hat{p}$ leads to the following formula for n when sampling is with replacement, when sampling is from an infinite population, or when the sampled population is large enough to make the use of the finite population correction unnecessary;

$$n = \frac{z^2 pq}{d^2} \tag{5.8.1}$$

where $q = 1 - p$.

If the finite population correction can not be disregarded the proper formula for n is

$$n = \frac{Nz^2pq}{d^2(N - 1) + z^2pq} \tag{5.8.2}$$

When N is large in comparison to n (that is, $n/N \leq .05$) the finite population correction may be ignored, and Equation 5.8.2 reduces to Equation 5.8.1.

As we see, both formulas require a knowledge of p, the proportion in the population possessing the characteristic of interest. Since this is the parameter we are trying to estimate, it, obviously, will be unknown. One solution to this problem is to take a pilot sample and compute an estimate to be used in place of p in the formula for n. Sometimes an investigator will have some notion of an upper bound for p which can be used in the formula. For example, if it is desired to estimate the proportion of some population who have a certain condition, we may feel that the true proportion cannot be greater than, say, .30. We then substitute .30 for p in the formula for n. If it is impossible to come up with a better estimate, one may set p equal to .5 and solve for n. Since $p = .5$ in the formula yields the maximum value of n, this procedure will give a large enough sample for the desired reliability and interval width. It may, however, be larger than needed and result in a more expensive sample than if a better estimate of p had been available. This procedure should be used only if one is unable to come up with a better estimate of p.

Example 5.8.1

A survey is being planned to determine what proportion of families in a certain area are medically indigent. It is felt that the proportion cannot be greater than .35. A 95 percent confidence interval is desired with $d = .05$. What size sample of families should be selected?

If the finite population correction can be ignored, we have

$$n = \frac{(1.96)^2(.35)(.65)}{(.05)^2} = 349.6$$

The necessary sample size, then, is 350.

Exercises

5.8.1. An epidemiologist wishes to know what proportion of adults living in a large metropolitan area have subtype ay hepatitis B virus. Determine the size sample that would be required to estimate the true proportion to within .03 with 95 percent confidence. In a similar metropolitan area the proportion of adults, with the characteristic is reported to be .20. If data from another metropolitan area were not available, and a pilot sample could not be drawn, what size sample would be required?

5.8.2. A survey is planned to determine what proportion of the high school students in a metropolitan school system have regularly smoked marijuana. If no estimate of p is available from previous studies, a pilot sample cannot be drawn, a confidence coefficient of .95 is desired, and $d = .04$ is to be used, determine the appropriate sample size. What size sample would be required if 99 percent confidence were desired?

5.8.3. A hospital administrator wishes to know what proportion of discharged patients are unhappy with the care received during hospitalization. How large a sample should be drawn if we let $d = .05$, the confidence coefficient is .95, and no other information is available? How large should the sample be if p is approximated by .25?

5.9 CONFIDENCE INTERVAL FOR THE VARIANCE OF A NORMALLY DISTRIBUTED POPULATION

Point Estimation of the Population Variance. In previous sections it has been suggested that when a population variance is unknown, the sample variance may be used as an estimator. The reader may have wondered about the quality of this estimator. We have discussed only one criterion of goodness—unbiasedness—so let us see if the sample variance is an unbiased estimator of the population variance. To be unbiased, the average value of the sample variance over all possible samples must be equal to the population variance. That is, the expression $E(s^2) = \sigma^2$ must hold. To see if this condition holds for a particular situation, let us refer to the example of constructing a sampling distribution given in Section 4.4. In Table 4.4.1 we have all possible samples of size 2 from the population consisting of the values 6, 8, 10, 12, and 14. It will be recalled that two measures of dispersion for this population were computed as follows:

$$\sigma^2 = \frac{\sum(x_i - \mu)^2}{N} = 8 \qquad \text{and} \qquad S^2 = \frac{\sum(x_i - \mu)^2}{N - 1} = 10$$

If we compute the sample variance $s^2 = \sum(x_i - \bar{x})^2/(n - 1)$ for each of the possible samples shown in Table 4.4.1, we obtain the sample variances shown in Table 5.9.1.

Table 5.9.1

Variances Computed from Samples Shown in Table 4.4.1

		Second Draw				
		6	8	10	12	14
First Draw	6	0	2	8	18	32
	8	2	0	2	8	18
	10	8	2	0	2	8
	12	18	8	2	0	2
	14	32	18	8	2	0

If sampling is with replacement, the expected value of s^2 is obtained by taking the mean of all sample variances in Table 5.9.1. When we do this, we have

$$E(s^2) = \frac{\sum s_i^2}{N^n} = \frac{0 + 2 + \cdots + 2 + 0}{25} = \frac{200}{25} = 8$$

and we see, for this example, that when sampling with replacement $E(s^2) = \sigma^2$ where $s^2 = \sum(x_i - \bar{x})^2/(n-1)$ and $\sigma^2 = \sum(x_i - \mu)^2/N$.

If we consider the case where sampling is without replacement, the expected value of s^2 is obtained by taking the mean of all variances above (or below) the principal diagonal. That is,

$$E(s^2) = \frac{\sum s_i^2}{\binom{N}{n}} = \frac{2 + 8 + \cdots + 2}{10} = \frac{100}{10} = 10$$

which, we see, is not equal to σ^2, but is equal to $S^2 = \sum(x_i - \mu)^2/(N-1)$.

These results are examples of general principles, as it can be shown that, in general,

$E(s^2) = \sigma^2$ *when sampling is with replacement,*

$E(s^2) = S^2$ *when sampling is without replacement.*

When N is large, $N - 1$ and N will be approximately equal and, consequently, σ^2 and S^2 will be approximately equal.

These results justify our use of $s^2 = \sum(x_i - \bar{x})^2/(n-1)$ when computing the sample variance. In passing, let us note that although s^2 is an unbiased estimator of σ^2, s is not an unbaised estimator of σ. The bias, however, diminishes rapidly as n increases. Those interested in pursuing this point further are referred to the articles by Cureton (18), and Gurland and Tripathi (19).

Interval Estimation of a Population Variance. With a point estimate available to us, it is logical to inquire about the construction of a confidence interval for a population variance.

Whether we are successful in constructing a confidence interval for σ^2 will depend on our ability to find an appropriate sampling distribution.

Confidence intervals for σ^2 are usually based on the sampling distribution of $(n-1)s^2/\sigma^2$. If samples of size n are drawn from a normally distributed population, this quantity has a distribution known as the *chi-square distribution* with $n - 1$ degrees of freedom. As we shall say more about this distribution in a later chapter, we only say here that it is the distribution that the quantity $(n-1)s^2/\sigma^2$ follows, and that it is useful in finding confidence intervals for σ^2 when the assumption that the population is normally distributed holds true.

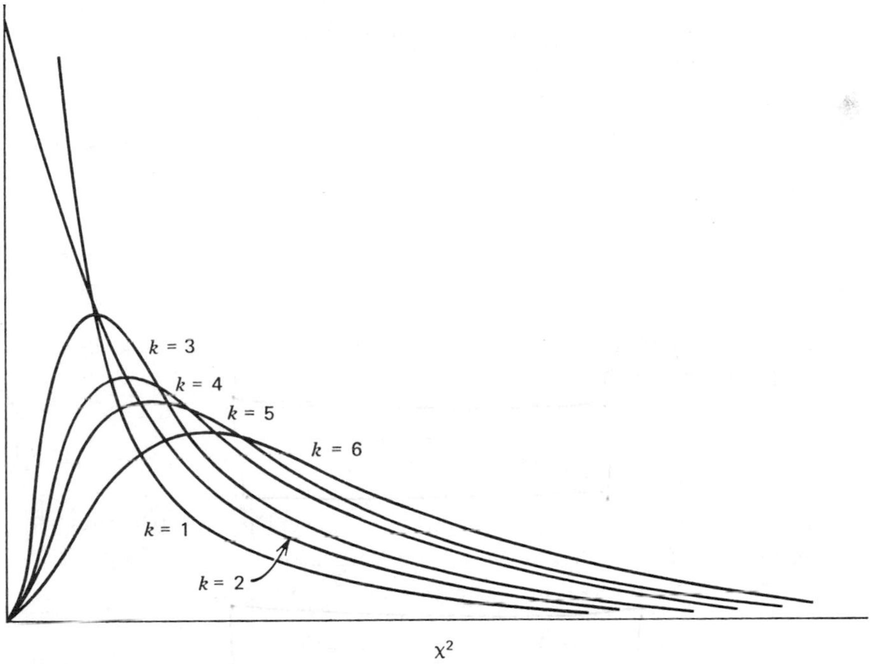

Figure 5.9.1. Chi-square distributions for several values of degrees of freedom k. (*Source. Paul G. Hoel and Raymond J. Jessen*, Basic Statistics for Business and Economics, *Wiley, 1971. Used by permission.*)

In Figure 5.9.1 are shown some chi-square distributions for several values of degrees of freedom. Percentiles of the chi-square distribution, designated by the Greek letter, χ^2, are given in Table I. The column headings give the values of χ^2 to the left of which lies a proportion of the total area under the curve equal to the subscript of χ^2. The row labels are the degrees of freedom.

To obtain a $100(1-\alpha)$ percent confidence interval for σ^2, we first obtain the $100(1-\alpha)$ confidence interval for $(n-1)s^2/\sigma^2$. To do this, we select the values of χ^2 from Table I in such a way that $\alpha/2$ is to the left of the smaller value and $\alpha/2$ is to the right of the larger value. In other words, the two values of χ^2 are selected in such a way that α is divided equally between the two tails of the distribution. We may designate these two values of χ^2 as $\chi^2_{\alpha/2}$ and $\chi^2_{(1-\alpha/2)}$, respectively. The $100(1-\alpha)$ percent confidence interval for $(n-1)s^2/\sigma^2$, then, is given by

$$\chi^2_{\alpha/2} < \frac{(n-1)s^2}{\sigma^2} < \chi^2_{(1-\alpha/2)}$$

We now manipulate this expression in such a way that we obtain an expression with σ^2 alone as the middle term. First, let us divide each term by $(n - 1)s^2$ to get

$$\frac{\chi^2_{\alpha/2}}{(n-1)s^2} < \frac{1}{\sigma^2} < \frac{\chi^2_{(1-\alpha/2)}}{(n-1)s^2}$$

If we take the reciprocal of this expression we have

$$\frac{(n-1)s^2}{\chi^2_{\alpha/2}} > \sigma^2 > \frac{(n-1)s^2}{\chi^2_{(1-\alpha/2)}}$$

Note that the direction of the inequalities changed when we took the reciprocals. If we reverse the order of the terms we have

$$\frac{(n-1)s^2}{\chi^2_{(1-\alpha/2)}} < \sigma^2 < \frac{(n-1)s^2}{\chi^2_{\alpha/2}} \qquad (5.9.1)$$

which is the $100(1 - \alpha)$ percent confidence interval for σ^2. If we take the square root of each term in Expression 5.9.1, we have the following $100(1 - \alpha)$ percent confidence interval for σ, the population standard deviation:

$$\sqrt{\frac{(n-1)s^2}{\chi^2_{(1-\alpha/2)}}} < \sigma < \sqrt{\frac{(n-1)s^2}{\chi^2_{\alpha/2}}} \qquad (5.9.2)$$

Example 5.9.1

Refer to Example 5.6.1 and assume that the population of serum amylase determinations from which the sample of size 15 was drawn is normally distributed. Let us construct the 95 percent confidence interval for σ^2.

The sample yielded a value of $s^2 = 1225$. The degrees of freedom are $n - 1 = 14$. The appropriate values of χ^2 from Table I are $\chi^2_{(1-\alpha/2)} = 26.119$ and $\chi^2_{\alpha/2} = 5.629$. Our 95 percent confidence interval for σ^2 is

$$\frac{(14)(1225)}{26.119} < \sigma^2 < \frac{14(1225)}{5.629}$$

$$656.61 < \sigma^2 < 3046.72$$

The 95 percent confidence interval for σ is

$$25.62 < \sigma < 55.20$$

We say we are 95 percent confident that the parameters being estimated are within the specified limits, because we know that in the long run, in repeated sampling, 95 percent of intervals constructed as illustrated would include the respective parameters.

Although this method of constructing confidence intervals for σ^2 is widely used, it is not without its drawbacks. First, the assumption of the normality of the population from which the sample is drawn is crucial, especially for small samples, and results may be misleading unless n is large.

Another difficulty with these intervals results from the fact that the estimator is not in the center of the confidence interval as is the case with the confidence interval for μ. This is because the chi-square distribution, unlike the normal, is not symmetric. The practical implication of this is that the method for the construction of confidence intervals for σ^2, which has just been described, does not yield the shortest possible confidence intervals. Tate and Klett (20) give tables that may be used to overcome this difficulty.

Exercises

5.9.1. Each of a sample of 51 nursing students was given a standardized test to measure his or her level of responsibility. A value of $s^2 = 12$ was computed. Construct 95 percent confidence intervals for σ^2 and σ.

5.9.2. White blood cell counts taken on a sample of 10 adult males with some type of leukemia yielded a variance of 25,000,000. Construct 95 percent confidence intervals for σ^2 and σ.

5.9.3. Forced vital capacity determinations were made on 20 healthy adult males. The sample variance was 1,000,000. Construct 90 percent confidence intervals for σ^2 and σ.

5.9.4. In a study of myocardial transit times, appearance transit times were obtained on a sample of 30 patients with coronary artery disease. The sample variance was found to be 1.03. Construct 99 percent confidence intervals for σ^2 and σ.

5.9.5. A sample of 25 physically and mentally healthy males participated in a sleep experiment in which the percentage of each participant's total sleeping time spent in a certain stage of sleep was recorded. The variance computed from the sample data was 2.25. Construct 95 percent confidence intervals for σ^2 and σ.

5.9.6. Hemoglobin determinations were made on 16 animals exposed to a harmful chemical. The following observations were recorded: 15.6, 14.8, 14.4, 16.6, 13.8, 14.0, 17.3, 17.4, 18.6, 16.2, 14.7, 15.7, 16.4, 13.9, 14.8, 17.5. Construct 95 percent confidence intervals for σ^2 and σ.

5.10 CONFIDENCE INTERVAL FOR THE RATIO OF THE VARIANCES OF TWO NORMALLY DISTRIBUTED POPULATIONS

It is frequently of interest to compare two variances, and one way to do this is to form their ratio, σ_1^2/σ_2^2. If two variances are equal, their ratio will be equal to 1. We usually will not know the variances of populations of interest and, consequently, any comparisons we make will have to be based on sample variances. To be specific, we may wish to estimate the ratio of two population variances. Again, since this is a form of inference, we must rely on some sampling distribution, and this time the distribution of $(s_1^2/\sigma_1^2)/(s_2^2/\sigma_2^2)$ is utilized provided certain assumptions are met. The assumptions are that s_1^2 and s_2^2 are computed from independent samples of size n_1 and n_2, respectively, drawn from two normally distributed populations.

If the assumptions are met $(s_1^2/\sigma_1^2)/(s_2^2/\sigma_2^2)$ follows a distribution known as the *F distribution*. We defer a more complete discussion of this distribution until a later chapter, but note that this distribution depends on two degrees of freedom values, one corresponding to the value of $n_1 - 1$ used in computing s_1^2, and the other corresponding to the value of $n_2 - 1$ used in computing s_2^2. These are usually referred to as the *numerator degrees of freedom* and *the denominator degrees of freedom.* Figure 5.10.1 shows some F distributions for several numerator and denominator degrees-of-freedom combinations. Table J contains, for specified combinations of degrees of freedom and values of α, F values to the right of which lies $\alpha/2$ of the area under the curve of F.

To find the $100(1 - \alpha)$ percent confidence interval for σ_1^2/σ_2^2, we begin with the expression

$$F_{\alpha/2} < \frac{s_1^2/\sigma_1^2}{s_2^2/\sigma_2^2} < F_{(1-\alpha/2)}$$

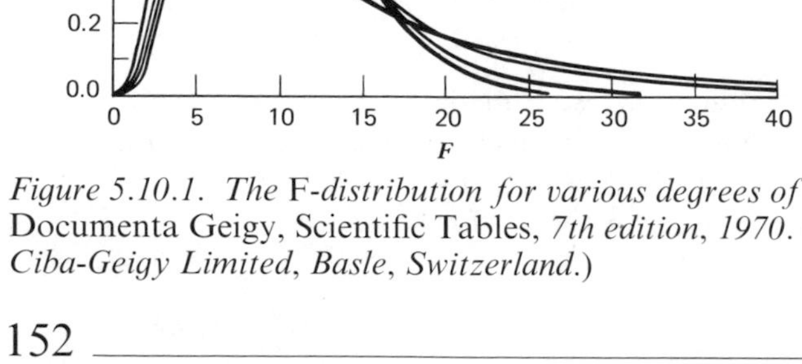

Figure 5.10.1. The F*-distribution for various degrees of freedom.* (*From* Documenta Geigy, Scientific Tables, *7th edition, 1970. Courtesy of Ciba-Geigy Limited, Basle, Switzerland.*)

where $F_{\alpha/2}$ and $F_{(1-\alpha/2)}$ are the values from the F table to the left and right of which, respectively, lies $\alpha/2$ of the area under the curve. The middle term of this expression may be rewritten so that the entire expression is

$$F_{\alpha/2} < \frac{s_1^2}{s_2^2} \cdot \frac{\sigma_2^2}{\sigma_1^2} < F_{(1-\alpha/2)}$$

If we divide through by s_1^2/s_2^2, we have

$$\frac{F_{\alpha/2}}{s_1^2/s_2^2} < \frac{\sigma_2^2}{\sigma_1^2} < \frac{F_{(1-\alpha/2)}}{s_1^2/s_2^2}$$

Taking the reciprocals of the three terms gives

$$\frac{s_1^2/s_2^2}{F_{\alpha/2}} > \frac{\sigma_1^2}{\sigma_2^2} > \frac{s_1^2/s_2^2}{F_{(1-\alpha/2)}}$$

and if we reverse the order we have the following $100(1-\alpha)$ percent confidence interval for σ_1^2/σ_2^2:

$$\boxed{\frac{s_1^2/s_2^2}{F_{(1-\alpha/2)}} < \frac{\sigma_1^2}{\sigma_2^2} < \frac{s_1^2/s_2^2}{F_{\alpha/2}}} \qquad (5.10.1)$$

Example 5.10.1

Let us refer to Example 5.6.2 and compute the 95 percent confidence interval for σ_1^2/σ_2^2. We have the following information:

$$n_1 = 22, \qquad n_2 = 15$$
$$s_1^2 = 1600, \qquad s_2^2 = 1225$$
$$\text{numerator degrees of freedom} = 21$$
$$\text{denominator degrees of freedom} = 14$$
$$\alpha = .05$$
$$F_{.025} = .395 \qquad F_{.975} = 2.84$$

At this point we must make a cumbersome, but unavoidable, digression and explain how the values $F_{.975} = 2.84$ and $F_{.025} = .395$ were obtained. First, it will be noted that in Table J we do not have a column headed 21 for numerator degrees of freedom. We took the closest value, 20. The value of $F_{.975}$ at the intersection of the column headed 20 and the row labeled 14 is 2.84. If we had a more extensive table of the F distribution, finding $F_{.025}$ would be no trouble; we would simply find $F_{.025}$ as we found $F_{.975}$. We would take the value at the intersection of the column headed 21 and the row headed 14. To include every possible percentile of F would make for a very lengthy table. Fortunately, however, there exists a relationship that enables us to compute the lower percentile values from our limited table. We proceed as follows.

Interchange the numerator and denominator degrees of freedom and locate the appropriate value of F. For the problem at hand we locate 2.53 which is at the intersection of the column headed 15 (the closest value to our 14 degrees of freedom) and the row labeled 21. We now take the reciprocal of this value, $1/2.53 = .395$.

We are now ready to obtain our 95 percent confidence interval for σ_1^2/σ_2^2 by substituting appropriate values into Expression 5.10.1:

$$\frac{1600/1225}{2.84} < \frac{\sigma_1^2}{\sigma_2^2} < \frac{1600/1225}{.395}$$

$$.460 < \frac{\sigma_1^2}{\sigma_2^2} < 3.31$$

We give this interval the appropriate probabilistic and practical interpretations.

Exercises

5.10.1 Oxytocin concentrations (picograms per milliliter) in the amniotic fluid of two samples of women were recorded. The first sample consisted of 25 parturient women with labor contractions. The second sample consisted of 16 women with no labor contractions. The sample variances were $s_1^2 = 40{,}000$ and $s_2^2 = 10{,}000$. Construct the 95 percent confidence interval for the ratio of the two population variances.

5.10.2. A measure of the nicotine content was obtained for urine specimens collected from two groups of adult males. Group 1 consisted of 25 apparently healthy cigarette smokers, and Group 2 was composed of 31 cigarette smokers with cancer of the urinary bladder. The sample variances were $s_1^2 = 1.00$ and $s_2^2 = 3.5$. Construct the 90 percent confidence interval for σ_2^2/σ_1^2.

5.10.3. Stroke index values were statistically analyzed for two samples of patients suffering from myocardial infarction. The sample variances were 12 and 10. There were 21 patients in each sample. Construct the 95 percent confidence interval for the ratio of the two population variances.

5.10.4. Thirty-two adult aphasics seeking speech therapy were divided equally into two groups. Group 1 received Treatment 1, and Group 2 received Treatment 2. Statistical analysis of the treatment effectiveness scores yielded the following variances: $s_1^2 = 8$, $s_2^2 = 15$. Construct the 90 percent confidence interval for σ_2^2/σ_1^2.

5.10.5. Sample variances were computed for the tidal volumes (ml) of two groups of patients suffering from atrial septal defect. The results and sample sizes were as follows:

$$n_1 = 31, \; s_1^2 = 35{,}000$$
$$n_2 = 41, \; s_2^2 = 20{,}000$$

Construct the 95 percent confidence interval for the ratio of the two variances.

5.10.6. Glucose responses to oral glucose were recorded for 11 patients with Huntington's disease (Group 1) and 13 control subjects (Group 2). Statistical analysis of the results yielded the following sample variances: $s_1^2 = 105$, $s_2^2 = 148$. Construct the 95 percent confidence interval for the ratio of the two variances.

5.11 SUMMARY

This chapter is concerned with one of the major areas of statistical inference—estimation. Both point and interval estimation are covered. The concepts and methods involved in the construction of confidence intervals are illustrated for the following parameters: means, the difference between two means, proportions, the difference between two proportions, variances, and the ratio of two variances.

Review Questions and Exercises

1. What is statistical inference?
2. Why is estimation an important type of inference?
3. What is a point estimate?
4. Explain the meaning of unbiasedness.
5. Define the following:
   (a) Reliability coefficient
   (b) Confidence coefficient
   (c) Standard error
   (d) Estimator
6. Give the general formula for a confidence interval.
7. State the probabilistic and practical interpretations of a confidence interval.
8. Of what use is the central limit theorem in estimation?

9. Describe the t distribution.

10. What are the assumptions underlying the use of the t distribution in estimating a single population mean?

11. What is the finite population correction? When can it be ignored?

12. What are the assumptions underlying the use of the t distribution in estimating the difference between two population means?

13. Arterial blood gas analyses performed on a sample of 15 physically active adult males yielded the following resting PaO_2 values:

    75, 80, 80, 74, 84, 78, 89, 72, 83, 76, 75, 87, 78, 79, 88

    Compute the 95 percent confidence interval for the mean of the population.

14. In a sample of 140 asthma patients, 35 percent had positive skin reactions to house dust. Construct the 95 percent confidence interval for the population proportion.

15. An industrial hygiene survey was conducted in a large metropolitan area. Of 70 manufacturing plants of a certain type visited, 21 received a "poor" rating with respect to absence of safety hazards. Construct a 95 percent confidence interval for the population proportion deserving a "poor" rating.

16. Refer to the previous problem. How large a sample would be required to estimate the population proportion to within .05 with 95 percent confidence (.30 is the best available estimate of p):
    (a) If the fpc can be ignored?
    (b) If the fpc is not ignored and $N = 1500$?

17. In a dental survey conducted by a county dental health team, 500 adults were asked to give the reason for their last visit to a dentist. Of the 220 who had less than a high school education, 44 said they went for preventive reasons. Of the remaining 280, who had a high school education or better, 150 stated that they went for preventive reasons. Construct a 95 percent confidence interval for the difference between the two population proportions.

18. A breast cancer research team collected the following data on tumor size:

Type of Tumor	n	$\bar{x}$	s
A	21	3.85 cm	1.95 cm
B	16	2.80 cm	1.70 cm

Construct a 95 percent confidence interval for the difference between population means.

19. A certain drug was found to be effective in the treatment of pulmonary disease in 180 out of 200 cases treated. Construct the 90 percent confidence interval for the population proportion.

20. Seventy patients with stasis ulcers of the leg were randomly divided into two equal groups. Each group received a different treatment for edema. At the end of the experiment, treatment effectiveness was measured in terms of reduction in leg volume as determined by water displacement. The means and standard deviations for the two groups were as follows:

Group (Treatment)	$\bar{x}$	s
A	95 cc	25
B	125 cc	30

Construct a 95 percent confidence interval for the difference in population means.

21. The following are the serum bilirubin values of a sample of 10 patients admitted to a hospital for treatment of hepatitis.

20.5, 14.8, 21.3, 12.7, 15.2, 26.6, 23.4, 22.9, 15.7, 19.2

Construct a 95 percent confidence interval for the population mean.

References

References cited

1. John E. Freund, *Mathematical Statistics*, Prentice-Hall, Englewood Cliffs, N.J., 1962.
2. Alexander M. Mood and Franklin A. Graybill, *Introduction to the Theory of Statistics*, Second Edition, McGraw-Hill, New York, 1963.
3. Taro Yamane, *Statistics: An Introductory Analysis*, Second Edition, Harper & Row, New York, 1967.
4. W. S. Gosset, ("Student"), "The Probable Error of a Mean," *Biometrika*, *6* (1908), 1–25.
5. W. V. Behrens, "Ein Beitrag zu Fehlerberechnung bei wenige Beobachtungen," *Landwirtsschaftliche Jahrbücher*, *68* (1929), 807–837.
6. R. A. Fisher, "The Comparison of Samples with Possibly Unequal Variances," *Annals of Eugenics*, *9* (1939), 174–180.
7. ______, "The Asymptotic Approach to Behrens' Integral with Further Tables for the *d* Test of Signficance," *Annals of Eugenics*, *11* (1941), 141–172.

8. J. Neyman, "Fiducial Argument and the Theory of Confidence Intervals," *Biometrika, 32* (1941), 128–150.

9. H. Scheffé, "On Solutions of the Behrens-Fisher Problem Based on the t-Distribution," *The Annals of Mathematical Statistics, 14* (1943), 35–44.

10. ______, "A Note on the Behrens-Fisher Problem," *The Annals of Mathematical Statistics, 15* (1944), 430–432.

11. B. L. Welch, "The Significance of the Difference Between Two Means When the Population Variances Are Unequal," *Biometrika, 29* (1937), 350–361.

12. ______, "The Generalization of 'Student's' Problem When Several Different Population Variances Are Involved," *Biometrika, 34* (1947), 28–35.

13. Alice A. Aspin, "Tables for Use in Comparisons Whose Accuracy Involves Two Variances s, Separately Estimated," *Biometrika, 36* (1949), 290–296.

14. W. H. Trickett, B. L. Welch, and G. S. James, "Further Critical Values for the Two-means Problem," *Biometrika, 43* (1956), 203–205.

15. William G. Cochran, "Approximate Significance Levels of the Behrens–Fisher Test," *Biometrics, 20* (1964), 191–195.

16. George W. Snedecor and William G. Cochran, *Statistical Methods*, Sixth Edition, The Iowa State University Press, Ames, 1967.

17. Wilfred J. Dixon and Frank J. Massey, Jr., *Introduction to Statistical Analysis*, Third Edition, McGraw-Hill, New York, 1969.

18. Edward E. Cureton, "Unbiased Estimation of the Standard Deviation," *The American Statistician, 22* (February 1968) 22.

19. John Gurland and Ran C. Tripathi, "A Simple Approximation for Unbiased Estimation of the Standard Deviation," *The American Statistician, 25* (October 1971), 30–32.

20. R. F. Tate and G. W. Klett, "Optimal Confidence Intervals for the Variance of a Normal Distribution," *Journal of the American Statistical Association, 54* (1959), 674–682.

Other references

1. H. A. Al-Bayyati, "A Rule of Thumb for Determining a Sample Size in Comparing Two Proportions," *Technometrics, 13* (1971), 675–677.

2. F. F. Ractliffe, "The Effect on the t Distribution of Nonnormality in the Sampled Population," *Applied Statistics, 17* (1968), 42–48.

6

HYPOTHESIS TESTING

6.1 INTRODUCTION

One type of statistical inference, estimation, is discussed in the preceding chapter. The other type, hypothesis testing, is the subject of the present chapter. As is true with estimation, the *purpose of hypothesis testing is to aid the clinician, researcher, or administrator in reaching a decision concerning a population by examining a sample from that population.* Estimation and hypothesis testing are not as different as they are made to appear by the fact that most textbooks devote a separate chapter to each. As we will explain later, one may use confidence intervals to arrive at the same conclusions that are reached by using the hypothesis testing procedures discussed in this chapter.

In this section some of the basic concepts essential to an understanding of hypothesis testing are presented. The specific details of particular tests will be given in succeeding sections.

A *hypothesis* may be defined simply as *a statement about one or more populations.* The hypothesis is usually concerned with the parameters of the populations about which the statement is made. A hospital administrator may hypothesize that the average length of stay of patients admitted to the hospital is five days; a public health nurse may hypothesize that a particular educational program will result in improved communication between nurse and patient; a physician may hypothesize that a certain drug will be effective in 90 percent of the cases with which it is used. By means of hypothesis testing one determines whether or not such statements are compatible with available data.

Researchers are concerned with two types of hypotheses—*research hypotheses* and *statistical hypotheses.* The research hypothesis is the conjecture or supposition that motivates the research. It may be the result of years of observation on the part of the researcher. A public health nurse, for example, may have noted that certain clients responded more readily to a particular type of health education program. A physician may recall numerous instances in which certain combinations of therapeutic measures were more effective than any one of them alone. Research projects often result from the desire of such health practitioners to determine whether or not their theories or suspicions can be verified when subjected to the rigors of scientific investigation.

Research hypotheses lead directly to statistical hypotheses. Statistical hypotheses are stated in such a way that they may be evaluated by appropriate statistical techniques. In this book the hypotheses that we shall focus on are statistical hypotheses. We shall assume that the research hypotheses for the examples and exercises have already been considered.

For convenience, hypothesis testing will be presented as a nine-step procedure. There is nothing magical or sacred about this particular format, although it does break the process down into a logical sequence of actions and decisions.

1. *Data.* The nature of the data that form the basis of the testing procedures must be understood, since this determines the particular test to be employed. Whether the data consist of counts or measurements, for example, must be determined.
2. *Assumptions.* As we learned in the chapter on estimation, different assumptions led to modifications of confidence intervals. The same is true in hypothesis testing: a general procedure is modified depending on the assumptions. In fact, the same assumptions that are of importance in estimation are also important in hypothesis testing. We have seen that these include, among others, assumptions about the normality of the population distribution, equality of variances, and independence of samples.
3. *Hypotheses.* There are two statistical hypotheses involved in hypothesis testing and these should be explicitly stated. The first is the *hypothesis to be tested*, usually referred to as the *null hypothesis*, and designated by the symbol H_0. The null hypothesis is sometimes referred to as a *hypothesis of no difference*, since it is a statement of agreement with (or no difference from) true conditions in the population of interest. In general, the null hypothesis is set up for the express purpose of being discredited. Consequently, the opposite of the conclusion that the researcher is seeking to reach becomes the statement of the null hypothesis. In the testing process the null hypothesis either is rejected or is not rejected. If the null hypothesis is not rejected, we will say that the data on which the test is based do not provide sufficient evidence to cause rejection. If the testing procedure leads to rejection, we will conclude that the data at hand are not compatible with the null hypothesis, but are supportive of some other hy-

pothesis. This other hypothesis is known as the *alternative hypothesis*, and may be designated by the symbol H_A.

It should be pointed out that neither hypothesis testing, nor statistical inference, in general, leads to the proof of a hypothesis, but merely indicates whether the hypothesis is supported or is not supported by the available data. When we fail to reject a null hypothesis, therefore, we do not say that it is true, but that it may be true. When we speak of accepting a null hypothesis, we have this limitation in mind, and do not wish to convey the idea that accepting implies proof.

4. *Test Statistic.* The test statistic is some statistic that may be computed from the data of the sample. As a rule, there are many possible values that the test statistic may assume, the particular value observed depending on the particular sample drawn. As we shall see, the test statistic serves as a decision maker, since the decision to reject or not to reject the null hypothesis depends on the magnitude of the test statistic. An example of a test statistic is the quantity

$$z = \frac{\bar{x} - \mu_0}{\sigma/\sqrt{n}}$$

where μ_0 is a hypothesized value of a population mean. This test statistic is related to the statistic

$$z = \frac{\bar{x} - \mu}{\sigma/\sqrt{n}}$$

The following is a general formula for a test statistic that will be applicable in many of the hypothesis tests discussed in this book:

$$\text{test statistic} = \frac{\text{relevant statistic} - \text{hypothesized parameter}}{\text{standard error of the relevant statistic}}$$

In the present example, $\bar{x}$ is the relevant statistic, μ_0 is the hypothesized parameter, and $\sigma/\sqrt{n}$ is the standard error of $\bar{x}$, the relevant statistic.

5. *Distribution of the Test Statistic.* It has been pointed out that the key to statistical inference is the sampling distribution. We are reminded of this again when it becomes necessary to specify the probability distribution of the test statistic. The distribution of the test statistic,

$$z = \frac{\bar{x} - \mu_0}{\sigma/\sqrt{n}}$$

for example, follows the unit normal distribution if the null hypothesis is true and the assumptions are met.

6. *Decision Rule.* All possible values that the test statistic can assume are points on the horizontal axis of the graph of the distribution of the test statistic and are divided into two groups, one group constitutes what is known as the *rejection region* and the other group makes up the *acceptance region.* The values of the test statistic comprising the rejection region are those values that are less likely to occur if the null hypothesis is true, while the values making up the acceptance region are more likely to occur if the null hypothesis is true. *The decision rule tells us to reject the null hypothesis if the value of the test statistic that we compute from our sample is one of the values in the rejection region, and to not reject (or "accept") the null hypothesis if the computed value of the test statistic is one of the values in the acceptance region.*

The decision as to which values go into the rejection region and which ones go into the acceptance region is made on the basis of the desired *level of significance*, designated by α. The term, level of significance, reflects the fact that hypothesis tests are sometimes called significance tests, and a computed value of the test statistic that falls in the rejection region is said to be *significant*. The level of significance, α, specifies the area under the curve of the distribution of the test statistic that is above the values on the horizontal axis constituting the rejection region. It is seen, then, that α is a probability and, in fact, is the *probability of rejecting a true null hypothesis.* Since to reject a true null hypothesis would constitute an error, it seems only reasonable that we should make the probability of rejecting a true null hypothesis small and, in fact, that is what is done. The more frequently encountered values of α are .01, .05, and .10.

The error committed when a true null hypothesis is rejected is called the *Type I error*. The *Type II error* is the error committed when a false null hypothesis is accepted. The probability of committing a Type II error is designated by β.

Whenever we reject a null hypothesis there is always the concomitant risk of committing a Type I error, rejecting a true null hypothesis. Whenever we "accept" a null hypothesis the risk of accepting a false null hypothesis is always present. We make α small, but we generally exercise no control over β, although we know that in most practical situations it is larger than α.

We never know whether we have committed one of these errors when we reject or fail to reject a null hypothesis, since the true state of affairs is unknown. If the testing procedure leads to rejection of the null hypothesis, we can take comfort from the fact that we made α small and, therefore, the probability of committing a Type I error was small. If we "accept" the null hypothesis, we do not know the concurrent risk of committing a Type II error, since β is usually unknown but, as has been pointed out, we do know that, in general, it is larger than α.

7. *Computed Test Statistic.* From the data contained in the sample we compute a value of the test statistic and compare it with the acceptance and rejection regions that have already been specified.

8. *Statistical Decision.* The statistical decision consists of rejecting or of not rejecting the null hypothesis. It is rejected if the computed value of the test statistic falls in the rejection region, and it is not rejected if the computed value of the test statistic falls in the acceptance region.
9. *Administrative or Clinical Decision.* The administrative or clinical decision usually depends on the statistical decision. If the null hypothesis is rejected, the administrative or clinical decision usually reflects this, in that the decision is compatible with the alternative hypothesis. The reverse is usually true if the null hypothesis is not rejected. The administrative or clinical decision, however, may take other forms, such as a decision to gather more data.

We must emphasize at this point, however, that the outcome of the statistical test is only one piece of evidence that influences the administrative or clinical decision. The statistical decision should not be interpreted as definitive, but should be considered along with all the other relevant information available to the experimenter.

With these general comments as background, we now discuss specific hypothesis tests.

6.2 HYPOTHESIS TESTING: A SINGLE POPULATION MEAN

In this section we consider the testing of a hypothesis about a population mean under three different conditions: (1) when sampling is from a normally distributed population of values with known variance, (2) when sampling is from a normally distributed population with unknown variance, and (3) when sampling is from a population that is not normally distributed. Although the theory for conditions 1 and 2 depend on normally distributed populations, it is common practice to make use of the theory when relevant populations are only approximately normally distributed. This is satisfactory so long as the departure from normality is not drastic.

Sampling from Normally Distributed Populations: Population Variances Known

Example 6.2.1

Researchers are interested in the mean level of some enzyme in a certain population. Let us say that they are asking the following question: Can we conclude that the mean enzyme level in this population is different from 25?

Based on our knowledge of hypothesis testing, we reply that they can conclude that the mean enzyme level is different from 25 if they can reject the null hypothesis that the mean is equal to 25. Let us use the information from Example 5.2.1 and the nine-step hypothesis testing procedure given in the previous section to help the researchers reach a decision.

1. *Data.* The data available to the researchers are the enzyme determinations made on a sample of 10 individuals from the population of interest. From this sample a mean of $\bar{x} = 22$ has been computed.
2. *Assumptions.* It is assumed that the sample comes from a population of normally distributed enzyme values with a known variance, $\sigma^2 = 45$.
3. *Hypotheses.* The hypothesis to be tested, or null hypothesis, is that the population mean enzyme level is equal to 25. The alternate hypothesis is that the population mean enzyme level is not equal to 25. Notice that we are identifying the conclusion they wish to reach with the alternative hypothesis, so that if the data permit rejection of the null hypothesis, the researchers' conclusion will carry more weight, since the accompanying probability of rejecting a true null hypothesis will be small. We will make sure of this by assigning a small value to α, the probability of committing a Type I error. We may present the relevant hypotheses in compact form as follows:

$$H_0: \mu = 25$$
$$H_A: \mu \neq 25$$

4. *Test Statistic.* Since we are testing a hypothesis about a population mean, since we assume that the population is normally distributed, and since the population variance is known, our test statistic is

$$z = \frac{\bar{x} - \mu_0}{\sigma/\sqrt{n}}$$

5. *Distribution of Test Statistic.* Based on our knowledge of sampling distributions and the normal distribution, we know that

$$z = \frac{\bar{x} - \mu_0}{\sigma/\sqrt{n}}$$

is normally distributed with a mean of 0 and a variance of 1, if H_0 is true. There are many possible values of the test statistic that the present situation can generate; one for every possible sample of size 10 that can be drawn from the population. Since we draw only one sample, we have only one of these possible values on which to base a decision.
6. *Decision Rule.* The decision rule tells us to reject H_0 if the computed value of the test statistic falls in the rejection region and to accept H_0 if it falls in the acceptance region. We must now specify the rejection and accep-

tance regions. We can begin by asking ourselves what magnitude of values of the test statistic will cause rejection of H_0. If the null hypothesis is false, it may be so either because the true mean is less than 25 or because the true mean is greater than 25. Therefore, either extremely small values or extremely large values of the test statistic will cause rejection of the null hypothesis. These extreme values we want to constitute the rejection region. How extreme must a possible value of the test statistic be to qualify for the rejection region? The answer depends on the significance level we choose, that is, the size of the probability of committing a Type I error. Let us say that we want the probability of rejecting a true null hypothesis to be $\alpha = .05$. Since our rejection region is to consist of two parts, extremely small values and extremely large values of the test statistic, part of α will have to be associated with the large values and part with the small values. It seems reasonable that we should divide α equally and let $\alpha/2 = .025$ be associated with extremely small values and $\alpha/2 = .025$ be associated with extremely large values.

What value of the test statistic is so large that, when the null hypothesis is true, the probability of obtaining a value this large or larger is .025? In other words, what is the value of z to the right of which lies .025 of the area under the unit normal distribution? The value of z to the right of which lies .025 of the area is the same value between zero and which lies .475 of the area. We look in the body of Table F until we find .475 or its closest value, and read the corresponding marginal entries to obtain our z value. In the present example the value of z is 1.96. Similar reasoning will lead us to find -1.96 as the value of the test statistic so small that when the null hypothesis is true, the probability of obtaining a value this small or smaller is .025. Our rejection region, then, consists of all values of the test statistic equal to or greater than 1.96, or less than or equal to -1.96. The acceptance region consists of all values in between. The acceptance and rejection regions are shown in Figure 6.2.1. The values of the test statistic that separate the rejection and

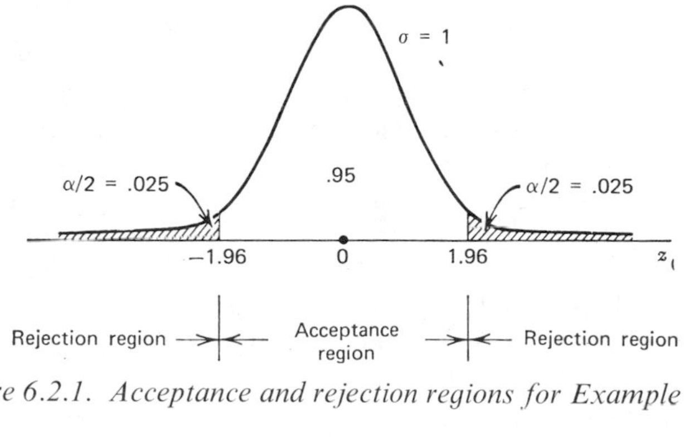

Figure 6.2.1. Acceptance and rejection regions for Example 6.2.1.

acceptance regions are sometimes called *critical values* of the test statistic, and the rejection region is sometimes referred to as the *critical region.*

The decision rule tells us to compute a value of the test statistic from the data of our sample and to reject H_0 if we get a value equal to or greater than 1.96 or equal to or less than -1.96, and to accept H_0 if we get any other value. The value of α and, hence, the decision rule, should be decided on prior to gathering the data. This prevents our being accused of allowing the sample results to influence our decision. This condition of objectivity is highly desirable and should be preserved in all tests.

7. *Computed Test Statistic.* From our sample we compute

$$z = \frac{22 - 25}{\sqrt{45/10}} = \frac{-3}{2.1213} = -1.41$$

8. *Statistical Decision.* Abiding by the decision rule, we are unable to reject the null hypothesis since -1.41 is not in the rejection region. We can say that the computed value of the test statistic is not significant at the .05 level.

9. *Administrative or Clinical Decision.* We conclude that μ *may be* equal to 25, and let our administrative or clinical actions be in accordance with this conclusion.

***p*-values.** Instead of saying that an observed value of the test statistic is significant or is not significant, most writers in the research literature prefer to report the exact probability of getting a value as extreme or more extreme than that observed if the null hypothesis is true. In the present instance these writers would give the computed value of the test statistic along with the statement $p = .1586$. The statement $p = .1586$ means that the probability of getting a value as extreme as 1.41 in either direction, when the null hypothesis is true, is .1586. The value .1586 is obtained from Table F and is the probability of observing a $z \geq 1.41$ or a $z \leq -1.41$ when the null hypothesis is true. That is, when H_0 is true, the probability of obtaining a value of z as large as or larger than 1.41 is .0793, and the probability of observing a value of z as small as or smaller than -1.41 is .0793. The probability of one or the other of these events occurring, when H_0 is true, is equal to the sum of the two individual probabilities, and hence, in the present example, we say that $p = .0793 + .0793 = .1586$. The quantity p is referred to as the *p-value* for the test. The p-value for a test is the smallest value of α for which the null hypothesis can be rejected.

The reporting of p-values as part of the results of an investigation is more informative to the reader than such statements as "the null hypothesis is rejected at the .05 level of significance" or "the results were not significant at the .05 level." Reporting the p-value associated with a test lets the reader know just how common or how rare is the computed value of the test statistic given that H_0 is true. Gibbons and Pratt (1) and Bahn (2) may be consulted for a more extensive treatment of the subject of p-values.

Testing H_0 by Means of a Confidence Interval. Earlier we stated that one can use confidence intervals to test hypotheses. In Example 6.2.1 we used a hypothesis testing procedure to test $H_0: \mu = 25$ against the alternative, $H_A: \mu \neq 25$. We were unable to reject H_0 because the computed value of the test statistic fell in the acceptance region.

Let us see how we might have arrived at this same conclusion by using a $100(1 - \alpha)$ percent confidence interval. The 95 percent confidence interval for μ is

$$22 \pm 1.96\sqrt{45}/\sqrt{10}$$
$$22 \pm 1.96(2.12)$$
$$22 \pm 4.16$$
$$17.84, 26.16$$

Since this interval includes 25, we say that 25 is a candidate for the mean we are estimating and, therefore, μ may be equal to 25. This is the same conclusion reached by means of the hypothesis testing procedure.

If the hypothesized parameter, 25, had not been included in the 95 percent confidence interval; that is, if the lower limit of the computed interval had been larger than 25, or if the upper limit had been smaller than 25, we would have said that H_0 is rejected at the .05 level of significance. In general, *when testing a null hypothesis by means of a two-sided confidence interval, we reject* H_0 *at the α level of significance if the hypothesized parameter is not contained within the* $100(1 - \alpha)$ *percent confidence interval. If the hypothesized parameter is contained within the interval,* H_0 *cannot be rejected at the α level of significance.*

The hypothesis test that we have just completed is an example of a *two-sided test*, so called because the rejection region is split between the two sides or tails of the distribution of the test statistic. A hypothesis test may be *one-sided*, in which case all of the rejection region is in one or the other tail of the distribution. Whether a one-sided or a two-sided test is used depends on the nature of the question being asked by the researcher.

If both large and small values will cause rejection of the null hypothesis, a two-sided test is indicated. When either relatively "small" values only or relatively "large" values only will cause rejection of the null hypothesis, a one-sided test is indicated.

Example 6.2.2

Suppose, instead of asking if they could conclude that $\mu \neq 25$, the researchers had asked: Can we conclude that $\mu < 25$? To this question we would reply that they can so conclude if they can reject the null hypothesis that $\mu \geq 25$. Let us go through the nine-step procedure to reach a decision based on a one-sided test.

1. *Data.* See the previous example.

2. *Assumptions.* See the previous example.

3. *Hypotheses.*

$$H_0 : \mu \geq 25$$
$$H_A : \mu < 25$$

The inequality in the null hypothesis implies that the null hypothesis consists of an infinite number of hypotheses. The test will be made only at the point of equality, since it can be shown that if H_0 is rejected at the point of equality it would be rejected if the test were done for any other value of μ indicated in the null hypothesis.

4. *Test statistic.*

$$z = \frac{\bar{x} - \mu_0}{\sigma/\sqrt{n}}$$

5. *Distribution of Test Statistic.* See the previous example.

6. *Decision Rule.* Let us again let $\alpha = .05$. To determine where to place the rejection region, let us ask ourselves what magnitude of values would cause rejection of the null hypothesis. If we look at the hypotheses, we see that small values would cause rejection, and that large values would tend to reinforce the null hypothesis. We will want our rejection region to be where the small values are—at the lower tail of the distribution. This time, since we have a one-sided test, all of α will go in the one tail of the distribution. By consulting Table F, we find that the value of z to the left of which lies .05 of the area under the unit normal curve is -1.645. Our rejection and acceptance regions are now specified and are shown in Figure 6.2.2.

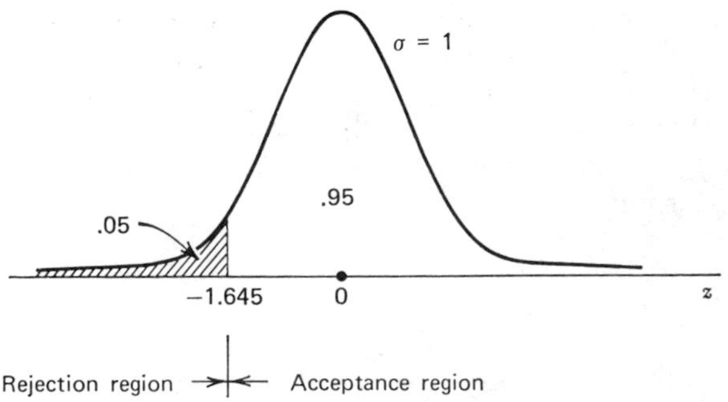

Figure 6.2.2. Acceptance and rejection regions for Example 6.2.2.

Our decision rule tells us to reject H_0 if the computed value of the test statistic is less than or equal to -1.645.

7. *Computed Test Statistic.* From our data we compute

$$z = \frac{22 - 25}{\sqrt{45}/\sqrt{10}} = -1.41$$

8. *Statistical Decision.* We are unable to reject the null hypothesis, since $-1.41 > -1.645$.
9. *Administrative or Clinical Decision.* We conclude that the true mean may be greater than or equal to 25 and act accordingly.

The *p*-value for this test is .0793, since $P(z \leq -1.41)$, when H_0 is true, is .0793 as given by Table F when we determine the magnitude of the area to the left of -1.41 under the unit normal curve. One can test a one-sided null hypothesis by means of a one-sided confidence interval. However, we shall not cover the construction and interpretation of this type of confidence interval in this book. The interested reader is referred to a discussion of the topic in the book by Daniel (3).

If the researchers' question had been, "Can we conclude that the mean is greater than 25?", following the above nine-step procedure would have led to a one-sided test with all of the rejection region at the upper tail of the distribution of the test statistic and a critical value of $+1.645$.

Sampling from a Normally Distributed Population: Population Variance Unknown. As we have already noted, the population variance is usually unknown in actual situations involving statistical inference about a population mean. The following example illustrates the hypothesis testing procedure when this is the case.

Example 6.2.3

The data for this example are taken from Example 5.6.1. Suppose we want to know whether we can conclude that the mean of the population from which the sample of serum amylase determinations came is different from 120. We can so conclude if we reject the null hypothesis that the true mean is equal to 120. This suggests a two-sided hypothesis test that we now make by using the familiar nine steps.

1. *Data.* The data consist of serum amylase determinations made on 15 apparently healthy subjects. The mean and standard deviation computed from the sample are 96 and 35 units/100 ml, respectively.
2. *Assumptions.* The 15 determinations constitute a random sample from a population of determinations that are normally distributed. The population variance is unknown.

3. *Hypotheses.*

$$H_0: \mu = 120$$
$$H_A: \mu \neq 120$$

4. *Test Statistic.* Since the population variance is unknown, our test statistic is

$$t = \frac{\bar{x} - \mu_0}{s/\sqrt{n}}$$

5. *Distribution of Test Statistic.* Our test statistic is distributed as Student's t with $n - 1$ degrees of freedom if H_0 is true.
6. *Decision Rule.* Let $\alpha = .05$. Since we have a two-sided test, we put $\alpha/2 = .025$ in each tail of the distribution of our test statistic. The t values to the right and left of which lies .025 of the area are 2.1448 and -2.1448. These values are obtained from Table H. The acceptance and rejection regions are shown in Figure 6.2.3.

   The decision rule tells us to compute a value of the test statistic and reject H_0 if the computed t is greater than or equal to 2.1448 or less than or equal to -2.1448.
7. *Computed Test Statistic.*

$$t = \frac{96 - 120}{35/\sqrt{15}} = \frac{-24}{9.04} = -2.65$$

8. *Statistical Decision.* Reject H_0, since -2.65 falls in the rejection region.
9. *Administrative or Clinical Decision.* Our conclusion, based on these data is that the mean of the population from which the sample came is not 120.

The exact p-value for this test cannot be obtained from Table H since it gives t-values only for selected percentiles. The p-value can be stated as an interval, however. In the present example, -2.65 is less than -2.624, the value of t to the left of which lies .01 of the area under the t with 14 degrees of freedom. Consequently, when H_0 is true, the probability of obtaining a

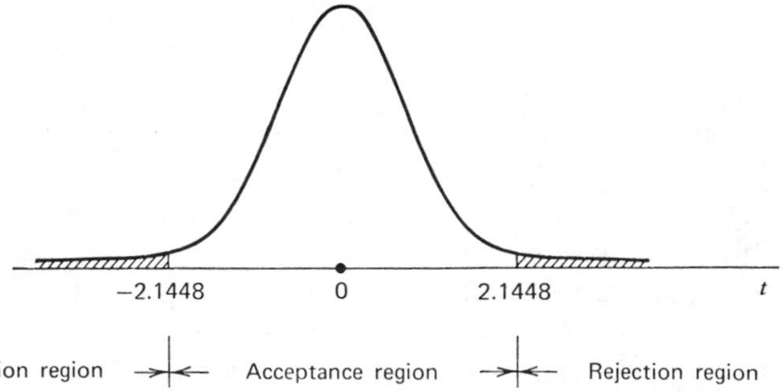

Figure 6.2.3. Acceptance and rejection regions for Example 6.2.3.

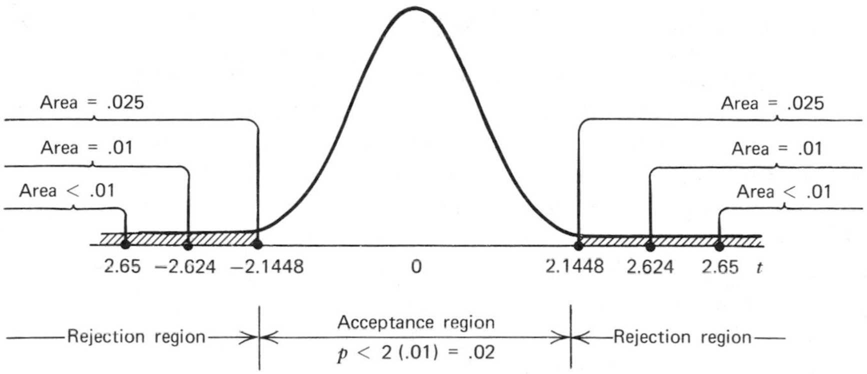

Figure 6.2.4. Determination of p-*value for Example 6.2.3 and its relationship to the rejection and acceptance regions.*

value of t as small as or smaller than -2.65 is less than .01. Since the test was two-sided, we must allow for the possibility of a computed value of the test statistic as large in the opposite direction as that observed. Table H reveals that $P(t \geq 2.65) < .01$. The p-value, then, is less than $2(.01) = .02$. This result would be reported in most journal articles as $p < .02$. Figure 6.2.4 shows the relationship between the p-value and the rejection and acceptance regions for this example.

If in the previous example the hypotheses had been

$$H_0: \mu \geq 120$$
$$H_A: \mu < 120$$

the testing procedure would have led to a one-sided test with all of the rejection region at the lower tail of the distribution, and if the hypotheses had been

$$H_0: \mu \leq 120$$
$$H_A: \mu > 120$$

we would have had a one-sided test with all of the rejection region at the upper tail of the distribution.

Sampling from a Population That Is Not Normally Distributed. If the sample on which we base our hypothesis test comes from a population that is not normally distributed, we may, if our sample is large, take advantage of the central limit theorem and use $z = (\bar{x} - \mu_0)/(\sigma/\sqrt{n})$ as the test statistic. If the population standard deviation is not known, the usual practice is to use the sample standard deviation as an estimate. The rationale is that the large sample, necessary for the central limit theorem to apply, will yield a close approximation of σ.

Example 6.2.4

In a health survey of a certain community 150 persons were interviewed. One of the items of information obtained was the number of prescriptions each person had had filled during the past year. The average number for the 150 people was 5.8 with a standard deviation of 3.1. The investigator wishes to know if these data provide sufficient evidence to indicate that the population mean is greater than 5. We say that the data do provide that evidence if we can reject the null hypothesis that the mean is less than or equal to 5. The following test may be carried out:

1. *Data.* The data consist of the number of prescriptions filled for 150 persons with $\bar{x} = 5.8$ and $s = 3.1$.
2. *Assumptions.* The data constitute a random sample from a population of unknown functional form.
3. *Hypotheses.*

$$H_0: \mu \leq 5$$
$$H_A: \mu > 5$$

4. *Test Statistic.*

$$z = \frac{\bar{x} - \mu_0}{\sigma/\sqrt{n}}$$

Since σ is unknown the sample standard deviation will be used as an estimate.

5. *Distribution of Test Statistic.* Because of the central limit theorem, the test statistic is approximately normally distributed with $\mu = 0$ if H_0 is true.
6. *Decision Rule.* Let $\alpha = .05$. The critical value of the test statistic is 1.645. The acceptance and rejection regions are shown in Figure 6.2.5. Reject H_0 if computed $z \geq 1.645$.
7. *Computed Test Statistic.*

$$z = \frac{5.8 - 5.0}{3.1/\sqrt{150}} = \frac{.8}{.25} = 3.2$$

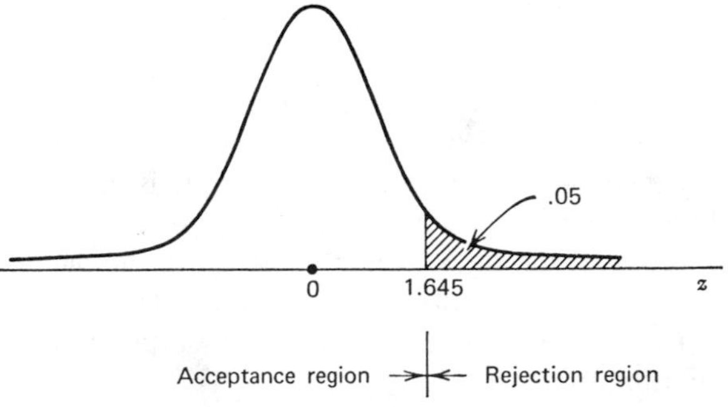

Figure 6.2.5. Acceptance and rejection regions for Example 6.2.4.

8. *Statistical Decision.* Reject H_0 since $3.2 > 1.645$.
9. *Administrative or Clinical Decision.* Conclude that the mean number of prescriptions filled per person per year for this population is greater than 5.

If the population variance had been known, the procedure would have been identical to the above except that the known value of σ, instead of the sample value, would have been used in the denominator of the computed test statistic. The p-value for this test is less than .001.

Depending on what the investigators wished to conclude, either a two-sided test or a one-sided test, with the rejection region at the lower tail of the distribution, could have been made by using the above data.

Exercises

For each of the following exercises carry out the nine-step hypothesis testing procedure for the given significance level. Compute the p-value for each test.

6.2.1. As part of a time and motion study conducted at a health care center, a sample of 100 patients spent, on the average, 23 minutes in the waiting room between registering and being seen by a member of the health team. The sample standard deviation was 10. Do these data provide sufficient evidence to indicate that the mean time spent in the waiting room is greater than 20 minutes? Let $\alpha = .05$.

6.2.2. An experiment was conducted to study the effect on rats of a certain type of brain surgery. Following surgery the rats were trained to perform a series of tasks. After the training period the rats were stimulated to perform the task and each was scored on the basis of the quality of its performance. The mean score for the 16 rats used in the experiment was 90 with a standard deviation of 10. Do these data provide sufficient evidence to indicate that the population mean is less than 95? Let $\alpha = .10$.

6.2.3. A survey of 64 medical laboratories revealed that the mean price charged for a certain test was \$12 with a standard deviation of \$6. Do these data provide sufficient evidence to indicate that the population mean is greater than \$10? Let $\alpha = .05$.

6.2.4. A study was made of a sample of 25 records of patients seen at a chronic disease hospital on an outpatient basis. The mean number of outpatient visits per patient was 4.8, and the sample standard deviation was 2. Can it be concluded from these data that the population mean is greater than four visits per patient? Let the probability of committing a Type I error be .05.

6.2.5. In a sample of 49 adolescents who served as the subjects in an immunologic study, one variable of interest was the diameter of skin test reaction to an antigen. The sample mean and standard deviation were 21 and 11 mm erythema, respectively. Can it be concluded from these data that the population mean is less than 30? Let $\alpha = .05$.

6.2.6. Nine laboratory animals were infected with a certain bacterium and then immunosuppressed. The mean number of organisms later recovered from tissue specimens was 6.5 (coded data) with a standard deviation of .6. Can one conclude from these data that the population mean is greater than 6? Let $\alpha = .05$.

6.2.7. A sample of 25 freshman nursing students made a mean score of 77 on a test designed to measure attitude toward the dying patient. The sample standard deviation was 10. Do these data provide sufficient evidence to indicate, at the .05 level of significance, that the population mean is less than 80?

6.2.8. A nutrition survey was conducted in a developing country. A sample of 500 rural adults reported a mean minimum daily caloric intake of 1985 with a standard deviation of 210. Can one conclude from these data that the population mean is less than 2,000? Let $\alpha = .05$.

6.2.9. A survey of 100 similar sized hospitals revealed a mean average daily census in the pediatrics service of 27 with a standard deviation of 6.5. Do these data provide sufficient evidence to indicate that the population mean is greater than 25? Let $\alpha = .05$.

6.2.10. Following a week-long hospital supervisory training program, 16 assistant hospital administrators made a mean score of 74 on a test administered as part of the evaluation of the training program. The sample standard deviation was 12. Can it be concluded from these data that the population mean is greater than 70? Let $\alpha = .05$.

6.3 HYPOTHESIS TESTING: THE DIFFERENCE BETWEEN TWO POPULATION MEANS

Hypothesis testing involving the difference between two population means is most frequently employed to determine whether or not it is reasonable to conclude that the two are unequal. In such cases, one or the other of the following hypotheses are tested:

$$\begin{aligned}
&(1)\quad H_0: \mu_1 - \mu_2 = 0, &&H_A: \mu_1 - \mu_2 \neq 0\\
&(2)\quad H_0: \mu_1 - \mu_2 \geq 0, &&H_A: \mu_1 - \mu_2 < 0\\
&(3)\quad H_0: \mu_1 - \mu_2 \leq 0, &&H_A: \mu_1 - \mu_2 > 0
\end{aligned}$$

It is possible, however, to test the hypothesis that the difference is equal to, greater than or equal to, or less than or equal to some value other than zero.

As was done in the previous section, hypothesis testing involving the difference between two population means will be discussed in three different contexts: (1) when sampling is from normally distributed populations with known population variances, (2) when sampling is from normally distributed populations with unknown population variances, and (3) when sampling is from populations that are not normally distributed.

Sampling from Normally Distributed Populations: Population Variances Known

Example 6.3.1

Refer to Example 5.3.1. Do these data provide sufficient evidence to indicate a difference in mean serum uric acid levels between normal individuals and individuals with mongolism? We may answer this question in the affirmative if we can reject the null hypothesis that the means are equal. Let us reach a decision by means of the nine-step hypothesis testing procedure.

1. *Data.* The data consist of serum uric acid readings on 12 mongoloid individuals and 15 normal individuals. The means are $\bar{x}_1 = 4.5$ mg/100 ml and $\bar{x}_2 = 3.4$ mg/100 ml.
2. *Assumptions.* The data constitute two independent random samples each drawn from a normally distributed population with a variance equal to 1.
3. *Hypotheses.*

$$H_0: \mu_1 - \mu_2 = 0$$
$$H_A: \mu_1 - \mu_2 \neq 0$$

   An alternative way of stating the hypotheses is as follows:

$$H_0: \mu_1 = \mu_2$$
$$H_A: \mu_1 \neq \mu_2$$

4. *Test Statistic.*

$$z = \frac{(\bar{x}_1 - \bar{x}_2) - (\mu_1 - \mu_2)}{\sqrt{\dfrac{\sigma_1^2}{n_1} + \dfrac{\sigma_2^2}{n_2}}}$$

   The hypothesized parameter in this case would be more correctly written as $(\mu_1 - \mu_2)_0$ where the subscript 0 indicates that the difference is a hypothesized parameter. To avoid cumbersome notation, however, we are deleting the subscript in the formula for the test statistic.
5. *Distribution of Test Statistic.* When the null hypothesis is true, the test statistic follows the unit normal distribution.
6. *Decision Rule.* Let $\alpha = .05$. The critical values of z are ± 1.96. Reject H_0 unless $-1.96 < z_{\text{computed}} < 1.96$. The acceptance and rejection regions are shown in Figure 6.3.1.

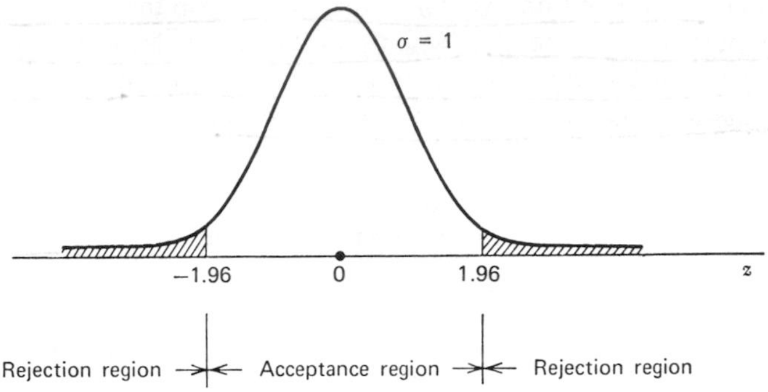

Figure 6.3.1. Acceptance and rejection regions for Example 6.3.1.

7. *Computed Test Statistic.*

$$z = \frac{(4.5 - 3.4) - 0}{\sqrt{\frac{1}{12} + \frac{1}{15}}} = \frac{1.1}{.39} = 2.82$$

8. *Statistical Decision.* Reject H_0, since $2.82 > 1.96$.

9. *Administrative or Clinical Decision.* Conclude that, on the basis of these data, there is an indication that the means are not equal. For this test, $p = .0048$.

In the previous chapter the 95 percent confidence interval for $\mu_1 - \mu_2$ was computed as .3 to 1.9. Since this interval does not include 0, we say that 0 is not a candidate for the true difference, and we conclude that the difference is not zero. Thus we arrive at the same conclusion by means of a confidence interval.

Although the population variances were equal in this example, this is not a requirement when population variances are known, and if they had been unequal, the same hypothesis testing procedure would have been followed.

Sampling from Normally Distributed Populations: Population Variances Unknown. As we have learned, when the population variances are unknown, two possibilities exist. The two population variances may be equal or they may be unequal. We consider first the case where it is known, or it is reasonable to assume, that they are equal.

Example 6.3.2

On the basis of the data presented in Example 5.6.2, would we be justified in concluding that the population means are different? We would if we can reject the null hypothesis that they are equal.

1. *Data.* The data consist of serum amylase determinations on 15 healthy subjects and 22 hospitalized subjects. The sample means and standard deviations are as follows:

$$\bar{x}_1 = 120 \text{ units/ml}, \qquad s_1 = 40 \text{ units/ml}$$
$$\bar{x}_2 = 96 \text{ units/ml}, \qquad s_2 = 35 \text{ units/ml}$$

2. *Assumptions.* The data constitute two independent random samples, each drawn from a normally distributed population. The population variances are unknown, but are assumed to be equal.
3. *Hypotheses.* $H_0: \mu_1 - \mu_2 = 0$, $H_A: \mu_1 - \mu_2 \neq 0$.
4. *Test Statistic.*

$$t = \frac{(\bar{x}_1 - \bar{x}_2) - (\mu_1 - \mu_2)}{\sqrt{\dfrac{s_p^2}{n_1} + \dfrac{s_p^2}{n_2}}}$$

It will be recalled that s_p^2 is the pooled estimate of the common population variance.

5. *Distribution of Test Statistic.* When the null hypothesis is true, the test statistic follows Student's t distribution with $n_1 + n_2 - 2$ degrees of freedom.
6. *Decision Rule.* Let $\alpha = .05$. The critical values of t are ± 2.0301. Reject H_0 unless $-2.0301 < t_{\text{computed}} < 2.0301$.
7. *Computed Test Statistic.*

$$t = \frac{(120 - 96) - 0}{\sqrt{\frac{1450}{15} + \frac{1450}{22}}} = \frac{24}{12.75} = 1.88$$

8. *Statistical Decision.* We are unable to reject H_0, since $-2.0301 < 1.88 < 2.0301$, that is, 1.88 falls in the acceptance region.
9. *Administrative or Clinical Decision.* On the basis of these data we cannot conclude that the two population means are different. For this test $.10 > p > .05$, since $1.6896 < 1.88 < 2.0301$.

Example 6.3.3

Let us use the data of Example 5.6.3 to illustrate the hypothesis testing procedure when the population variances are unknown and unequal. We will test the null hypothesis that the population means are equal against the alternative that they are unequal.

1. *Data.* The data consist of total serum complement activity (C_{H50}) determinations on $n_2 = 20$ apparently normal subjects and $n_1 = 10$ subjects with disease. The sample means and standard deviations are

$$\bar{x}_1 = 62.6, \qquad s_1 = 33.8$$
$$\bar{x}_2 = 47.2, \qquad s_1 = 10.1$$

2. *Assumptions.* The data constitute two independent random samples, each drawn from a normally distributed population. The population variances are unknown and unequal.
3. *Hypotheses.*

$$H_0: \mu_1 - \mu_2 = 0$$
$$H_A: \mu_1 - \mu_2 \neq 0$$

4. *Test Statistic.*

$$t' = \frac{(\bar{x}_1 - \bar{x}_2) - (\mu_1 - \mu_2)}{\sqrt{\frac{s_1^2}{n_1} + \frac{s_2^2}{n_2}}}$$

5. *Distribution of Test Statistic.* When the null hypothesis is true, the test statistic is distributed approximately as Student's t distribution with degrees of freedom given by Equation 5.6.4.
6. *Decision Rule.* Let $\alpha = .05$. The degrees of freedom value, computed as a part of Example 5.6.3. was found to be 10.9, so that ± 2.2010, the critical values of t for 11 degrees of freedom, are used. Reject H_0 unless $-2.2010 < t'_{\text{computed}} < 2.2010$.
7. *Computed Test Statistic.*

$$t' = \frac{(62.6 - 47.2) - 0}{\sqrt{\frac{(33.8)^2}{10} + \frac{(10.1)^2}{20}}} = \frac{15.4}{10.92} = 1.41$$

8. *Statistical Decision.* H_0 cannot be rejected since $-2.2010 < 1.41 < 2.2010$.
9. *Administrative or Clinical Decision.* On the basis of these data, we cannot conclude that the population means are different.

Sampling from Populations That Are Not Normally Distributed. When sampling is from populations that are not normally distributed, the results of the central limit theorem may be employed if sample sizes are large. This will allow the use of normal theory. If the population variances are known, they are used; but if they are unknown, the sample variances, which are necessarily based on large samples, are used as estimates. Sample variances are not pooled, since equality of population variances is not a necessary assumption when the z statistic is used.

Example 6.3.4

Refer to Example 5.3.2. Do these data provide sufficient evidence to indicate that the population which patronizes hospital A has a larger mean family income than does the population which patronizes hospital B? The answer is, yes, if we can reject the null hypothesis that μ_1 is less than or equal to μ_2, where μ_1 and μ_2 are the parameters for the hospital A and hospital B populations, respectively.

1. *Data.* The data consist of the family incomes of 75 patients admitted to hospital A and of 80 patients admitted to hospital B. The sample means are $\bar{x}_1 = \$6800$ and $\bar{x}_2 = \$4450$.
2. *Assumptions.* The data constitute two independent random samples, each drawn from a nonnormally distributed population with standard deviations, $\sigma_1 = \$600$ and $\sigma_2 = \$500$.
3. *Hypotheses.*

$$H_0: \mu_1 - \mu_2 \leq 0$$
$$H_A: \mu_1 - \mu_2 > 0$$

   or, alternatively,

$$H_0: \mu_1 \leq \mu_2$$
$$H_A: \mu_1 > \mu_2$$

4. *Test Statistic.* Since we have large samples, the central limit theorem allows us to use as the test statistic

$$z = \frac{(\bar{x}_1 - \bar{x}_2) - (\mu_1 - \mu_2)}{\sqrt{\dfrac{\sigma_1^2}{n_1} + \dfrac{\sigma_2^2}{n_2}}}$$

5. *Distribution of Test Statistic.* When the null hypothesis is true, the test statistic is distributed approximately as the unit normal.
6. *Decision Rule.* Let $\alpha = .01$. This is a one-sided test with a critical value of z equal to 2.33. Reject H_0 if $z_{\text{computed}} \geq 2.33$.
7. *Computed Test Statistic.*

$$z = \frac{(6800 - 4450) - 0}{\sqrt{\dfrac{(600)^2}{75} + \dfrac{(500)^2}{80}}} = \frac{2350}{89} = 26.4$$

8. *Statistical Decision.* Reject H_0, since $z = 26.4$ is in the rejection region.
9. *Administrative or Clinical Decision.* These data indicate that the population patronizing hospital A has a larger mean family income than does the population patronizing hospital B. For this test $p < .001$, since $26.4 > 3.09$.

Exercises

In each of the following exercises complete the nine-step hypothesis testing procedure and compute the p-value for each test.

6.3.1. Seventy patients suffering from epilepsia were divided at random into two groups. Group A was placed on a treatment regimen that included daily doses of vitamin D. Group B received the same treatment with the exception that for this group a placebo was given in place of vitamin D. The means of the number of seizures experienced during the period of treatment by the two groups were $\bar{x}_A = 15$ and $\bar{x}_B = 24$. The sample variances were $s_A^2 = 8$ and $s_B^2 = 12$. Do these data provide sufficient evidence to indicate that vitamin D is effective in reducing the number of seizures? Let $\alpha = .05$.

6.3.2. An epidemiologist wished to compare two rabies vaccines. Subjects who had previously received rabies vaccine were divided into two groups. Group 1 received a booster dose of Type 1 vaccine, and Group 2 received a booster dose of Type 2 vaccine. Antibody responses were recorded two weeks later. The means, standard deviations, and sample sizes for the two groups were as follows:

Group	Sample Size	$\bar{x}$	s
1	10	4.5	2.5
2	9	2.5	2.0

Do these data indicate that there is a difference in the effectiveness of the two vaccines used for booster doses? Let $\alpha = .05$.

6.3.3. Median nerve motor conduction velocity values were recorded for 10 subjects admitted to the poison control center of a metropolitan hospital with a diagnosis of methylmercury poisoning. Similar determinations also were made on 15 apparently healthy subjects. The means and standard deviations were as follows:

	$\bar{x}$	s
Poisoned Group:	55	6
Normal Subjects:	63	5

Do these data provide sufficient evidence to indicate that the means of the populations represented by the samples differ? Let $\alpha = .05$.

6.3.4. A test designed to measure self-confidence was administered to 16 chronically ill and 20 healthy children. The mean scores and standard deviations were as follows:

	$\bar{x}$	s
Ill Group	22.5	4.1
Well Group:	26.9	3.2

Can one conclude from these data that chronically ill children tend, on the average, to make lower scores on the test than do healthy children? Let $\alpha = .05$.

6.3.5. A nurse researcher wished to know if graduates of baccalaureate nursing programs and graduates of associate degree nursing programs differ with respect to mean scores on a personality inventory. A sample of 50 baccalaureate graduates (Group A) and a sample of 60 associate degree graduates (Group B) yielded the following means and standard deviations.

Group	$\bar{x}$	s
A	52.5	10.5
B	49.6	11.2

On the basis of these data what should the researcher conclude? Let $\alpha = .05$.

6.3.6. A test designed to measure mothers' attitudes toward their labor and delivery experiences was given to two groups of new mothers. Group 1 (attenders) had attended prenatal classes held at the local health department. Group 2 (nonattenders) did not attend the classes. The group sizes and means and standard deviations of the test scores were as follows:

Group	n	$\bar{x}$	s
1	15	4.75	1.0
2	20	3.00	1.5

Do these data provide sufficient evidence to indicate that attenders, on the average, score higher than nonattenders? Let $\alpha = .05$.

6.3.7. Cortisol level determinations were made on two groups of women at childbirth. Group 1 subjects underwent emergency Caesarean section following induced labor. Group 2 subjects delivered by either Caesarean section or the vaginal route following spontaneous labor. The group sizes, mean cortisol levels and standard deviations were as follows:

Group	n	$\bar{x}$	s
1	10	435	65
2	12	645	80

Do these data provide sufficient evidence to indicate a difference in the mean cortisol levels in the populations represented? Let $\alpha = .05$.

6.3.8. Protoporphyrin levels were measured in two groups of subjects. Group 1 consisted of 50 adult male alcoholics with ring sideroblasts in the bone marrow. Group 2 consisted of 40 apparently normal adult nonalcoholic males. The mean protoporphyrin levels and standard deviations for the two groups were as follows:

Group	$\bar{x}$	s
1	340	250
2	45	25

Can one conclude on the basis of these data that protoporphyrin levels are higher in the represented alcoholic population than in the nonalcoholic population? Let $\alpha = .01$.

6.3.9. A researcher was interested in knowing if preterm infants with late metabolic acidosis and preterm infants without the condition differed with respect to urine levels of a certain chemical. The mean levels, standard deviations, and sample sizes for the two groups studied were as follows:

Group	n	$\bar{x}$	s
With condition	35	8.5	5.5
Without condition	40	4.8	3.6

What should the researcher conclude on the basis of these results? Let $\alpha = .05$.

6.4 PAIRED COMPARISONS

In our previous discussion involving the difference between two population means, it has been assumed that the samples were independent. A method frequently employed for assessing the effectiveness of a treatment or experimental procedure is one that makes use of related observations resulting from nonindependent samples. A hypothesis test based on this type data is known as a *paired comparisons* test.

It frequently happens that true differences do not exist between two populations with respect to the variable of interest, but the presence of extraneous sources of variation may cause rejection of the null hypothesis of no difference. On the other hand, true differences also may be masked by the presence of extraneous factors.

The objective in paired comparisons tests is to eliminate a maximum number of sources of extraneous variation, by making the pairs similar with respect to as many variables as possible.

Related or paired observations may be obtained in a number of ways. The same subjects may be measured before and after receiving some treatment. Litter mates of the same sex may be randomly assigned to receive either a treatment or a placebo. Pairs of twins or siblings may be randomly assigned to two treatments in such a way that members of a single pair receive different treatments. In comparing two methods of analysis, the material to be analyzed may be equally divided, so that one half is analyzed by one method, and one half is analyzed by the other. Or pairs may be formed by matching individuals on some characteristic, for example, digital dexterity, which is closely related to the measurement of interest, say, posttreatment scores on some test requiring digital manipulation.

Instead of performing the analysis with individual observations, we use the difference between individual pairs of observations as the variable of interest.

Example 6.4.1

Twelve subjects participated in an experiment to study the effectiveness of a certain diet, combined with a program of exercise, in reducing serum cholesterol levels. Table 6.4.1 shows the serum cholesterol levels for the 12 subjects at the beginning of the program (Before) and at the end of the program (After).

Table 6.4.1

Serum Cholesterol Levels for 12 Subjects Before and After Diet-Exercise Program

	Serum Cholesterol		**Difference (After-Before)**
Subject	**Before** (X_1)	**After** (X_2)	d_i
1	201	200	−1
2	231	236	+5
3	221	216	−5
4	260	233	−27
5	228	224	−4
6	237	216	−21
7	326	296	−30
8	235	195	−40
9	240	207	−33
10	267	247	−20
11	284	210	−74
12	201	209	+8

Concentrating on the differences, d_i, the following descriptive measures may be computed:

$$\bar{d} = \frac{\sum d_i}{n} = \frac{(-1) + (5) + (-5) + \cdots + (8)}{12} = \frac{-242}{12} = -20.17$$

$$s_d^2 = \frac{n\sum d_i^2 - (\sum d_i)^2}{n(n-1)} = \frac{12(10766) - (-242)^2}{12(11)} = 535.06$$

Notice that $\bar{d} = \bar{x}_2 - \bar{x}_1$.

The question to be asked is: Do the data provide sufficient evidence for us to conclude that the diet-exercise program is effective in reducing serum cholesterol levels? We will say that such evidence is provided if we can reject the null hypothesis that the true average change is zero or positive. We may reach a decision by means of the nine-step hypothesis testing procedure.

1. *Data.* The data consist of serum cholesterol levels in 12 individuals, before and after an experimental diet-exercise program.
2. *Assumptions.* The observed differences constitute a random sample from a normally distributed population of differences that could be generated under the same circumstances.
3. *Hypotheses.* The null hypothesis to be tested is that $\mu_2 - \mu_1 \geq 0$. If we let $\mu_d = \mu_2 - \mu_1$, we may state the null and alternate hypotheses as follows:

$$H_0: \mu_d \geq 0$$
$$H_A: \mu_d < 0$$

4. *Test Statistic.* In light of the assumptions, the appropriate test statistic is

$$t = \frac{\bar{d} - \mu_d}{s_{\bar{d}}} \qquad (6.4.1)$$

where $s_{\bar{d}} = s_d/\sqrt{n}$.

Again, the hypothesized parameter in Equation 6.4.1 would be more correctly specified by a symbol such as μ_{d0}. But, again, to avoid cumbersome notation we are eliminating the zero.

Although, in a sense, we have two samples, before levels and after levels, we do not have to worry about equality of variances, as with independent samples, since our variable is the difference between readings in the same individual and, hence, only one variance is involved.

5. *Distribution of Test Statistic.* If the null hypothesis is true, the test statistic is distributed as Student's t with $n - 1$ degrees of freedom.
6. *Decision Rule.* Let $\alpha = .05$. The critical value of t is -1.7959. Reject H_0 if computed t is less than the critical value. The acceptance and rejection regions are shown in Figure 6.4.1.
7. *Computed Test Statistic.*

$$t = \frac{-20.17 - 0}{\sqrt{535.06/12}} = \frac{-20.17}{6.68} = -3.02$$

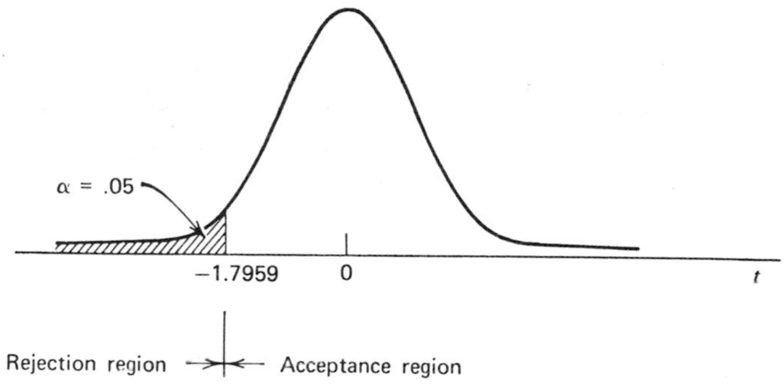

Figure 6.4.1. Acceptance and rejection regions for Example 6.4.1.

8. *Statistical Decision.* Reject H_0, since -3.02 is in the rejection region.
9. *Administrative or Clinical Decision.* We may conclude that the diet-exercise program is effective. For this test, $.01 > p > .005$, since $-2.718 > -3.02 > -3.1058$.

A 95 percent confidence interval for μ_d may be obtained as follows:

$$\bar{d} \pm t_{(1-\alpha/2)} s_{\bar{d}}$$

$$-20.17 \pm 2.2010(6.68)$$

$$-20.17 \pm 14.70$$

$$-34.87, \; -5.47$$

If, in the analysis of paired data, the population variance of the differences is known, the appropriate test statistic is

$$z = \frac{\bar{d} - \mu_d}{\sigma_d/\sqrt{n}} \qquad (6.4.2)$$

It is unlikely that σ_d will be known in practice.

If the assumption of normally distributed d_i's cannot be made, the central limit theorem may be employed if n is large. In such cases the test statistic is Equation 6.4.2, with s_d used to estimate σ_d when, as is generally the case, the latter is unknown.

The use of the paired comparisons test is not without its problems. If different subjects are used and randomly assigned to two treatments, considerable time and expense may be involved in our trying to match individuals on one or more relevant variables. A further price we pay for using paired comparisons is a loss of degrees of freedom. If we do not use paired observations we have $2n - 2$ degrees of freedom available as compared to $n - 1$ when we use the paired comparisons procedure.

In general, in deciding whether or not to use the paired comparisons procedure, one should be guided by the economics involved, as well as by a consideration of the gains to be realized in terms of controlling extraneous variation.

Exercises

In the following exercises carry out the nine-step hypothesis testing procedure at the specified significance level. Determine the p-value for each test.

6.4.1. Ten experimental animals were subjected to conditions simulating disease. The number of heartbeats per minute, before and after the experiment, were recorded as follows.

	Heartbeats per Minute			Heartbeats per Minute	
Animal	Before	After	Animal	Before	After
1	70	115	6	100	178
2	84	148	7	110	179
3	88	176	8	67	140
4	110	191	9	79	161
5	105	158	10	86	157

Do these data provide sufficient evidence to indicate that the experimental condition increases the number of heartbeats per minute? Let $\alpha = .05$.

6.4.2. A study was conducted to test the effectiveness of a new therapeutic procedure in improving the digital dexterity of certain handicapped persons. Twenty-four pairs of individuals were used in the study, and each pair was matched on degree of impairment, intelligence, and age. One member of each pair was randomly assigned to receive the new treatment, while the other member of the pair received the standard therapy. At the end of the experimental period each individual was given a digital dexterity test with scores as follows.

Pair	New	Standard	Pair	New	Standard
1	49	54	13	52	41
2	56	42	14	73	67
3	70	63	15	52	57
4	83	77	16	73	70
5	83	83	17	78	72
6	68	51	18	64	62
7	84	82	19	71	64
8	63	54	20	42	44
9	67	62	21	51	44
10	79	71	22	56	42
11	88	82	23	40	35
12	48	50	24	81	73

Do these data provide sufficient evidence for concluding at the .05 level of significance that the new therapy is more effective than the standard?

6.4.3. A group of 15 twelve-year-old boys were measured by two different nurses. The results were as follows:

Subject	Nurse 1	Nurse 2	Subject	Nurse 1	Nurse 2
1	142.9	143.0	9	142.1	142.5
2	150.9	151.5	10	159.9	160.0
3	151.9	152.1	11	141.9	142.0
4	158.1	158.0	12	140.8	141.0
5	151.2	151.5	13	147.1	148.0
6	160.2	160.5	14	143.6	144.0
7	157.8	158.0	15	139.9	141.0
8	150.1	150.0			

Do these data justify the conclusion that there is a difference in the accuracy of the two nurses? Let $\alpha = .05$. Construct a 95 percent confidence interval for μ_d.

6.4.4. Ten 16-year-old males were measured at time of arising in the morning and at time of retiring in the evening with the following results.

	Height (Centimeters)			Height (Centimeters)	
Subject	Morning	Evening	Subject	Morning	Evening
1	169.7	168.2	6	168.8	166.5
2	168.5	165.5	7	169.2	167.4
3	165.9	164.4	8	167.9	166.3
4	177.7	175.7	9	181.8	179.7
5	179.6	176.6	10	163.3	161.5

Do these data provide sufficient evidence to indicate that 16-year-old males are shorter in the evening than in the morning? Construct the 95 percent confidence interval for μ_d.

6.5 HYPOTHESIS TESTING: A SINGLE POPULATION PROPORTION

Testing hypotheses about population proportions is carried out in much the same way as for means when the conditions necessary for using the normal curve are met. One-sided or two-sided tests may be made, depending on the question being asked.

Example 6.5.1

Let us refer to the survey discussed in Example 5.4.1 and test the null hypothesis that $p = .50$.

1. *Data.* The data are obtained from the responses of 300 individuals of which 123 possessed the characteristic of interest, that is, $\tilde{p} = .41$.
2. *Assumptions.* The sampling distribution of $\tilde{p}$ is approximately normally distributed in accordance with the central limit theorem. If H_0 is true, $p = .5$ and the standard error, $\sigma_{\tilde{p}} = \sqrt{(.5)(.5)/300}$. Note that we use the hypothesized value of p in computing $\sigma_{\tilde{p}}$. We do this because the entire test is based on the assumption that the null hypothesis is true. To use the sample proportion, $\tilde{p}$, in computing $\sigma_{\tilde{p}}$ would not be consistent with this concept.
3. *Hypotheses.*

$$H_0: p = .50$$
$$H_A: p \neq .50$$

4. *Test Statistic.*

$$z = \frac{\tilde{p} - p_0}{\sqrt{\dfrac{p_0 q_0}{n}}}$$

5. *Distribution of Test Statistic.* If the null hypothesis is true the test statistic is approximately normally distributed with a mean of zero.
6. *Decision Rule.* Let $\alpha = .05$. Critical values of z are ± 1.96. Reject H_0 unless $-1.96 < z_{\text{computed}} < 1.96$.
7. *Computed Test Statistic.*

$$z = \frac{.41 - .50}{\sqrt{\dfrac{(.5)(.5)}{300}}} = \frac{-.09}{.0289} = -3.11$$

8. *Statistical Decision.* Reject H_0 since $-3.11 < -1.96$.
9. *Administrative or Clinical Decision.* We conclude that not 50 percent of the population regularly have a dental checkup twice a year. For this test, $p < .002$, since $-3.11 < -3.09$.

Exercises

For each of the following exercises, carry out the nine-step hypothesis testing procedure at the designated level of significance. Compute the p-value for each test.

6.5.1. In a sample of 1500 residents of an inner city neighborhood who participated in a health screening program, 125 tests yielded positive results for sickle cell anemia. Do these data provide sufficient evidence to indicate that the proportion of individuals with sickle cell anemia in the sampled population is greater than .06? Let $\alpha = .05$.

6.5.2. A sample of 100 hospital employees who have frequent contact with blood or blood products was screened for serologic evidence of hepatitis B infection. Twenty-three were found to be positive. Can it be concluded from these data that the proportion of positives in the sampled population is greater than .15? Let $\alpha = .05$.

6.5.3. Prior to initiation of a rubella immunization program in a metropolitan county a survey revealed that 150 out of a sample of 500 elementary school children in the county had been immunized against the disease. Are these data compatible with the contention that less than 50 percent of the elementary school children in the county had been immunized against rubella? Let $\alpha = .05$.

6.6 HYPOTHESIS TESTING: THE DIFFERENCE BETWEEN TWO POPULATION PROPORTIONS

The most frequent test employed relative to the difference between two population proportions is that their difference is zero. It is possible, however, to test that the difference is equal to some other value. Both one-sided and two-sided tests may be made.

When the null hypothesis to be tested is $p_1 - p_2 = 0$, we are hypothesizing that the two population proportions are equal. We use this as justification for combining the results of the two samples to come up with a pooled estimate of the hypothesized common proportion. If this procedure is adopted, one computes

$$\bar{p} = \frac{x_1 + x_2}{n_1 + n_2}$$

where x_1 and x_2 are the number in the first and second sample, respectively, possessing the characteristic of interest. This pooled estimate of $p = p_1 = p_2$ is used in computing $\hat{\sigma}_{\hat{p}_1 - \hat{p}_2}$

$$\hat{\sigma}_{\hat{p}_1 - \hat{p}_2} = \sqrt{\frac{\bar{p}(1-\bar{p})}{n_1} + \frac{\bar{p}(1-\bar{p})}{n_2}}$$

and the test statistic becomes

$$z = \frac{(\hat{p}_1 - \hat{p}_2) - (p_1 - p_2)}{\hat{\sigma}_{\hat{p}_1 - \hat{p}_2}}$$

which is approximately distributed as the unit normal if the null hypothesis is true.

Example 6.6.1

The data from this example are taken from Example 5.5.1. Suppose that we are asked the question: Do these data provide sufficient evidence to indicate that the new treatment is more effective than the standard? The answer is yes, if we can reject the null hypothesis that the new treatment is no more effective than the standard.

The hypothesis testing procedure for this example consists of the following steps.

1. *Data.* The data consist of the responses of 100 individuals to the standard treatment and the responses of 100 individuals to the new treatment. The number of favorable responses were 78 and 90, respectively. Let us compute $\tilde{p}_1 = 78/100 = .78$, $\tilde{p}_2 = 90/100 = .90$, and
$$\bar{p} = \frac{90 + 78}{100 + 100} = .84$$
2. *Assumptions.* It is assumed that the sampling distribution of $\tilde{p}_2 - \tilde{p}_1$ is approximately normally distributed with mean, $p_2 - p_1 \leq 0$ and estimated standard error
$$\hat{\sigma}_{\tilde{p}_2 - \tilde{p}_1} = \sqrt{\frac{\bar{p}(1-\bar{p})}{n_2} + \frac{\bar{p}(1-\bar{p})}{n_1}}$$
when the null hypothesis is true and the sample estimates are pooled.
3. *Hypotheses.*
$$H_0: p_2 - p_1 \leq 0$$
$$H_A: p_2 - p_1 > 0$$
4. *Test Statistic.* The test statistic is
$$z = \frac{(\tilde{p}_2 - \tilde{p}_1) - (p_2 - p_1)}{\sqrt{\dfrac{\bar{p}(1-\bar{p})}{n_2} + \dfrac{\bar{p}(1-\bar{p})}{n_1}}}$$
5. *Distribution of the Test Statistic.* If the null hypothesis is true the test statistic is distributed approximately as the unit normal.
6. *Decision Rule.* Let $\alpha = .05$. The critical value of z is 1.645. Reject H_0 if computed z is greater than 1.645.
7. *Computed Test Statistic.*
$$z = \frac{(.90 - .78) - 0}{\sqrt{\dfrac{(.84)(.16)}{100} + \dfrac{(.84)(.16)}{100}}} = \frac{.12}{.0518} = 2.32$$

8. *Statistical Decision.* Reject H_0 since $2.32 > 1.645$.

9. *Administrative or Clinical Decision.* These data suggest that the new treatment is more effective than the standard ($p = .0102$).

Exercises

In each of the exercises below use the nine-step hypothesis testing procedure. Determine the p-value for each test.

6.6.1. A sample of patients discharged from a state mental hospital within six months after admission and a sample of those who were discharged after six months but within a year of admission were compared with respect to distance of residence from the hospital. The results were as follows:

Length of Stay	n	Number Who Live More than 20 mi from Hospital
≤ 6 mo.	100	75
Longer than 6 mo.	150	90

Do these data provide sufficient evidence to indicate that the proportion who live more than 20 miles from the hospital is different in the two represented populations? Let $\alpha = .05$.

6.6.2. An epidemiologist in a developing country compared a sample of 90 adult subjects suffering from a certain neurologic disease with a sample of 100 comparable control subjects who were free of the disease. It was found that 69 of the subjects with the disease and 67 of the controls were employed in subsistence occupations. Can the epidemiologist conclude from these data that the two populations represented by the samples differ with respect to the proportion employed in subsistence occupations? Let $\alpha = .05$.

6.6.3. A sample of one-year-old children seen in a certain group of county health departments during a year was selected from each of the two predominant ethnic groups composing the departments' clientele. The following information regarding anemia was revealed.

Ethnic Group	Number in Sample	Number Anemic
1	450	105
2	375	120

Do these data provide sufficient evidence to indicate a difference in the two populations with respect to the proportion who are anemic? Let $\alpha = .05$.

6.7 HYPOTHESIS TESTING: A SINGLE POPULATION VARIANCE

In Section 5.9 we examine how it is possible to construct a confidence interval for the variance of a normally distributed population. The general principles presented in that section may be employed to test a hypothesis about a population variance. Let us refer to Example 5.9.1 and test the null hypothesis that $\sigma^2 = 2500$.

Example 6.7.1

1. *Data.* The data consist of serum amylase determinations on 15 apparently healthy subjects. The sample variance was computed as $s^2 = 1225$.
2. *Assumptions.* The data constitute a random sample of size 15 from a normally distributed population.
3. *Hypotheses*:

$$H_0: \sigma^2 = 2500$$
$$H_A: \sigma^2 \neq 2500$$

4. *Test Statistic.*

$$\chi^2 = (n-1)s^2/\sigma^2$$

5. *Distribution of Test Statistic.* When the null hypothesis is true the test statistic is distributed as χ^2 with $n - 1$ degrees of freedom.
6. *Decision Rule.* Let $\alpha = .05$. Critical values of χ^2 are 5.629 and 26.119. Reject H_0 unless the computed value of the test statistic is between 5.629 and 26.119. The acceptance and rejection regions are shown in Figure 6.7.1.

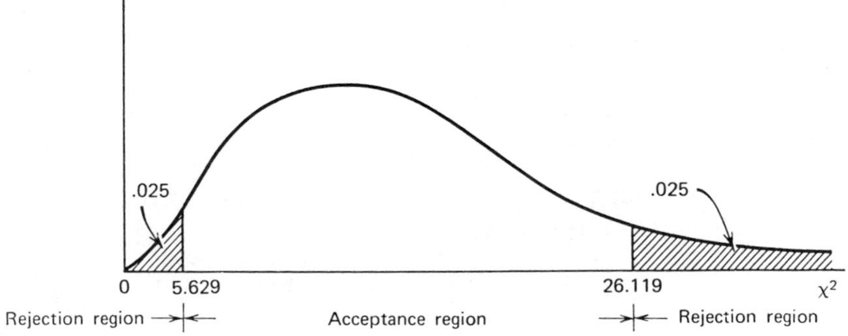

Figure 6.7.1. Acceptance and rejection regions for Example 6.7.1.

$\chi^2 = \frac{(n-1)(s^2)}{\sigma^2}$

7. *Computed Test Statistic.*

$$\chi^2 = \frac{(14)(1225)}{2500} = 6.86$$

8. *Statistical Decision.* Do not reject H_0 since $5.629 < 6.86 < 26.119$.

9. *Administrative or Clinical Decision.* Based on these data we are unable to conclude that the population variance is not 2500.

Although this was an example of a two-sided test, one-sided tests may also be made by the logical modification of the procedure given here.

The determination of the p-value for this test is complicated by the fact that we have a two-sided test and an asymmetric sampling distribution. When we have a two-sided test and a symmetric sampling distribution such as the unit normal or t, we may, as we have seen, double the one-sided p-value. Problems arise when we attempt to do this with an asymmetric sampling distribution such as the chi-square distribution. Gibbons and Pratt (1) suggest that, in this situation, the one-sided p-value be reported along with the direction of the observed departure from the null hypothesis. In fact this procedure may be followed in the case of symmetric sampling distributions. Precedent, however, seems to favor doubling the one-sided p-value when the test is two-sided and involves a symmetric sampling distribution.

For the present example, then, we may report the p-value as follows:

$p > .05$ (two-sided test). A population variance less than 2500 is suggested by the sample data, but this hypothesis is not strongly supported by the test.

If the problem is stated in terms of the population standard deviation, one may square the sample standard deviation and perform the test as indicated above.

Exercises

In each of the following exercises carry out the nine-step testing procedure. Determine the p-value for each test.

6.7.1. As part of a research project, a sample of 25 infants was selected from those born in hospitals in a metropolitan area. The standard deviation of the weights of the infants in the sample was 150 grams. Do these data provide sufficient evidence to indicate that the population variance is greater than 10,000? Let $\alpha = .05$.

6.7.2. Each of a random sample of 30 student nurses who participated in a research project was given a test designed to measure degree of creative thinking. The standard deviation of the scores was 11. Can one conclude from these data that the population variance is less than 400? Let $\alpha = .05$.

6.7.3. Vital capacity values were recorded for a sample of ten patients with severe chronic airway obstruction. The variance of the ten observations was .75. Test the null hypothesis that the population variance is 1.00. Let $\alpha = .05$.

6.7.4. Hemoglobin (gm %) values were recorded for a sample of 20 children who were part of a study of acute leukemia. The variance of the observations was 5. Do these data provide sufficient evidence to indicate that the population variance is greater than 4? $\alpha = .05$.

6.7.5. A sample of 25 administrators of large hospitals participated in a study to investigate the nature and extent of frustration and emotional tension associated with the job. Each participant was given a test designed to measure the extent of emotional tension he or she experienced as a result of the duties and responsibilities associated with the job. The variance of the scores was 30. Can it be concluded from these data that the population variance is greater than 25? Let $\alpha = .05$.

6.7.6. In a study in which the subjects were 15 patients suffering from pulmonary sarcoid disease, blood gas determinations were made. The variance of the PaO_2 (mm Hg) values was 450. Test the null hypothesis that the population variance is greater than 250. Let $\alpha = .05$.

6.8 HYPOTHESIS TESTING: THE RATIO OF TWO POPULATION VARIANCES

As we have seen, the use of the t distribution in constructing confidence intervals and in testing hypotheses for the difference between two population means assumes that the population variances are equal. As a rule, the only hints available about the magnitudes of the respective variances are the variances computed from samples taken from the populations. We would like to know if the difference that, undoubtedly, will exist between the sample variances is indicative of a real difference in population variances, or if the difference is of such magnitude that it could have come about as a result of chance alone when the population variances are equal.

Two methods of chemical analysis may give the same results on the average. It may be, however, that the results produced by one method are more variable than the results of the other. We would like some method of determining whether this is likely to be true.

These are two examples of the many instances in which interest focuses on the question of whether or not two population variances are equal.

Decisions regarding the comparability of two population variances are usually based on the *variance ratio test*, which is a test of the null hypothesis that two population variances are equal. When we test the hypothesis that two population variances are equal, we are, in effect, testing the hypothesis that their ratio is equal to 1.

We learned in the preceding chapter that, when certain assumptions are met, the quantity $(s_1^2/\sigma_1^2)/(s_2^2/\sigma_2^2)$ is distributed as F with $n_1 - 1$ numerator degrees of freedom and $n_2 - 1$ denominator degrees of freedom. If we are hypothesizing that $\sigma_1^2 = \sigma_2^2$, we assume that the hypothesis is true, and they cancel out in the above expression leaving s_1^2/s_2^2, which follows the same F distribution. The ratio s_1^2/s_2^2 will be designated V. R. for variance ratio. In comparing two variances, we will follow the convention of always placing the larger sample variance in the numerator, so that the ratio of the sample variances always will be equal to or greater than 1. We will then be trying to determine if we can conclude that the variance in the numerator is significantly larger than the variance in the denominator.

Example 6.8.1

Let us refer to Example 5.6.2 and see if the data presented there provide sufficient evidence for us to conclude that the variance of serum amylase determinations for the population represented by the hospitalized subjects is greater than the variance for the population represented by the sample of healthy subjects.

1. *Data.* The data consist of serum amylase determinations for 22 hospitalized subjects and 15 healthy subjects. The sample variances were 1600 and 1225, respectively.
2. *Assumptions.* The data constitute independent random samples each drawn from a normally distributed population. These are general assumptions that must be met for the following test to be valid.
3. *Hypotheses:*

$$H_0: \sigma_1^2 \leq \sigma_2^2$$
$$H_A: \sigma_1^2 > \sigma_2^2$$

4. *Test Statistic.*

$$\text{V. R.} = s_1^2/s_2^2$$

5. *Distribution of Test Statistic.* When the null hypothesis is true, the test statistic is distributed as F with $n_1 - 1$ and $n_2 - 1$ degrees of freedom.
6. *Decision Rule.* Let $\alpha = .05$. The critical value of F, from Table J, is 2.39. Note that Table J does not contain an entry for 21 numerator degrees of freedom and, therefore, 2.39 is obtained by using 20, the closest value to 21 in the table. Reject H_0 if V. R. ≥ 2.39. The acceptance and rejection regions are shown in Figure 6.8.1.
7. *Computed Test Statistic.*

$$\text{V. R.} = \tfrac{1600}{1225} = 1.31$$

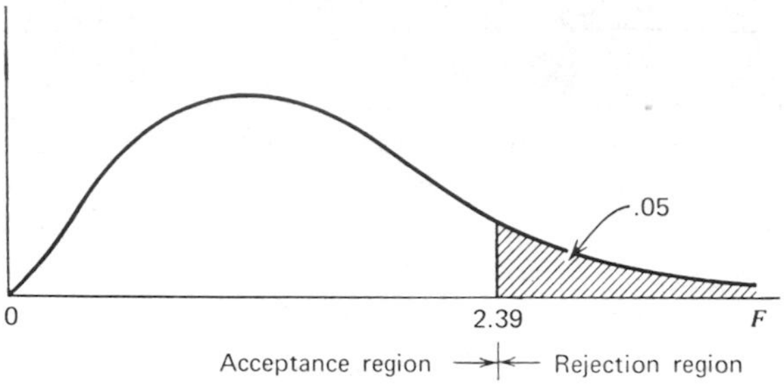

Figure 6.8.1. Acceptance and rejection regions, Example 6.8.1.

8. *Statistical Decision.* We cannot reject H_0, since $1.31 < 2.39$, that is, the computed ratio falls in the acceptance region.

9. *Administrative or Clinical Decision.* We are unable to conclude that the two variances are not equal. Since the computed V. R. of 1.31 is less than 1.96, the p-value for this test is greater than .10.

Exercises

In the following exercises perform the nine-step test. Determine the p-value for each test.

6.8.1. Cardiac index values (liters/minute/M^2) were analyzed in two groups of patients following prosthetic valve replacement. The sample sizes and variances were as follows: $n_1 = 16$, ${s_1}^2 = 3.75$, $n_2 = 10$, ${s_2}^2 = 1.8$. Do these data provide sufficient evidence to indicate a difference in population variances? Let $\alpha = .05$.

6.8.2. Viable *Toxoplasma gondii* organisms were injected into 21 normal guinea pigs and 21 guinea pigs chronically infected with toxoplasma. Twenty-four hours later erythema diameter measurements were taken at the reaction site. Sample variances computed from these observations were 10 mm^2 for the infected group and 3 mm^2 for the normal group. Can it be concluded from these data that the population variance for the infected group is greater than that for the normal group? Let $\alpha = .05$.

6.8.3. A test designed to measure level of anxiety was administered to a sample of male and a sample of female patients just prior to undergoing the same surgical procedure. The sample sizes and the variances computed from the scores were as follows:

$$\text{Males:} \quad n = 16, \quad s^2 = 150$$
$$\text{Females:} \quad n = 21, \quad s^2 = 275$$

Do these data provide sufficient evidence to indicate that in the represented populations, the scores made by females are more variable than those made by males? Let $\alpha = .05$.

6.8.4. In an experiment to assess the effects on rats of exposure to cigarette smoke, 11 animals were exposed and 11 control animals were not exposed to smoke from unfiltered cigarettes. At the end of the experiment measurements were made of the frequency of the ciliary beat (beats/min at 20°C) in each animal. The variance for the exposed group was 3400 and 1200 for the unexposed group. Do these data indicate that in the populations represented the variances are different? Let $\alpha = .05$.

6.8.5. Two pain relieving drugs were compared for effectiveness on the basis of length of time elapsing between administration of the drug and cessation of pain. Thirteen patients received Drug 1 and 13 received Drug 2. The sample variances were $s_1^2 = 64$ and $s_2^2 = 16$. Test the null hypothesis that the two population variances are equal. Let $\alpha = .05$.

6.8.6. Packed cell volume determinations were made on two groups of children with cyanotic congenital heart disease. The sample sizes and variances were as follows:

Group	n	s^2
1	10	40
2	16	85

Do these data provide sufficient evidence to indicate that the variance of population 2 is larger than the variance of population 1? Let $\alpha = .05$.

6.9 SUMMARY

In this chapter the general concepts of hypothesis testing are discussed. A general procedure for carrying out a hypothesis test consisting of the following nine steps is suggested.

1. Description of data.
2. Statement of necessary assumptions.
3. Statement of null and alternate hypotheses.
4. Specification of the test statistic.
5. Specification of the distribution of the test statistic.
6. Statement of the decision rule.
7. Computation of test statistic from sample data.
8. The statistical decision based on sample results.
9. Administrative or clinical decision based on sample results.

A number of specific hypothesis tests are described in detail and are illustrated with appropriate examples. These include tests concerning population means, the difference between two population means, paired comparisons, population proportions, the difference between two population proportions, a population variance, and the ratio of two population variances.

Review Questions and Exercises

1. What is the purpose of hypothesis testing?
2. What is a hypothesis?
3. List and explain each step in the nine-step hypothesis testing procedure.
4. What is a Type I error?
5. What is a Type II error?
6. Explain how one decides what statement goes into the null hypothesis and what statement goes into the alternate hypothesis.
7. What are the assumptions underlying the use of the t statistic in testing hypotheses about a single mean? The difference between two means?
8. When may the z statistic be used in testing hypotheses about
   (a) A single population mean?
   (b) The difference between two population means?
   (c) A single population proportion?
   (d) The difference between two population proportions?
9. In testing a hypothesis about the difference between two population means, what is the rationale behind pooling the sample variances?
10. Explain the rationale behind the use of the paired comparisons test.
11. Give an example from your field of interest where a paired comparisons test would be appropriate. Use real or realistic data and perform an appropriate hypothesis test.
12. Give an example from your field of interest where it would be appropriate to test a hypothesis about the difference between two population means. Use real or realistic data and carry out the nine-step hypothesis testing procedure.
13. Do Exercise 12 for a single population mean.
14. Do Exercise 12 for a single population proportion.
15. Do Exercise 12 for the difference between two population proportions.
16. Do Exercise 12 for a population variance.
17. Do Exercise 12 for the ratio of two population variances.

18. A health survey of urban and rural adults, residents of a developing country, revealed the following information:

Group	Number in Sample	Number Blind
Rural	300	24
Urban	500	15

Do these data provide sufficient evidence to indicate a difference in the prevalence of blindness in the two populations? Let $\alpha = .05$. Determine the p-value.

19. During an experiment using laboratory animals the following data on renal cortical blood flow during control conditions and during the administration of a certain anesthetic were recorded.

	Renal Cortical Blood Flow (ml/g/min)	
Animal Number	Control	During Administration of Anesthetic
1	2.35	2.00
2	2.55	1.71
3	1.95	2.22
4	2.79	2.71
5	3.21	1.83
6	2.97	2.14
7	3.44	3.72
8	2.58	2.10
9	2.66	2.58
10	2.31	1.32
11	3.43	3.70
12	2.37	1.59
13	1.82	2.07
14	2.98	2.15
15	2.53	2.05

Can one conclude on the basis of these data that the anesthetic retards renal cortical blood flow? Let $\alpha = .05$. Determne the p-value.

20. An allergy research team conducted a study in which two groups of subjects were used. As part of the research, blood eosinophil determinations were made on each subject with the following results:

Group	n	Mean Eosinophil Value (No./mm^3)	s
A	14	584	225
B	16	695	185

Do these data provide sufficient evidence to indicate that the population means are different? Let $\alpha = .05$. Determine the p-value.

21. A survey of 90 recently delivered women on the rolls of a county welfare department revealed that 27 had a history of intrapartum or postpartum infection. Test the null hypothesis that the population proportion with a history of intrapartum or postpartum infection is less than or equal to .25. Let $\alpha = .05$. Determine the p-value.

22. In a sample of 150 hospital emergency admissions with a certain diagnosis, 128 listed vomiting as a presenting symptom. Do these data provide sufficient evidence to indicate, at the .01 level of significance, that the population proportion is less than .92? Determine the p-value.

23. A research team measured tidal volume in 15 experimental animals. The mean and standard deviation were 45 and 5 cc, respectively. Do these data provide sufficient evidence to indicate that the population mean is greater than 40 cc? Let $\alpha = .05$.

24. A sample of eight patients admitted to a hospital with a diagnosis of biliary cirrhosis had a mean Ig M level of 160.55 units per ml. The sample standard deviation was 50. Do these data provide sufficient evidence to indicate that the population mean is greater than 150? Let $\alpha = .05$. Determine the p-value.

25. Some researchers have observed a greater airway resistance in smokers than in nonsmokers. Suppose a study, conducted to compare the percent tracheobronchial retention of particles in smoking-discordant monozygotic twins, yielded the following results:

Percent Retention	
Smoking Twin	Nonsmoking Twin
60.6	47.5
12.0	13.3
56.0	33.0
75.2	55.2
12.5	21.9
29.7	27.9
57.2	54.3
62.7	13.9
28.7	8.9
66.0	46.1
25.2	29.8
40.1	36.2

Do these data support the hypothesis that tracheobronchial clearance is slower in smokers? Let $\alpha = .05$. Determine the p-value for this test.

References

References cited

1. Jean D. Gibbons and John W. Pratt, "*P*-values: Interpretation and Methodology," *The American Statistician, 29* (1975), 20–25.
2. Anita K. Bahn, "*P* and the Null Hypothesis," *Annals of Internal Medicine, 76* (1972), 674.
3. Wayne W. Daniel, *Introductory Statistics with Applications*, Houghton Mifflin, Boston, 1977.

Other references, journal articles

1. Arnold Binder, "Further Considerations of Testing the Null Hypothesis and the Strategy and Tactics of Investigating Theoretical Models," *Psychological Review, 70* (1963), 107–115.
2. C. Allen Boneau, "The Effects of Violations of Assumptions Underlying the *t* Test," *Psychological Bulletin, 57* (1960), 49–64.
3. C. J. Burke, "A Brief Note on One-tailed Tests," *Psychological Bulletin, 50* (1953), 384–387.
4. C. J. Burke, "Further Remarks on One-tailed Tests," *Psychological Bulletin, 51* (1954), 587–590.
5. Eugene S. Edgington, "Statistical Inference and Nonrandom Samples," *Psychological Bulletin, 66* (1966), 485–487.
6. Ward Edwards, "Tactical Note on the Relation Between Scientific and Statistical Hypotheses," *Psychological Bulletin, 63* (1965), 400–402.
7. William E. Feinberg, "Teaching the Type I and Type II Errors: The Judical Process," *The American Statistician, 25* (June 1971), 30–32.
8. I. J. Good, "What Are Degrees of Freedom?" *The American Statistician, 27* (1973), 227–228.
9. David A. Grant, "Testing the Null Hypothesis and the Strategy and Tactics of Investigating Theoretical Models," *Psychological Review, 69* (1962), 54–61.
10. W. E. Hick, "A Note on One-tailed and Two-tailed Tests," *Psychological Review, 59* (1952), 316–318.
11. L. V. Jones, "Tests of Hypotheses: One-sided vs. Two-sided Alternatives," *Psychological Bulletin, 46* (1949), 43–46.
12. L. V. Jones, "A Rejoinder on One-tailed Tests," *Psychological Bulletin, 51* (1954), 585–586.
13. Sanford Labovitz, "Criteria for Selecting a Significance Level: A Note on the Sacredness of .05," *The American Sociologist, 3* (1968), 220–222.
14. William Lurie, "The Impertinent Questioner: The Scientist's Guide to the Statistician's Mind," *American Scientist, 46* (1958), 57–61.

15. M. R. Marks, "One- and Two-tailed Tests," *Psychological Review, 60* (1953), 207–208.

16. C. A. McGilchrist and J. Y. Harrison, "Testing of Means with Different Alternatives," *Technometrics, 10* (1968), 195–198.

17. Mary G. Natrella, "The Relation Between Confidence Intervals and Tests of Significance," *American Statistician, 14* (1960), 20–22, 33.

18. O. B. Ross, Jr., "Use of Controls in Medical Research," *Journal of the American Medical Association, 145* (1951), 72–75.

19. William W. Rozeboom, "The Fallacy of the Null-Hypothesis Significance Test," *Psychological Bulletin, 57* (1960), 416–428.

20. H. C. Selvin, "A Critique of Tests of Significance in Survey Research," *American Sociological Review, 22* (1957), 519–527.

21. James K. Skipper, Anthony L. Guenther, and Gilbert Nass, "The Sacredness of .05: A Note Concerning the Uses of Significance in Social Science," *The American Sociologist, 2* (1967), 16–18.

22. Warren R. Wilson and Howard Miller, "A Note on the Inconclusiveness of Accepting the Null Hypothesis," *Psychological Review, 71* (1964), 238–242.

23. Warren Wilson, Howard L. Miller, and Jerold S. Lower, "Much Ado About the Null Hypothesis," *Psychological Bulletin, 67* (1967), 188–196.

24. R. F. Winch and D. T. Campbell, "Proof? No. Evidence? Yes. The Significance of Tests of Significance," *American Sociologist, 4* (1969), 140–143.

Other references, books

1. W. I. B. Beveridge, *The Art of Scientific Investigation*, Third Edition, W. W. Norton, New York, 1957.

2. Dwight J. Ingle, *Principles of Research in Biology and Medicine*, J. B. Lippincott, Philadelphia, 1958.

3. E. L. Lehman, *Testing Statistical Hypotheses*, Wiley, New York, 1959.

Other references, other publications

1. David Bakan, "The Test of Significance in Psychological Research," in *On Method: Toward a Reconstruction of Psychological Investigation*, Jossey-Bass, San Francisco, 1967.

2. William H. Kruskal, "Tests of Significance," in *International Encyclopedia of the Social Sciences, 14* (1968), 238–250.

7

ANALYSIS OF VARIANCE

7.1 INTRODUCTION

In the preceding chapters the basic concepts of statistics have been examined, and they provide a foundation for the present and succeeding chapters.

The present chapter is concerned with *analysis of variance*, which may be defined as *a technique whereby the total variation present in a set of data is partitioned into several components. Associated with each of these components is a specific source of variation, so that in the analysis it is possible to ascertain the magnitude of the contributions of each of these sources to the total variation.*

The development of this subject is mainly due to the work of the late R. A. Fisher (1), whose contributions to statistics, spanning the years 1912 to 1962, have had a tremendous influence on modern statistical thought (2, 3).

Analysis of variance finds its widest application in the analysis of data derived from experiments. The principles of the design of experiments are well covered in several books, including those of Cochran and Cox (4), Cox (5), Davies (6), Federer (7), Finney (8), Fisher (1), John (9), Kempthorne (10), Li (11), and Mendenhall (12). We do not study this topic in detail, since to do it justice would require a minimum of an additional chapter. Some of the important concepts in experimental design, however, will become apparent as we discuss analysis of variance.

The relationship between the two topics may be summarized by pointing out that when experiments are designed with the analysis in mind, researchers can, before conducting experiments, identify those sources of variation that they consider important and can choose a design that will allow them to measure the extent of the contribution of these sources to the total variation. Analysis of variance is used for two different purposes: (1) to estimate and test hypotheses about population variances, and (2) to estimate and test hypotheses about population means. We are concerned here with the latter use. However, as we shall see, our conclusions regarding the means will depend on the magnitudes of the observed variances.

Underlying the valid use of analysis of variance as a tool of statistical inference are a set of fundamental assumptions. For a detailed discussion of these assumptions, the reader is referred to the paper by Eisenhart (13). Although an experimenter must not expect to find all the assumptions met to perfection, it is important that the user of analysis of variance techniques be aware of the underlying assumptions and be able to recognize when they are substantially unsatisfied. The consequences of the failure to meet the assumptions are discussed by Cochran (14) in a companion paper to that of Eisenhart's. Because experiments in which all the assumptions are perfectly met are rare, Cochran suggests that analysis of variance results be considered as approximate rather than exact. These assumptions are pointed out at appropriate points in the following sections.

We discuss analysis of variance as it is used to analyze the results of two different experimental designs, the completely randomized and the randomized complete block designs. In addition to these, the concept of a factorial experiment is given through its use in a completely randomized design. These do not exhaust the possibilities. A discussion of additional designs will be found in the references (4–12).

In our presentation of the analysis of variance for the different designs, this format is followed:

1. *Model*. The model will consist of a symbolic representation of a typical value from the data being analyzed.
2. *Assumptions*. The assumptions underlying the model will be specified.
3. *Hypotheses*. The hypotheses that may be tested under the model will be indicated. Appropriate null and alternate hypotheses will be stated.
4. *Calculations*. The necessary arithmetic calculations will be explained.
5. *ANOVA Table*. The results of the arithmetic calculations will be summarized in a table that will allow for quick and convenient assessment of the results.
6. *Decision*. A statistical decision will be made as to whether or not a null hypothesis should be rejected. Any administrative or clinical decision will be influenced by the statistical decision.

7.2 THE COMPLETELY RANDOMIZED DESIGN

We have seen in Chapter 6 how it is possible to test the null hypothesis of no difference between two population means. It is not unusual for the investigator to be interested in testing the null hypothesis of no difference among several population means. The student first encountering this problem might be inclined to suggest that all possible pairs of sample means be tested separately by means of the Student t test. Suppose there are five populations involved. The number of possible pairs of sample means is $\binom{5}{2} = 10$. As the amount of work involved in carrying out this many t tests is substantial, it would be worthwhile if a more efficient alternative for analysis were available. A more important consequence of performing all possible t tests, however, is that it is very likely to lead to a false conclusion.

Suppose we draw five samples from populations having equal means. As we have seen, there would be 10 tests if we were to do each of the possible tests separately. If we select a significance level of $\alpha = .05$ for each test, the probability of failing to reject a hypothesis of no difference in each case would be .95. By the multiplication rule of probability, if the tests were independent of one another, the probability of failing to reject a hypothesis of no difference in all 10 cases would be $(.95)^{10} = .5987$. The probability of rejecting, at least, one hypothesis of no difference, then, would be $1 - .5987 = .4013$. Since we know that the null hypothesis is true in every case in this illustrative example, rejecting the null hypothesis constitutes the committing of a Type I error. In the long run, then, in testing all possible pairs of means from five samples, we would commit a Type I error 40 percent of the time. The problem becomes even more complicated in practice, since three or more t tests would not be independent of one another.

It becomes clear, then, that some other method for testing for a significant difference among several means is needed. Analysis of variance provides such a method, and to illustrate its use let us consider the following example.

Example 7.2.1

In a study of the effect of glucose on insulin release, specimens of pancreatic tissue from experimental animals were treated with five different stimulants. Later, a determination was made on the amount of insulin released. The results are shown in Table 7.2.1. The experimenter wished to know if it was valid to conclude that there is a difference among the five populations with respect to the mean amount of insulin released.

1. *Model.* To write down the model for this example, let us begin by identifying a typical value from the set of data represented by the sample displayed in Table 7.2.1; and let us use the symbol x_{ij} to represent this typical value. The subscript ij indicates that this typical value is the ith observation in the jth group. Alternatively, since our stimulants represent different treatments, we may say that x_{ij} is the ith observation receiving the jth treatment. In our present example the subscript i may assume any value

Table 7.2.1

Insulin Released						
			Stimulant			
	1	2	3	4	5	
	1.53	3.15	3.89	8.18	5.86	
	1.61	3.96	4.80	5.64	5.46	
	3.75	3.59	3.68	7.36	5.69	
	2.89	1.89	5.70	5.33	6.49	
	3.26	1.45	5.62	8.82	7.81	
	2.83	3.49	5.79	5.26	9.03	
	2.86	1.56	4.75	8.75	7.49	
	2.59	2.44	5.33	7.10	8.98	
Total	21.32	21.53	39.56	56.44	56.81	195.66
Mean	2.66	2.69	4.94	7.06	7.10	4.89

between 1 and 8 (the number of observations in each group) and j runs from 1 to 5 (the number of groups or treatments).

Within each group (or population) represented by our data, any particular value bears this relationship to the true mean, μ_j, of that group: it is equal to the true group mean plus some amount that is either zero, a positive amount, or a negative amount. This means that a particular value in a given group may be equal to the group mean, larger than the group mean, or smaller than the group mean. Let us call the amount by which any value differs from its group mean the *error* and represent this error by the symbol e_{ij}. By the term error, we do not mean a mistake. The term is used to refer to the uncontrolled variation that exists among members of any population. Given a population of adult males, for example, we know that the heights of some individuals are above the true mean height of the population, while some heights are below the population mean. This variation is caused by a myriad of hereditary and environmental factors. If to any group mean, μ_j, we add a given error, e_{ij}, the result will be x_{ij}, the observation that deviates from the group mean by the amount e_{ij}.

We may write this relationship symbolically as

μ_j = group mean

$$x_{ij} = \mu_j + e_{ij} \tag{7.2.1}$$

e_{ij} = a given error

Solving for e_{ij} we have

x_{ij} = observation that deviates from the mean by e_{ij}

$$e_{ij} = x_{ij} - \mu_j \tag{7.2.2}$$

If we have k populations (in the present example $k = 5$), we may refer to the grand mean of all the observations in all the populations as μ. Given k

μ = grand mean of all populations

populations, we could compute μ by taking the average of the k population means, that is,

$$\mu = \frac{\sum \mu_j}{k} \tag{7.2.3}$$

Just as a particular observation within a group, in general, differs from its group mean by some amount, a particular group mean differs from the grand mean by some amount. The amount by which a group mean differs from the grand mean we refer to as the *treatment effect*. We may write the jth treatment effect as

$$\tau_j = \mu_j - \mu \tag{7.2.4}$$

τ_j: treatment effect for jth treatment

τ_j is a measure of the effect on μ_j of having been computed from observations receiving the jth treatment.

We may solve Equation 7.2.4 for μ_j to obtain

$$\mu_j = \mu + \tau_j \tag{7.2.5}$$

If we substitute the right-hand portion of Equation 7.2.5 for μ_j in Equation 7.2.1 we have

$$x_{ij} = \mu + \tau_j + e_{ij}, \qquad i = 1, 2, \ldots n_j; \quad j = 1, 2, \ldots k \tag{7.2.6}$$

and our model is specified.

By looking at our model we can see that a typical observation from the total set of data under study is composed of the grand mean, a treatment effect, and an error term representing the deviation of the observation from its group mean.

2. *Assumptions.* The set of assumptions adopted in a particular case depends on the manner in which the treatments are selected. There are two cases, usually referred to as the *Fixed Effects Model*, or *Model I*, and the *Random Effects Model*, or *Model II*.

The calculations are the same for both models; the distinction comes only in the interpretation of the results when the parameters of interest are means. The Fixed Effects Model will be assumed in the examples and exercises of this chapter. Refer to the papers by Eisenhart (13) and Wilk and Kempthorne (15) for further information.

Fixed Effects Model. The assumptions for this model are as follows.

1. The k sets of observed data constitute k independent random samples from the respective populations.
2. Each of the populations from which the samples come is normally distributed with mean, μ_j, and variance σ_j^2.

3. Each of the populations has the same variance. That is, $\sigma_1{}^2 = \sigma_2{}^2 = \cdots = \sigma_k{}^2 = \sigma^2$, the common variance.

4. The τ_j's are unknown constants and $\sum \tau_j = 0$, since the sum of all deviations of the μ_j from their mean, μ, is zero.

Three consequences of the relationship

$$e_{ij} = x_{ij} - \mu_j$$

specified in Equation 7.2.2 are

(a) The e_{ij} have a mean of 0, since the mean of x_{ij} is μ_j

(b) The e_{ij} have a variance equal to the variance of the x_{ij}, since the e_{ij} and x_{ij} differ only by a constant, that is, the error variance is equal to σ^2, the common variance specified in assumption 3 above.

(c) The e_{ij} are normally (and independently) distributed.

Use of the Fixed Effects Model implies that we are interested only in the k populations represented by our sample data. Any inferences that we make apply only to these populations. For example, if the treatments consisted of three weight-reducing regimens, any inferences we might make under Model I are limited to these three regimens. We could not extend our inferences to any larger collection of weight-reducing regimens.

Random Effects Model. The assumptions underlying the Random Effects model may be summarized as follows.

1. The k sets of observed data constitute k random samples from the respective populations.

2. The e_{ij} are normally and independently distributed with mean, 0, and equal variances, σ^2.

3. The τ_i's are normally and independently distributed with mean, 0, and variance, $\sigma_\tau{}^2$.

The significance of the last assumption is that the treatments under investigation are considered to be a random sample of treatments from some population of treatments in which we have an interest. For example, suppose more weight-reducing regimens are available than we have resources to study. We could assume Model II and randomly select, from this population of regimens, a sample of regimens for investigation. The analysis of variance computational procedure would be the same as for Model I. We could test hypotheses concerning the equality of group means, and we could draw inferences regarding the entire population of weight-reducing regimens from which we drew our sample. Under Model II we may also test hypotheses about, and construct confidence intervals for the treatment variances.

Model II is sometimes referred to as the *components of variance model.* Additional information on it will be found in the articles by Crump (16),

Cunningham and Henderson (17), Henderson (18), Rutherford (19), Schultz (20), and Searle (21).

3. *Hypotheses.* We may test the null hypothesis that all group (population) or treatment means are equal against the alternative that the members of, at least, one pair are not equal. We may state the hypotheses formally as follows:

$$H_0: \mu_1 = \mu_2 = \cdots = \mu_k$$
$$H_A: \text{not all } \mu_j \text{ are equal}$$

If the population means are equal, each treatment effect is equal to zero, so that, alternatively, the hypotheses may be stated as

$$H_0: \tau_j = 0, \qquad j = 1, 2, \ldots, k$$
$$H_A: \text{not all } \tau_j = 0$$

At this point a level of significance, α, is chosen.
For our present example we have

$$H_0: \mu_1 = \mu_2 = \mu_3 = \mu_4 = \mu_5$$
$$H_A: \text{not all } \mu_j \text{ are equal.}$$

Let us use a .05 level of significance.

4. *Calculations.* Our discussion of the calculations will be facilitated if we prepare a table for displaying sample data as was done in Table 7.2.1. In general, such a table would contain the information shown in Table 7.2.2.

Table 7.2.2

Table of Sample Values for the Completely Randomized Design

	Treatment					
	1	2	3	$\cdots$	k	
	x_{11}	x_{12}	x_{13}	$\cdots$	x_{1k}	
	x_{21}	x_{22}	x_{23}	$\cdots$	x_{2k}	
	x_{31}	x_{32}	x_{33}	$\cdots$	x_{3k}	
	$\vdots$	$\vdots$	$\vdots$	$\vdots$	$\vdots$	
	$x_{n_1 1}$	$x_{n_2 2}$	$x_{n_3 3}$	$\cdots$	$x_{n_k k}$	
Total	$T_{.1}$	$T_{.2}$	$T_{.3}$		$T_{.k}$	$T_{..}$
Mean	$\bar{x}_{.1}$	$\bar{x}_{.2}$	$\bar{x}_{.3}$		$\bar{x}_{.k}$	$\bar{x}_{..}$

The symbols used in this table are defined as follows:

$$x_{ij} = \text{the } i\text{th observation receiving the } j\text{th treatment},$$
$$i = 1, 2, \ldots, n_j, \quad j = 1, 2, \ldots, k$$

$$T_{.j} = \sum_{i=1}^{n_j} x_{ij} = \text{total of the } j\text{th column}$$

$$\bar{x}_{.j} = \frac{T_{.j}}{n_j} = \text{mean of the } j\text{th column}$$

$$T_{..} = \sum_{j=1}^{k} T_{.j} = \sum_{j=1}^{k} \sum_{i=1}^{n_j} x_{ij} = \text{total of all observations}$$

$$\bar{x}_{..} = \frac{T_{..}}{N}, \qquad N = \sum_{j=1}^{k} n_j$$

We have defined analysis of variance as a process whereby the total variation present in a set of data is partitioned into components that are attributable to different sources. The term *variation* used in this context refers to the *sum of squared deviations of observations from their mean*, or *sum of squares* for short.

The Total Sum of Squares. Before we can do any partitioning, we must first obtain the total sum of squares. The total sum of squares is the sum of the squares of the deviations of each observation from the mean of all the observations taken together. This *total sum of squares* is defined as

$$SS_{\text{total}} = \sum_{j=1}^{k} \sum_{i=1}^{n_j} (x_{ij} - \bar{x}_{..})^2 \tag{7.2.7}$$

where $\sum_{i=1}^{n_j}$ tells us to sum the squared deviations for each group, and $\sum_{j=1}^{k}$ tells us to add the k group totals obtained by applying $\sum_{i=1}^{n_j}$. The reader will recognize Equation 7.2.7 as the numerator of the variance that may be computed from the complete set of observations taken together.

We may rewrite Equation 7.2.7. as

total sum of squares

$$SS_{\text{total}} = \sum_{j=1}^{k} \sum_{i=1}^{n_j} x_{ij}^2 - \frac{T_{..}^2}{N} \tag{7.2.8}$$

which is more convenient for computational purposes.

The total sum of squares for our illustrative example is

$$SS_{\text{total}} = (1.53)^2 + (1.61)^2 + \cdots + (8.98)^2 - \frac{(195.66)^2}{40}$$

$$= 1157.5482 - \frac{38282.8356}{40}$$

$$= 1157.5482 - 957.0709$$
$$= 200.4773$$

We now proceed with the partitioning of the total sum of squares. We may, without changing its value, insert $-\bar{x}_{.j} + \bar{x}_{.j}$ in the parentheses of Equation 7.2.7. The reader will recognize this added quantity as a well chosen zero that does not change the value of the expression. The result of this addition is

$$SS_{\text{total}} = \sum_{j=1}^{k} \sum_{i=1}^{n_j} (x_{ij} - \bar{x}_{.j} + \bar{x}_{.j} - \bar{x}_{..})^2 \tag{7.2.9}$$

If we group terms and expand, we have

$$SS_{\text{total}} = \sum_{j=1}^{k} \sum_{i=1}^{n_j} [(x_{ij} - \bar{x}_{.j}) + (\bar{x}_{.j} - \bar{x}_{..})]^2$$

$$= \sum_{j=1}^{k} \sum_{i=1}^{n_j} (x_{ij} - \bar{x}_{.j})^2 + 2 \sum_{j=1}^{k} \sum_{i=1}^{n_j} (x_{ij} - \bar{x}_{.j})(\bar{x}_{.j} - \bar{x}_{..})$$

$$+ \sum_{j=1}^{k} \sum_{i=1}^{n_j} (\bar{x}_{.j} - \bar{x}_{..})^2 \tag{7.2.10}$$

The middle term above may be written as

$$2 \sum_{j=1}^{k} (\bar{x}_{.j} - \bar{x}_{..}) \sum_{i=1}^{n_j} (x_{ij} - \bar{x}_{.j}) \tag{7.2.11}$$

Examination of Equation 7.2.11 reveals that this term is equal to zero, since the sum of the deviations of a set of values from their mean as in $\sum_{i=1}^{n_j} (x_{ij} - \bar{x}_{.j})$, is equal to zero.

We now may write Equation 7.2.10 as

$$SS_{\text{total}} = \sum_{j=1}^{k} \sum_{i=1}^{n_j} (x_{ij} - \bar{x}_{.j})^2 + \sum_{j=1}^{k} \sum_{i=1}^{n_j} (\bar{x}_{.j} - \bar{x}_{..})^2$$

$$= \sum_{j=1}^{k} \sum_{i=1}^{n_j} (x_{ij} - \bar{x}_{.j})^2 + \sum_{j=1}^{k} n_j(\bar{x}_{.j} - \bar{x}_{..})^2 \tag{7.2.12}$$

When the number of observations is the same in each group the last term on the right may be rewritten to give

$$SS_{\text{total}} = \sum_{j=1}^{k} \sum_{i=1}^{n_j} (x_{ij} - \bar{x}_{.j})^2 + n \sum_{j=1}^{k} (\bar{x}_{.j} - \bar{x}_{..})^2 \qquad (7.2.13)$$

where $n = n_1 = n_2 = \cdots = n_k$.

The Within Groups Sum of Squares. The partitioning of the total sum of squares is now complete, and we see that in the present case there are two components. Let us now investigate the nature and source of these two components of variation.

If we look at the first term on the right of Equation 7.2.12, we see that the first step in the indicated computation calls for performing certain calculations *within* each group. These calculations involve computing within each group the sum of the squared deviations of the individual observations from their mean. When these calculations have been performed within each group, the symbol, $\sum_{j=1}^{k}$, tells us to obtain the sum of the individual group results. This component of variation is called the *within groups sum of squares* and may be designated SS_{within}. This quantity is sometimes referred to as the residual or error sum of squares. The expression may be written in a computationally more convenient form as follows:

$$SS_{\text{within}} = \sum_{j=1}^{k} \sum_{i=1}^{n_j} (x_{ij} - \bar{x}_{.j})^2 = \sum_{j=1}^{k} \sum_{i=1}^{n_j} x_{ij}^2 - \sum_{j=1}^{k} \frac{(T_{.j})^2}{n_j} \qquad (7.2.14)$$

By using the data from Table 7.2.1, we find the within sum of squares to be

$$\begin{aligned}
SS_{\text{within}} &= (1.53)^2 + (1.61)^2 + \cdots + (8.98)^2 \\
&\quad - \left[\frac{(21.32)^2}{8} + \frac{(21.53)^2}{8} + \frac{(39.56)^2}{8} + \frac{(56.44)^2}{8} + \frac{(56.81)^2}{8}\right] \\
&= 1157.5482 - (56.8178 + 57.9426 \\
&\quad + 195.6242 + 398.1842 + 403.4220) \\
&= 1157.5482 - 1111.9908 \\
&= 45.5574
\end{aligned}$$

The Among Groups Sum of Squares. Now let us examine the second term on the right in Equation 7.2.12. The operation called for by this term is to obtain for each group the squared deviation of the group mean from the grand mean and to multiply the result by the size of the group. Finally, we must add these results over all groups. This quantity is a measure of the variation among groups and is referred to as the *sum of squares among groups* or SS_{among}. The computing formula is as follows:

$$SS_{\text{among}} = \sum_{j=1}^{k} n_j(\bar{x}_{.j} - \bar{x}_{..})^2 = \sum_{j=1}^{k} \frac{T_{.j}^2}{n_j} - T_{..}^2/N \qquad (7.2.15)$$

The SS_{among} for our illustrative example is computed as follows:

$$SS_{\text{among}} = \frac{(21.32)^2}{8} + \frac{(21.53)^2}{8} + \frac{(39.56)^2}{8} + \frac{(56.44)^2}{8} + \frac{(56.81)^2}{8} - \frac{(195.66)^2}{40}$$

$$= 1111.9908 - 957.0709$$

$$= 154.9199$$

In summary, then, we have found that the total sum of squares is equal to the sum of the among sum of squares and the within sum of squares. We express this relationship as follows:

$$SS_{\text{total}} = SS_{\text{among}} + SS_{\text{within}}$$

For our illustrative example we have

$$200.4773 = 154.9199 + 45.5574$$

$$200.4773 = 200.4773$$

5. *The Analysis of Variance Table.* From the sums of squares that we have just computed, it is possible to obtain two estimates of the population variance, σ^2. It can be shown that when the true group means are all equal, both the among sum of squares and the within sum of squares, when divided by their respective degrees of freedom, yield independent and unbiased estimates of σ^2.

The First Estimate of σ^2**.** Within any group

$$\frac{\sum_{i=1}^{n_j} (x_{ij} - \bar{x}_{.j})^2}{n_j - 1}$$

provides an unbiased estimate of the true variance of that group. Under the assumption that the true group variances are all equal, we may pool the k estimates to obtain

$$\frac{\sum_{j=1}^{k} \sum_{i=1}^{n_j} (x_{ij} - \bar{x}_{.j})^2}{\sum_{j=1}^{k} (n_j - 1)} \qquad (7.2.16)$$

This is our first estimate of σ^2 and may be called the *within groups variance*, since it is the within groups sum of squares of Equation 7.2.14 divided by the appropriate degrees of freedom. The student will recognize this as an extension to k samples of the pooling of variances procedure encountered in Chapters 5 and 6 when the variances from two samples were pooled in order to use the t distribution. The quantity in Equation 7.2.16 is customarily referred to as the within groups *mean square* rather than the within groups variance. The within groups mean square for our illustrative example is

$$\frac{SS_{\text{within}}}{5(7)} = \frac{45.5574}{35} = 1.3016$$

The Second Estimate of σ^2**.** The second estimate of σ^2 may be obtained from the familiar formula for the variance of sample means, $\sigma_{\bar{x}}^2 = \sigma^2/n$. If we solve this equation for σ^2, the variance of the population from which the samples were drawn, we have

$$\sigma^2 = n\sigma_{\bar{x}}^2 \tag{7.2.17}$$

An unbiased estimate of $\sigma_{\bar{x}}^2$, computed from sample data, is provided by

$$\frac{\sum_{j=1}^{k} (\bar{x}_{.j} - \bar{x}_{..})^2}{k - 1}$$

If we substitute this quantity into Equation 7.2.17, we obtain the desired estimate of σ^2,

$$\frac{n \sum_{j=1}^{k} (\bar{x}_{.j} - \bar{x}_{..})^2}{k - 1} \tag{7.2.18}$$

The reader will recognize the numerator of Equation 7.2.18 as the among groups sum of squares for the special case when all sample sizes are equal. This sum of squares when divided by the associated degrees of freedom $k - 1$ is referred to as the *among groups mean square.*

For our illustrative example we have the following among groups mean square:

$$\frac{SS_{\text{among}}}{(5 - 1)} = \frac{154.9199}{4} = 38.7300$$

If, indeed, the null hypothesis is true we would expect these two estimates of σ^2 to be fairly close in magnitude. If the null hypothesis is false, that is, if all true group means are not equal, we would expect the among groups mean square, which is computed by using the squared deviations of these means from the overall mean, to be larger than the within groups mean square.

The Variance Ratio. What we need to do, then, is to compare these two estimates of σ^2; and we do this by computing the following variance ratio:

$$\text{V. R.} = \frac{\text{among groups mean square}}{\text{within groups mean square}}$$

If the two estimates are about equal, the variance ratio (V. R.) will be close to 1. A ratio close to 1 tends to support the hypothesis of equal group means. If, on the other hand, the among groups mean square is considerably larger than the within groups mean square, V. R. will be considerably greater than 1. A value of V. R. considerably greater than 1 would cast doubt on the hypothesis of equal group means.

We know that because of the vagaries of sampling, even when the null hypothesis is true, it is unlikely that the among and within groups mean squares will be equal. We must decide, then, how big the observed difference has to be before we can conclude that the difference is due to something other than sampling fluctuation. In other words, how large a value of V. R. is required for us to be willing to conclude that the observed difference between our two estimates of σ^2 is not the result of chance alone?

The F Test. To answer the question posed above, we must consider the sampling distribution of the ratio of two sample variances. In Chapter 5 we learned that the quantity $(s_1^2/\sigma_1^2)/(s_2^2/\sigma_2^2)$ follows a distribution known as the F distribution when the sample variances are computed from random and independently drawn samples from normal populations. The F distribution, introduced by R. A. Fisher in the early 1920s, has become one of the most widely used distributions in modern statistics. We have already become acquainted with its use in constructing confidence intervals for, and testing hypotheses about, population variances. In this chapter we shall see that it is the distribution fundamental to analysis of variance.

In Chapter 6 we learned that when the population variances are the same, they cancel in the expression $(s_1^2/\sigma_1^2)/(s_2^2/\sigma_2^2)$, leaving s_1^2/s_2^2 which is itself distributed as F. The F distribution is really a family of distributions, and the particular F distribution we use in a given situation depends on the number of degrees of freedom associated with the sample variance in the numerator (*numerator degrees of freedom*) and the number of degrees of freedom associated with the sample variance in the denominator (*denominator degrees of freedom*).

Once the appropriate F distribution has been determined, the size of the observed V. R. that will cause rejection of the hypothesis of equal population variances depends on the significance level chosen. The significance level chosen determines the critical value of F, the value that separates the acceptance region from the rejection region.

As we have seen, we compute V. R. in situations of this type by placing the among groups mean square in the numerator and the within groups mean square in the denominator, so that the numerator degrees of freedom is equal to the number of groups minus 1, $(k - 1)$, and the denominator degrees of freedom value is equal to $\sum_{j=1}^{k} (n_j - 1) = \sum_{j=1}^{k} n_j - k = N - k$. For our present example we have

$$\text{numerator degrees of freedom} = 5 - 1 = 4$$
$$\text{denominator degrees of freedom} = 40 - 5 = 35$$

The calculations that we have performed may be summarized and displayed in a table such as Table 7.2.3, which is called the ANOVA Table.

Table 7.2.4 is the ANOVA table for our illustrative example.

Table 7.2.3

Analsysis of Variance Table for the Completely Randomized Design

Source of Variation	**Sum of Squares**	**Degrees of Freedom**	**Mean Square**	**Variance Ratio**
Among groups	$SS_{\text{among}} = \sum_{j=1}^{k} n_j(\bar{x}_{.j} - \bar{x}_{..})^2 = \sum_{j=1}^{k} \frac{T_{.j}^2}{n_j} - \frac{T_{..}^2}{N}$	$k - 1$	$MS_{\text{among}} = SS_{\text{among}}/(k - 1)$	$\text{V. R.} = \frac{MS_{\text{among}}}{MS_{\text{within}}}$
Within groups	$SS_{\text{within}} = \sum_{j=1}^{k} \sum_{i=1}^{n_j} (x_{ij} - \bar{x}_{.j})^2 = \sum_{j=1}^{k} \sum_{i=1}^{n_j} x_{ij}^2 - \sum_{i=1}^{k} \frac{(T_{.j})^2}{n_j}$	$N - k$	$MS_{\text{within}} = SS_{\text{within}}/(N - k)$	
Total	$SS_{\text{total}} = \sum_{j=1}^{k} \sum_{i=1}^{n_j} (x_{ij} - \bar{x}_{..})^2 = \sum_{j=1}^{k} \sum_{i=1}^{n_j} x_{ij}^2 - \frac{T_{..}^2}{N}$	$N - 1$		

Table 7.2.4

ANOVA Table, Example 7.2.1

Source	*SS*	**d. f.**	*MS*	**V. R.**
Among groups	154.9199	4	38.7300	29.76
Within groups	45.5574	35	1.3016	
Total	200.4773	39		

Notice that in Table 7.2.3 the term $\sum_{j=1}^{k} \sum_{i=1}^{n_j} x_{ij}^2/N = T_{..}^2/N$ occurs in both the expression for SS_{among} and SS_{total}. A savings in computational time and labor may be realized if we take advantage of this fact. We need only to compute this quantity, which is called the correction term and designated by the letter C, once, and use it as needed.

The computational burden may be lightened in still another way. Since SS_{total} is equal to the sum of SS_{among} and SS_{within}, and since SS_{among} is easier to compute than SS_{within}, we may compute SS_{total} and SS_{among} and subtract the latter from the former to obtain SS_{within}.

6. *The Decision.* To reach a decision we must compare our computed V. R. with the critical value of F, which we obtain from Table J. We find, by looking in Table J, that there is no entry for denominator degrees of freedom equal to 35. Since 35 is equidistant from the two entries 30 and 40, there is no "closest" value to select. An appropriate procedure is to select the conservative value of F, which is the value of F corresponding to the next smallest denominator degrees of freedom given in the table. Following this procedure, we take the value of F corresponding to 4 and 30 degrees of freedom. If we choose a .05 level of significance, the value of F we seek is 2.69. The resulting acceptance and rejection regions are shown in Figure 7.2.1.

Since our computed V. R., 29.83, is greater than our critical value of F, 2.69, we must try to explain the difference. There are two possible explanations.

If the null hypothesis is true, that is, if the two sample variances are estimates of a common variance, we know that the probability of getting a value as large or larger than 2.69 is .05. We obtained a value much greater than 2.69 which, if the null hypothesis is true, we would consider to be a very rare

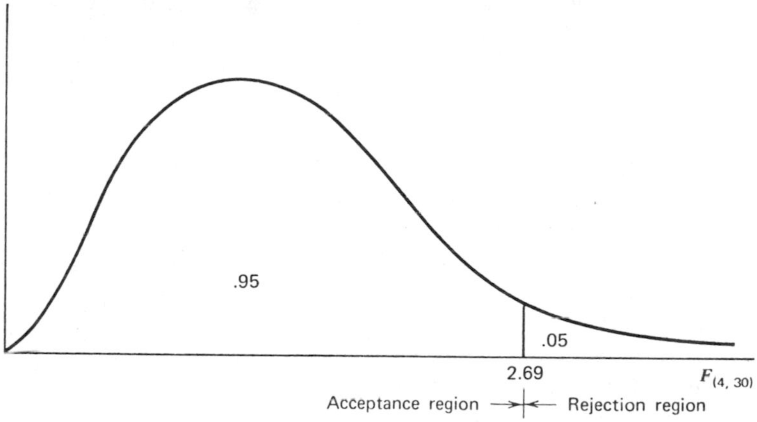

Figure 7.2.1., Acceptance and rejection regions, Example 7.2.1.

occurrence. We may, if we wish, conclude that the null hypothesis is true and assume that because of chance we got a set of data that gave rise to a rare event. On the other hand, we may prefer to take the position that our large computed V. R. value does not represent a rare event brought about by chance but, instead, reflects the fact that something other than chance is operative. This other something we conclude to be a false null hypothesis.

It is this latter explanation that we usually give for computed values of V. R. that exceed the critical value of F. In other words, if the computed value of V. R. is greater than the critical value of F, we reject the null hypothesis. Since, in our present example, 29.76 is greater than 2.69, we reject the hypothesis that the observed sample variances are estimates of a common variance. For this test, $p < .005$, since $29.76 > F_{.995} = 4.62$.

It will be recalled that the original hypothesis we set out to test was

$$H_0: \mu_1 = \mu_2 = \mu_3 = \mu_4 = \mu_5$$

Does rejection of the hypothesis about variances imply a rejection of the hypothesis of equal population means? The answer is, yes. A large value of V. R. resulted from the fact that the among groups mean square was considerably larger than the within groups mean square. Since the among groups mean square is a measure of the dispersion of the group means about their mean, this quantity will be large when there is a large discrepancy among the sizes of the sample group means. Because of this, then, a significant value of V. R. tells us to reject the null hypothesis that all true group means are equal. In the present example, our decision is to reject the null hypothesis and to conclude that not all group means are equal.

This section is concerned with the analysis of variance that is appropriate for the *completely randomized experimental design.* A completely randomized design is a design in which the treatments are randomly assigned to the experimental units, or in which the experimental units are randomly assigned to the treatments. The design is simple and, therefore, widely used. It should be used, however, only when the units receiving the treatments are homogeneous. If the experimental units are not homogeneous, the researcher should consider an alternate design such as one of those to be discussed later in this chapter.

Although, in our illustrative example, the sample sizes were equal, this is not a requirement, as the completely randomized design and its analysis may be used when the sample sizes are not equal.

In our illustrative example the five treatments are treatments in the usual sense of the word. This is not always the case, however, as the term "treatment" as used in experimental design is quite general. We might, for example, wish to study the response to the same treatment (in the usual sense of the word) of several breeds of animal. We would, however, refer to the breed of animal as the "treatment."

We must also point out that, although the techniques of analysis of variance are more often applied to data resulting from controlled experiments, the techniques also may be used to analyze data collected by a survey, provided that the underlying assumptions are reasonably met.

Testing for Significant Differences Between Individual Pairs of Means. Whenever the analysis of variance leads to a rejection of the null hypothesis of no difference among group means, the question naturally arises regarding just which pairs of means are different. In fact, the desire, more often than not, is to carry out a significance test on each and every pair of treatment means. For instance, in Example 7.2.1, where there are five treatments, we may wish to know, after rejecting $H_0: \mu_1 = \mu_2 = \mu_3 = \mu_4 = \mu_5$, which of the 10 possible individual hypotheses should be rejected. The experimenter, however, must exercise caution in testing for significant differences between individual means, and must always make certain that his procedure is valid. The critical point in the procedure is the level of significance. Although the probability, α, of rejecting a true null hypothesis for the test as a whole is made small, the probability of rejecting, at least, one true hypothesis when several pairs of means are tested is, as we have seen, greater than α.

Over the years several procedures for making individual comparisons have been suggested. The oldest procedure, and perhaps the one most widely used in the past, is the *least significant difference* (LSD) procedure due to Fisher, who first discussed it in the 1935 edition of his book, *The Design of Experiments* (1). The LSD procedure which is a Student's t test using a pooled error variance, is valid only when making independent comparisons or comparisons planned before the data are analyzed. A difference between any two means that exceeds a least significant difference is considered significant at the level of significance used in computing the LSD. The LSD procedure usually is used only when the overall analysis of variance leads to a significant V. R. For an example of the use of the LSD, see Steel and Torrie (22).

Duncan (23–26) has contributed a considerable amount of research to the subject of multiple comparisons with the result that at the present time a widely used procedure is *Duncan's new multiple range test.* The extension of the test to the case of unequal sample sizes is discussed by Kramer (27).

When the objective of an experiment is to compare several treatments with a control, and not with each other, a procedure due to Dunnett (28, 29) for comparing the control against each of the other treatments is usually followed.

Other multiple comparison procedures in use are those proposed by Tukey (30, 31), Newman (32), Keuls (33), and Scheffé (34, 35). The advantages and disadvantages of the various procedures are discussed by Bancroft (36) and Winer (37).

Tukey's HSD Test. A multiple comparison procedure developed by Tukey (31) is frequently used for testing the null hypotheses that all possible pairs of treatment means are equal. When this test is employed we select an overall significance level of α. The probability is α, then, that one or more of the null hypotheses is false.

Tukey's test, which is usually referred to as the HSD (*honestly significant difference*) test, makes use of a single value against which all differences are compared. This value, called the HSD, is given by

$$\text{HSD} = q_{\alpha,k,N-k}\sqrt{\frac{\text{MSE}}{n}} \tag{7.2.19}$$

where α is the chosen level of significance, k is the number of means in the experiment, N is the total number of observations in the experiment, n is the number of observations in a treatment, MSE is the error mean square from the ANOVA table, and q is obtained by entering Appendix Table K with α, k, and $N - k$.

All possible differences between pairs of means are computed, and any difference (absolute value) that exceeds HSD is declared to be significant.

Example 7.2.2

Let us illustrate the use of the HSD test with the data from Example 7.2.1. The first step is to prepare a table of all possible differences between means. The results of this step for the present example are displayed in Table 7.2.5.

Suppose we let $\alpha = .05$. Entering Table K with $\alpha = .05$, $k = 5$, and $N - k = 35$, we find that q is about 4.07, if we interpolate. In Table 7.2.4, we have MSE = 1.3016, so that

$$\text{HSD} = 4.07\sqrt{\frac{1.3016}{8}} = 1.64$$

Table 7.2.5

Differences Between Means for Example 7.2.2
(Means are Taken from Table 7.2.1)

	$\bar{x}_{.1}$	$\bar{x}_{.2}$	$\bar{x}_{.3}$	$\bar{x}_{.4}$	$\bar{x}_{.5}$
$\bar{x}_{.1} = 2.66$	—	.03	2.28	4.40	4.44
$\bar{x}_{.2} = 2.69$		—	2.25	4.37	4.41
$\bar{x}_{.3} = 4.94$			—	2.12	2.16
$\bar{x}_{.4} = 7.06$				—	.04
$\bar{x}_{.5} = 7.10$					—

Since all the differences between sample means, except .03 and .04, exceed 1.64 we conclude that all pairs of treatment means are different except one and two and four and five.

Exercises

In each of the following exercises go through the six steps of analysis of variance. Determine the p-value for each test.

7.2.1. Four groups of physical therapy patients were subjected to different treatment regimens. At the end of a specified time period each was given a test to measure treatment effectiveness. The following scores were obtained.

Treatment			
1	2	3	4
64	76	58	95
88	70	74	90
72	90	66	80
80	80	60	87
79	75	82	88
71	82	75	85

Do these data present sufficient evidence to indicate a difference among the treatments? Let $\alpha = .05$.

7.2.2. An experiment was conducted to compare three methods of packaging a certain frozen food. The criterion was the ascorbic acid content (mg/100 gm) after a specified period of time. The following data were obtained.

Packaging Method		
A	B	C
14.29	20.06	20.04
19.10	20.64	26.23
19.09	18.00	22.74
16.25	19.56	24.04
15.09	19.47	23.37
16.61	19.07	25.02
19.63	18.38	23.27

Do these data provide sufficient evidence at the .01 level of significance to indicate a difference in packaging methods?

7.2.3. Three groups of animals were used in an experiment to compare response times, in seconds, to three different stimuli. The following results were obtained.

Stimulus		
I	II	III
16	6	8
14	7	10
14	7	9
13	8	10
13	4	6
12	8	7
12	9	10
17	6	9
17	8	11
17	6	11
19	4	9
14	9	10
15	5	9
20	5	5

Do these data provide sufficient evidence to indicate a true difference among group means? Let $\alpha = .05$.

7.2.4. Blood sugar determinations (mg/100 ml) were made on 10 specimens from each of five breeds of a certain experimental animal with the following results.

		Breed		
A	B	C	D	E
124	111	117	104	142
116	101	142	128	139
101	130	121	130	133
118	108	123	103	120
118	127	121	121	127
120	129	148	119	149
110	122	141	106	150
127	103	122	107	149
106	122	139	107	120
130	127	125	115	116

Do these data provide sufficient evidence to indicate a difference in mean blood sugar level among breeds? Let $\alpha = .05$.

7.2.5. It was desired to compare three physicians with regard to the length of stay in the hospital of their patients following a certain minor surgical procedure without complications. A sample of eight records were selected from the records of each physician, and the following lengths of stay were observed.

Physician		
A	B	C
4	4	5
5	5	3
5	4	3
4	3	3
6	4	3
6	5	3
4	3	4
5	3	5

Do these data suggest a difference in average length of stay among the three physicians? Let $\alpha = .01$.

7.2.6. Refer to Exercise 7.2.1 and apply Tukey's HSD test. Let $\alpha = .01$.

7.2.7. Refer to Exercise 7.2.2 and apply Tukey's HSD test. Let $\alpha = .05$.

7.2.8. Refer to Exercise 7.2.3 and apply Tukey's HSD test. Let $\alpha = .05$.

7.2.9. Refer to Exercise 7.2.4 and apply Tukey's HSD test. Let $\alpha = .01$.

7.2.10. Refer to Exercise 7.2.5 and apply Tukey's HSD test. Let $\alpha = .01$.

7.3 THE RANDOMIZED COMPLETE BLOCK DESIGN

Of all the experimental designs that are in use, the *randomized complete block* design appears to be the most widely used by far. This design was developed about 1925 by R. A. Fisher (3, 38), who was seeking methods of improving agricultural field experiments. The name of the design reflects its origin in agricultural experiments where the land was divided into *blocks* and the blocks were divided into *plots* that received the treatments under investigation.

The randomized complete block design is a design in which the units (called *experimental units*) to which the treatments are applied are subdivided into homogeneous groups called *blocks*, so that the number of experimental units in a block is equal to the number (or some multiple of the number) of treatments being studied. The treatments are then assigned at random to the experimental units within each block. It should be emphasized that each treatment appears in every block, and each block receives every treatment.

The objective in using the randomized complete block design is to isolate and remove from the error term the variation attributable to the blocks, while assuring that treatment means will be free of block effects. The effectiveness of the design depends on the ability to achieve homogeneous blocks of experimental units. The ability to form homogeneous blocks depends on the researcher's knowledge of the experimental material.

In animal experiments if it is felt that different breeds of animal will respond differently to the same treatment, the breed of animal may be used as a blocking factor. Litters may also be used as blocks, in which case an animal from each litter receives a treatment. In experiments involving human beings, if it is desired that differences resulting from age be eliminated, then subjects may be grouped according to age so that one person of each age receives each treatment. The randomized complete block design also may be employed effectively when an experiment must be carried out in more than one laboratory (block), or when several days (blocks) are required for completion.

Some of the advantages of the randomized complete block design include the fact that it is both easily understood and computationally simple. Furthermore, certain complications that may arise in the course of an experiment are easily handled when this design is employed.

It is instructive here to point out that the paired comparisons analysis presented in Chapter 6 is a special case of the randomized complete block design. Example 6.3.1, for example, may be treated as a randomized complete block design in which the two cholesterol levels are the treatment effects and the 12 individuals on whom the measurements were taken are the blocks.

In general, the data from an experiment utilizing the randomized complete block design may be displayed in a table such as Table 7.3.1. The following

Table 7.3.1

Table of Sample Values for the Randomized Complete Block Design

	Treatments						
Blocks	1	2	3	$\cdots$	k	**Total**	**Mean**
1	x_{11}	x_{12}	x_{13}	$\cdots$	x_{1k}	$T_{1.}$	$\bar{x}_{1.}$
2	x_{21}	x_{22}	x_{23}	$\cdots$	x_{2k}	$T_{2.}$	$\bar{x}_{2.}$
3	x_{31}	x_{32}	x_{33}	$\cdots$	x_{3k}	$T_{3.}$	$\bar{x}_{3.}$
$\vdots$	$\vdots$	$\vdots$	$\vdots$	$\vdots$	$\vdots$	$\vdots$	$\vdots$
n	x_{n1}	x_{n2}	x_{n3}	$\cdots$	x_{nk}	$T_{n.}$	$\bar{x}_{n.}$
Total	$T_{.1}$	$T_{.2}$	$T_{.3}$	$\cdots$	$T_{.k}$	$T_{..}$	
Mean	$\bar{x}_{.1}$	$\bar{x}_{.2}$	$\bar{x}_{.3}$	$\cdots$	$\bar{x}_{.k}$		$\bar{x}_{..}$

new notation in this table should be observed:

$$\text{the total of the } i\text{th block} = T_{i.} = \sum_{j=1}^{k} x_{ij}$$

$$\text{the mean of the } i\text{th block} = \bar{x}_{i.} = \frac{\sum_{j=1}^{k} x_{ij}}{k}$$

$$\text{and the grand total} = T_{..} = \sum_{j=1}^{k} T_{.j} = \sum_{i=1}^{n} T_{i.}$$

indicating that the grand total may be obtained either by adding row totals or by adding column totals.

Example 7.3.1

A physical therapist wished to compare three methods for teaching patients to use a certain prosthetic device. He felt that the rate of learning would be different for patients of different ages and wished to design an experiment in which the influence of age could be taken into account. The randomized complete block design is the appropriate design for achieving this goal. Consequently, three patients in each of five age groups were selected to participate in the experiment, and one patient in each age group was randomly assigned to each of the teaching methods. The methods of instruction constitute our three treatments, and the five age groups are the blocks. The data shown in Table 7.3.2 were obtained.

Table 7.3.2

Time (in Days) Required To Learn the Use of a Certain Prosthetic Device

	Teaching Method (Treatments)				
Age Group	**A**	**B**	**C**	**Total**	**Mean**
Under 20	7	9	10	26	8.67
20 to 29	8	9	10	27	9.00
30 to 39	9	9	12	30	10.00
40 to 49	10	9	12	31	10.33
50 and over	11	12	14	37	12.33
Total	45	48	58	151	
Mean	9.0	9.6	11.6		10.07

blocks

In analyzing the data from a randomized complete block design we can follow the six-step analysis of variance procedure given in Sections 7.1 and 7.2.

1. *The Model.* Following a line of reasoning similar to that used in Section 7.2 for deriving the model for the completely randomized design, we can develop the following model for the randomized complete block design:

$$x_{ij} = \mu + \beta_i + \tau_j + e_{ij} \tag{7.3.1}$$

$$i = 1, 2, \ldots, n; \qquad j = 1, 2, \ldots, k$$

In this model

x_{ij} is a typical value from the overall population.
μ is an unknown constant.
β_i represents a block effect reflecting the fact that the experimental unit fell in the ith block.
τ_j represents a treatment effect, reflecting the fact that the experimental unit received the jth treatment.
e_{ij} is a residual component representing all sources of variation other than treatments and blocks.

For our illustrative example we may say that the value of a particular observation is a result of a patient's being in the study, plus the effect of the method of treatment, plus the effect of his age, plus other factors that are not accounted for.

2. *Assumptions.* The following assumptions are made:
   (a) Each x_{ij} that is observed constitutes a random independent sample of size 1 from one of the kn populations represented.
   (b) Each of these kn populations is normally distributed with mean μ_{ij} and the same variance σ^2. This implies that the e_{ij} are independently and normally distributed with mean 0 and variance σ^2.
   (c) The block and treatment effects are additive. This assumption may be interpreted to mean that there is no *interaction* between treatments and blocks. In other words, a particular block-treatment combination does not produce an effect that is greater or less than the sum of their individual effects. It can be shown that when this assumption is met

$$\sum_{j=1}^{k} \tau_j = \sum_{i=1}^{n} \beta_i = 0$$

The consequences of a violation of this assumption are misleading results. Anderson and Bancroft (39) suggest that one need not become concerned over the violation of the additivity assumption unless the largest mean is more than 50 percent greater than the smallest. The nonadditivity problem is also dealt with by Tukey (40) and Mandel (41).

When these assumptions hold true, the τ_j and β_i are a set of fixed constants, and we have a situation that fits the fixed-effects model. Frequently the blocks are considered to be a sample of blocks from some population of blocks about which the experimenter wishes to draw inferences. When this is true, and when the treatments are fixed, we have a situation that fits what is known as the *mixed model.* If both blocks and treatments are considered to be random samples from populations of blocks and treatments, respectively, the random-effects model is applicable.

For our illustrative example we assume the fixed-effects model to be appropriate, since we do not wish to draw inferences to either a larger group of training methods or a larger collection of age groups.

3. *Hypotheses.* We may test

$$H_0: \tau_j = 0, \qquad j = 1, 2, \ldots, k$$

against the alternative

$$H_A: \text{not all } \tau_j = 0$$

A hypothesis test regarding block effects is not usually carried out under the assumptions of the fixed-effects model for two reasons. First, the primary interest is in treatment effects, the usual purpose of the blocks being to provide a means of eliminating an extraneous source of variation. Second, although the experimental units are randomly assigned to the treatments, the blocks are obtained in a nonrandom manner.

For our illustrative example we have the following hypotheses:

$$H_0: \tau_j = 0, \qquad j = 1, 2, 3$$

$$H_A: \text{not all } \tau_j = 0$$

$$\text{Let } \alpha = .05$$

4. *Calculations.* It can be shown that the total sum of squares for the randomized complete block design can be partitioned into three components, one each attributable to treatments, blocks, and error. The algebra is somewhat tedious and will be omitted. The partitioned sum of squares may be expressed by the following equation:

$$\sum_{j=1}^{k}\sum_{i=1}^{n}(x_{ij} - \bar{x}_{..})^2 = \sum_{j=1}^{k}\sum_{i=1}^{n}(\bar{x}_{i.} - \bar{x}_{..})^2 + \sum_{j=1}^{k}\sum_{i=1}^{n}(\bar{x}_{.j} - \bar{x}_{..})^2 + \sum_{j=1}^{k}\sum_{i=1}^{n}(x_{ij} - \bar{x}_{i.} - \bar{x}_{.j} + \bar{x}_{..})^2 \qquad (7.3.2)$$

that is,

$$SS_{\text{total}} = SS_{\text{blocks}} + SS_{\text{treatments}} + SS_{\text{residual}} \qquad (7.3.3)$$

The computing formulas for the quantities in Equations 7.3.2 and 7.3.3 are as follows:

$$SS_{\text{total}} = \sum_{j=1}^{k} \sum_{i=1}^{n} x_{ij}^2 - C \tag{7.3.4}$$

$$SS_{\text{blocks}} = \sum_{i=1}^{n} \frac{T_{i.}^2}{k} - C \tag{7.3.5}$$

$$SS_{\text{treatments}} = \sum_{j=1}^{k} \frac{T_{.j}^2}{n} - C \tag{7.3.6}$$

$$SS_{\text{residual}} = SS_{\text{total}} - SS_{\text{blocks}} - SS_{\text{treatments}} \tag{7.3.7}$$

It will be recalled that C is a correction term, and in the present situation it is computed as follows:

$$C = \left(\sum_{j=1}^{k} \sum_{i=1}^{n} x_{ij} \right)^2 \Big/ kn$$

$$= T_{..}^2/kn \tag{7.3.8}$$

The appropriate degrees of freedom for each component of Equation 7.3.3 are

$$\begin{array}{cccc} \text{total} & \text{blocks} & \text{treatments} & \text{residual} \\ kn - 1 = & (n-1) + & (k-1) & + (n-1)(k-1) \end{array}$$

The residual degrees of freedom, like the residual sum of squares, may be obtained by subtraction as follows:

$$\begin{aligned} (kn - 1) - (n - 1) - (k - 1) &= kn - 1 - n + 1 - k + 1 \\ &= n(k - 1) - 1(k - 1) = (n - 1)(k - 1) \end{aligned}$$

For our illustrative example we compute the following sums of squares:

$$C = \frac{(151)^2}{(3)(5)} = \frac{22801}{15} = 1520.0667$$

$$SS_{\text{total}} = 7^2 + 9^2 + \cdots + 14^2 - 1520.0667 = 46.9333$$

$$SS_{\text{blocks}} = \frac{26^2 + 27^2 + \cdots + 37^2}{3} - 1520.0667 = 24.9333$$

$$SS_{\text{treatments}} = \frac{45^2 + 48^2 + 58^2}{5} - 1520.0667 = 18.5333$$

$$SS_{\text{residual}} = 46.9333 - 24.9333 - 18.5333 = 3.4667$$

The degrees of freedom are total $= (3)(5) - 1 = 14$, blocks $= 5 - 1 = 4$, treatments $= 3 - 1 = 2$, and residual $= (5 - 1)(3 - 1) = 8$.

Table 7.3.3

ANOVA Table for the Randomized Complete Block Design

Source	*SS*	**d. f.**	*MS*	**V. R.**
Treatments	$SS_{\text{treatments}}$	$(k-1)$	$MS_{\text{treatments}} = SS_{\text{treatments}}/(k-1)$	$MS_{\text{treatments}}/MS_{\text{residual}}$
Blocks	SS_{blocks}	$(n-1)$	$MS_{\text{blocks}} = SS_{\text{blocks}}/(n-1)$	
Residual	SS_{residual}	$(n-1)(k-1)$	$MS_{\text{residual}} = SS_{\text{residual}}/(n-1)(k-1)$	
Total	SS_{total}	$kn-1$		

Table 7.3.4

ANOVA Table for Example 7.3.1

Source	*SS*	**d. f.**	*MS*	**V. R.**
Treatments	18.5333	2	9.2667	21.39
Blocks	24.9333	4	6.2333	
Residual	3.4667	8	.4333	
Total	46.9333	14		

5. *The ANOVA Table.* The results of the calculations for the randomized complete block design may be displayed in an analysis of variance table such as Table 7.3.3.

For our illustrative example we have the ANOVA table shown in Table 7.3.4.

6. *Decision.* It can be shown that when the fixed-effects model applies and the null hypothesis of no treatment effects (all $\tau_i = 0$) is true, both the error, or residual, mean square and the treatments mean square are estimates of the common variance σ^2. When the null hypothesis is true therefore, the quantity

$$MS_{\text{treatments}}/MS_{\text{residual}}$$

is distributed as F with $k-1$ numerator degrees of freedom and $(n-1) \times (k-1)$ denominator degrees of freedom. The computed variance ratio, therefore, is compared with the critical value of F. If the computed ratio is greater than the critical value of F, the null hypothesis is rejected.

For our illustrative example the critical value of F with 2 and 8 degrees of freedom and $\alpha = .05$ is 4.46. Since our computed variance ratio, 21.39, is greater than 4.46, we reject the null hypothesis of no treatment effects on the assumption that such a large V. R. reflects the fact that the two sample mean squares are not estimating the same quantity. The only other explanation for this large V. R. would be that the null hypothesis is really true, and we have just observed an unusual set of results. We rule out the second explanation in favor of the first.

We conclude, therefore, that not all treatment effects are equal to zero, or equivalently, that not all treatment means are equal. For this test $p < .005$.

Exercises

For each of the following exercises perform the analysis of variance following the six-step procedure. Determine the p-value for each exercise.

7.3.1. Three food service systems were studied in five hospitals. The variable of interest was time (in minutes) utilized per meal served. The noon meal was served by each hospital by each method with the following results.

	Method		
Hospital	A	B	C
1	7.56	9.68	11.65
2	9.98	9.69	10.69
3	7.23	10.49	11.77
4	8.22	8.55	10.72
5	7.59	8.30	12.36

After eliminating hospital effects, do these data suggest a difference among the methods in mean time utilized per meal served? Let $\alpha = .05$.

7.3.2. Sixteen overweight subjects participated in a study to compare four weight reducing regimens. Subjects were grouped according to initial weight, and each of four subjects from each initial weight group was randomly assigned to one of the four reducing regimens. At the end of the experimental period the following weight losses, in pounds, were recorded.

Initial	Regimen			
Weight (pounds)	A	B	C	D
150 to 174	12	26	24	23
175 to 199	15	29	23	25
200 to 225	15	27	25	24
Over 225	18	38	33	31

After eliminating differences due to initial weight, do these data provide sufficient evidence to indicate a difference in regimen effects? Let $\alpha = .01$.

7.3.3. A remotivation team in a psychiatric hospital conducted an experiment to compare five methods for remotivating patients. Patients were grouped according to level of initial motivation. Patients in each group were randomly assigned to the five methods. At the end of the experimental period the patients were evaluated by a team composed of a psychiatrist, a psychologist, a nurse, and a social worker, none of whom were aware of the method to which patients had been assigned. The team assigned each patient a composite score as a measure of his or her level of motivation. The results were as follows.

Level of Initial Motivation	Remotivation Method				
	A	B	C	D	E
Nil	58	68	60	68	64
Very low	62	70	65	80	69
Low	67	78	68	81	70
Average	70	81	70	89	74

Do these data provide sufficient evidence to indicate a difference in mean scores among methods? Let $\alpha = .05$.

7.3.4. The nursing supervisor in a local health department wished to study the influence of time of day on length of home visits by the nursing staff. It was felt that individual differences among nurses might be large, so the nurse was used as a blocking factor. The nursing supervisor collected the following data.

Nurse	Length of Home Visit by Time of Day			
	Early Morning	Late Morning	Early Afternoon	Late Afternoon
A	27	28	30	23
B	31	30	27	20
C	35	38	34	30
D	20	18	20	14

Do these data provide sufficient evidence to indicate a difference in length of home visit among the different times of day? Let $\alpha = .05$.

7.3.5. Analyze the data of Exercise 6.4.1 as a randomized block design.

7.4 THE FACTORIAL EXPERIMENT

In the experimental designs that we have considered up to this point we have been interested in the effects of only one variable, the treatments. Frequently, however, we may be interested in studying, simultaneously, the effects of two or more variables. We refer to the variables in which we are interested as *factors*. The experiment in which two or more factors are investigated simultaneously is called a *factorial experiment*.

The different designated categories of the factors are called *levels*. Suppose, for example, that we are studying the effect on reaction time of three dosages of some drug. The drug factor, then, is said to occur at three levels. Suppose the second factor of interest in the study is age, and it is felt that two age groups, under 65 years and 65 years and over, should be included. We then have two levels of the age factor. In general, we say that Factor A occurs at a levels and Factor B occurs at b levels.

In a factorial experiment we may study not only the effects of individual factors but, if the experiment is properly conducted, we can also study the *interaction* between factors. To illustrate the concept of interaction let us consider the following example.

Example 7.4.1

Suppose, in terms of effect on reaction time, that the true relationship between three dosage levels of some drug and the age of human subjects taking the drug is known. Suppose further that age occurs at two levels—"young" (under 65) and "old" (65 and over). If the true relationship between the two factors is known, we will know, for the three dosage levels, the mean effect on reaction time of subjects in the two age groups. Let us assume that effect is measured in terms of reduction in reaction time to some stimulus. Suppose these means are as shown in Table 7.4.1.

Table 7.4.1

Mean Reduction in Reaction Time (Milliseconds) of Subjects in Two Age Groups at Three Drug Dosage Levels

	Factor B—Drug Dosage		
Factor A—Age	$j = 1$	$j = 2$	$j = 3$
Young ($i = 1$)	$\mu_{11} = 5$	$\mu_{12} = 10$	$\mu_{13} = 20$
Old ($i = 2$)	$\mu_{21} = 10$	$\mu_{22} = 15$	$\mu_{23} = 25$

The following important features of the data in Table 7.4.1 should be noted:

1. For both levels of factor A the difference between the means for any two levels of factor B is the same. That is, for both levels of factor A, the difference between means for levels 1 and 2 is 5, for levels 2 and 3 the difference is 10, and for levels 1 and 3 the difference is 15.
2. For all levels of factor B the difference between means for the two levels of factor A is the same. In the present case the difference is 5 at all three levels of factor B.
3. A third characteristic is revealed when the data are plotted as in Figure 7.4.1. We note that the curves corresponding to the different levels of a factor are all parallel.

When population data possess the three characteristics listed above, we say that there is no interaction present.

The presence of interaction between two factors can affect the characteristics of the data in a variety of ways depending on the nature of the interaction. We illustrate the effect of one type of interaction by altering the data of Table 7.4.1 as shown in Table 7.4.2.

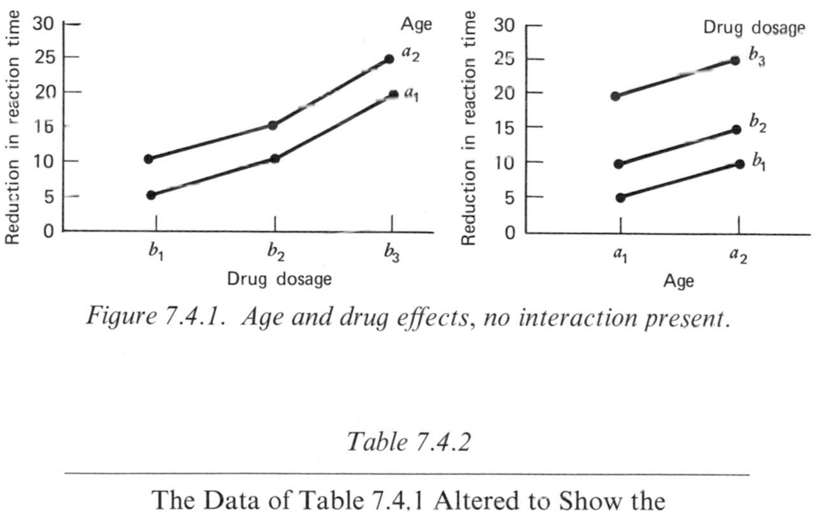

Figure 7.4.1. Age and drug effects, no interaction present.

Table 7.4.2

The Data of Table 7.4.1 Altered to Show the Effect of One Type of Interaction

Factor A—Age	Factor B—Drug Dosage $j = 1$	$j = 2$	$j = 3$
Young ($i = 1$)	$\mu_{11} = 5$	$\mu_{12} = 10$	$\mu_{13} = 20$
Old ($i = 2$)	$\mu_{21} = 15$	$\mu_{22} = 10$	$\mu_{23} = 5$

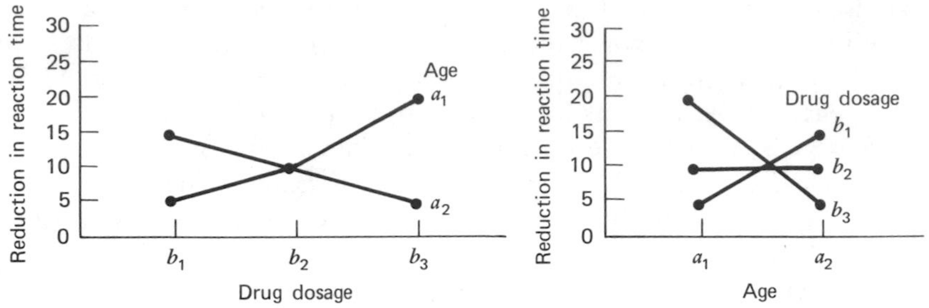

Figure 7.4.2. Age and drug effects, interaction present.

The important characteristics of the data in Table 7.4.2 are as follows:

1. The difference between means for any two levels of factor B is not the same for both levels of factor A. We note in Table 7.4.2, for example, that the difference between levels 1 and 2 of factor B is -5 for the young age group and $+5$ for the old age group.
2. The difference between means for both levels of factor A is not the same at all levels of factor B. The differences between factor A means are -10, 0, and 15 for levels 1, 2, and 3, respectively, of factor B.
3. The factor level curves are not parallel as shown in Figure 7.4.2.

When population data exhibit the characteristics illustrated by Table 7.4.2 and Figure 7.4.2 we say that there is interaction between the two factors. We emphasize that the kind of interaction illustrated by the present example is only one of many types of interaction that may occur between two factors.

In summary, then, we can say that *there is interaction between two factors if a change in one of the factors produces a change in response at one level of the other factor different from that produced at other levels of this factor.*

The advantages of the factorial experiment include the following.

1. The interaction of the factors may be studied.
2. There is a saving of time and effort.

In the factorial experiment all the observations may be used to study the effects of each of the factors under investigation. The alternative, when two factors are being investigated, would be to conduct two different experiments, one to study each of the two factors. If this were done, some of the observations would yield information only on one of the factors, and the remainder would yield information only on the other factor. To achieve the level of accuracy of the factorial experiment, more experimental units would be needed if the factors were studied through two experiments. It is seen, then, that 1 two-factor experiment is more economical than 2 one-factor experiments.

3. Since the various factors are combined in one experiment, the results have a wider range of application.

A factorial arrangement may be studied with either of the designs that have been discussed. We illustrate the analysis of a factorial experiment by means of a two-factor completely randomized design.

The results from a two-factor completely randomized design may be presented in tabular form as shown in Table 7.4.3.

Here we have a levels of factor A, b levels of factor B, and n observations for each combination of levels. Each of the ab combinations of levels of factor A with levels of factor B is a treatment. In addition to the totals and means shown in Table 7.4.3, we note that the total and mean of the ijth cell are $T_{ij.} = \sum_{k=1}^{n} x_{ijk}$ and $\bar{x}_{ij.} = T_{ij.}/n$, respectively. The subscript i runs from 1 to a and j runs from 1 to b. The total number of observations is nab.

To show that Table 7.4.3 represents data from a completely randomized design, we consider that each combination of factor levels is a treatment and that we have n observations for each treatment. An alternative arrangement of the data would be obtained by listing the observations of each treatment in a separate column. Table 7.4.3 may also be used to display data from a two-factor randomized block design if we consider the first observation in each cell as belonging to block 1, the second observation in each cell as belonging to block 2, and so on to the nth observation in each cell which may be considered as belonging to block n.

Table 7.4.3

Table of Sample Data from a Two-Factor Completely Randomized Experiment

Factor A	Factor B				Totals	Means
	1	2	$\cdots$	b		
1	x_{111} $\vdots$ x_{11n}	x_{121} $\vdots$ x_{12n}	$\cdots$ $\vdots$ $\cdots$	x_{1b1} $\vdots$ x_{1bn}	$T_{1..}$	$\bar{x}_{1..}$
2	x_{211} $\vdots$ x_{21n}	x_{221} $\vdots$ x_{22n}	$\cdots$ $\vdots$ $\cdots$	x_{2b1} $\vdots$ x_{2bn}	$T_{2..}$	$\bar{x}_{2..}$
$\vdots$	$\vdots$	$\vdots$	$\vdots$	$\vdots$	$\vdots$	$\vdots$
a	x_{a11} $\vdots$ x_{a1n}	x_{a21} $\vdots$ x_{a2n}	$\cdots$ $\vdots$ $\cdots$	x_{ab1} $\vdots$ x_{abn}	$T_{a..}$	$\bar{x}_{a..}$
Totals	$T_{.1.}$	$T_{.2.}$	$\cdots$	$T_{.b.}$	$T_{...}$	
Means	$\bar{x}_{.1.}$	$\bar{x}_{.2.}$	$\cdots$	$\bar{x}_{1b1}$		$\bar{x}_{...}$

Table 7.4.4

Length of Home Visit in Minutes by Public Health Nurses by Nurse's Age Group and Type of Patient

Factor A (Type of Patient) Levels	Factor B (Nurse's Age Group) Levels 1 (20 to 29)	2 (30 to 39)	3 (40 to 49)	4 (50 and over)	Totals	Means
1 (Cardiac)	20	25	24	28		
	25	30	28	31		
	22	29	24	26	534	26.70
	27	28	25	29		
	21	30	30	32		
2 (Cancer)	30	30	39	40		
	45	29	42	45		
	30	31	36	50	765	38.25
	35	30	42	45		
	36	30	40	60		
3 (C. V. A.)	31	32	41	42		
	30	35	45	50		
	40	30	40	40	766	38.30
	35	40	40	55		
	30	30	35	45		
4 (Tuberculosis)	20	23	24	29		
	21	25	25	30		
	20	28	30	28	509	25.45
	20	30	26	27		
	19	31	23	30		
Totals	557	596	659	762	2574	
Means	27.85	29.8	32.95	38.10		32.18

Cell	a_1b_1	a_1b_2	a_1b_3	a_1b_4	a_2b_1	a_2b_2	a_2b_3	a_2b_4
Totals	115	142	131	146	176	150	199	240
Means	23.0	28.4	26.2	29.2	35.2	30.0	39.8	48.0

Cell	a_3b_1	a_3b_2	a_3b_3	a_3b_4	a_4b_1	a_4b_2	a_4b_3	a_4b_4
Totals	166	167	201	232	100	137	128	144
Means	33.2	33.4	40.2	46.4	20.0	27.4	25.6	28.8

Example 7.4.2

In a study of length of time spent on individual home visits by public health nurses, the data on length of home visit, in minutes, cross tabulated by the nurse's age group and type of patient, were obtained as shown in Table 7.4.4.

To analyze these data we assume a fixed-effects model and a two-factor completely randomized design, and follow the familiar six-step procedure.

1. *The Model.* The fixed-effects model for the two-factor completely randomized design may be written as

$$x_{ijk} = \mu + \alpha_i + \beta_j + (\alpha\beta)_{ij} + e_{ijk}, \qquad i = 1, 2, \ldots, a; \quad j = 1, 2, \ldots, b; \quad k = 1, 2, \ldots, n \tag{7.4.1}$$

where x_{ijk} is a typical observation, μ is a constant, α represents an effect due to factor A, β represents an effect due to factor B, $(\alpha\beta)$ represents an effect due to the interaction of factors A and B, and e_{ijk} represents the experimental error.

2. *Assumptions.*

(a) The observations in each of the ab cells constitute a random independent sample of size n drawn from the population defined by the particular combination of the levels of the two factors. In our illustrative example we have a sample from 16 populations.

(b) Each of the ab populations is normally distributed.

(c) The populations all have the same variance.

3. *Hypotheses.*

The following hypotheses may be tested.

(1) $H_0: \alpha_i = 0 \qquad i = 1, 2, \ldots, a$
H_A: not all $\alpha_i = 0$

(2) $H_0: \beta_j = 0 \qquad j = 1, 2, \ldots, b$
H_A: not all $\beta_j = 0$

(3) $H_0: (\alpha\beta)_{ij} = 0 \qquad i = 1, 2, \ldots, a; \quad j = 1, 2, \ldots, b$
H_A: not all $(\alpha\beta)_{ij} = 0$

Before collecting data, the researchers may decide to test only one of the possible hypotheses. In this case they select the hypothesis they wish to test, choose a significance level, α, and proceed in the familiar, straightforward fashion. This procedure is free of the complications that arise if the researchers wish to test all three hypotheses.

When all three hypotheses are tested, the situation is complicated by the fact that the three tests are not independent in the probability sense. If we let α be the significance level associated with the test as a whole, and α', α'', and α''' the significance levels associated with hypotheses 1, 2, and 3, respectively, Kimball (42) has shown that

$$\alpha < 1 - (1 - \alpha')(1 - \alpha'')(1 - \alpha''') \tag{7.4.2}$$

If $\alpha' = \alpha'' = \alpha''' = .05$, then $\alpha < 1 - (.95)^3$, or $\alpha < .143$. This means that the probability of rejecting one or more of the three hypotheses is something less than .143 when a significance level of .05 has been chosen for the hypotheses and all are true. To demonstrate the hypothesis testing procedure for each case, we perform all three tests. The reader, however, should be aware of the problem involved in interpreting the results. The problem is discussed by Dixon and Massey (43) and Guenther (44).

For our illustrative example we may test the following hypotheses subject to the conditions mentioned above.

(1) $H_0: \alpha_1 = \alpha_2 = \alpha_3 = \alpha_4 = 0$

H_A: not all $\alpha_i = 0$

(2) $H_0: \beta_1 = \beta_2 = \beta_3 = \beta_4 = 0$

H_A: not all $\beta_j = 0$

(3) $H_0: (\alpha\beta)_{ij} = 0$

H_A: not all $(\alpha\beta)_{ij} = 0$

Let $\alpha = .05$

4. *Calculations.* By an adaptation of the procedure used in partitioning the total sum of squares for the completely randomized design, it can be shown that the total sum of squares under the present model can be partitioned into two parts as follows:

$$\sum_{i=1}^{a}\sum_{j=1}^{b}\sum_{k=1}^{n}(x_{ijk} - \bar{x}_{...})^2 = \sum_{i=1}^{a}\sum_{j=1}^{b}\sum_{k=1}^{n}(\bar{x}_{ij.} - \bar{x}_{...})^2 + \sum_{i=1}^{a}\sum_{j=1}^{b}\sum_{k=1}^{n}(x_{ijk} - \bar{x}_{ij.})^2 \tag{7.4.3}$$

or

$$SS_{\text{total}} = SS_{\text{treatments}} + SS_{\text{residual}} \tag{7.4.4}$$

The sum of squares for treatments can be partitioned into three parts as follows:

$$\sum_{i=1}^{a}\sum_{j=1}^{b}\sum_{k=1}^{n}(\bar{x}_{ij.} - \bar{x}_{...})^2 = \sum_{i=1}^{a}\sum_{j=1}^{b}\sum_{k=1}^{n}(\bar{x}_{i..} - \bar{x}_{...})^2 + \sum_{i=1}^{a}\sum_{j=1}^{b}\sum_{k=1}^{n}(\bar{x}_{.j.} - \bar{x}_{...})^2 + \sum_{i=1}^{a}\sum_{j=1}^{b}\sum_{k=1}^{n}(\bar{x}_{ij.} - \bar{x}_{i..} - \bar{x}_{.j.} + \bar{x}_{...})^2 \tag{7.4.5}$$

or

$$SS_{\text{treatments}} = SS_A + SS_B + SS_{AB}$$

The computing formulas for the various components are as follows:

$$SS_{\text{total}} = \sum_{i=1}^{a} \sum_{j=1}^{b} \sum_{k=1}^{n} x_{ijk}^2 - C \tag{7.4.6}$$

$$SS_{\text{treatments}} = \frac{\sum_{i=1}^{a} \sum_{j=1}^{b} T_{ij.}^2}{n} - C \tag{7.4.7}$$

$$SS_{\text{residual}} = SS_{\text{total}} - SS_{\text{treatments}} \tag{7.4.8}$$

$$SS_A = \frac{\sum_{i=1}^{a} T_{i..}^2}{bn} - C \tag{7.4.9}$$

$$SS_B = \frac{\sum_{j=1}^{b} T_{.j.}^2}{an} - C \tag{7.4.10}$$

and

$$SS_{AB} = SS_{\text{treatments}} - SS_A - SS_B \tag{7.4.11}$$

In the above equations

$$C = \left(\sum_{i=1}^{a} \sum_{j=1}^{b} \sum_{k=1}^{n} x_{ijk} \right)^2 \Big/ abn \tag{7.4.12}$$

For our illustrative example we have

$$C = (2574)^2/80 = 82818.45$$

$$SS_{\text{total}} = (20^2 + 25^2 + \cdots + 30^2) - 82818.45 = 5741.55$$

$$SS_{\text{treatments}} = \frac{115^2 + 142^2 + \cdots + 144^2}{5} - 82818.45 = 4801.95$$

$$SS_A = \frac{534^2 + 765^2 + 766^2 + 509^2}{20} - 82818.45 = 2992.45$$

$$SS_B = \frac{557^2 + 596^2 + 659^2 + 762^2}{20} - 82818.45 = 1201.05$$

$$SS_{AB} = 4801.95 - 2992.45 - 1201.05 = 608.45$$

$$SS_{\text{residual}} = 5741.55 - 4801.95 = 939.60$$

5. *The Analysis of Variance Table.* The results of the calculations for the fixed-effects model for a two-factor completely randomized experiment may, in general, be displayed as shown in Table 7.4.5.

The results for our illustrative example are displayed in Table 7.4.6.

Table 7.4.5

Analysis of Variance Table for a Two-Factor Completely Randomized Experiment (Fixed-Effects Model)

Source	*SS*	**d. f.**	*MS*	**V. R.**
A	SS_A	$a-1$	$MS_A = SS_A/(a-1)$	$MS_A/MS_{\text{residual}}$
B	SS_B	$b-1$	$MS_B = SS_B/(b-1)$	$MS_B/MS_{\text{residual}}$
AB	SS_{AB}	$(a-1)(b-1)$	$MS_{AB} = SS_{AB}/(a-1)(b-1)$	$MS_{AB}/MS_{\text{residual}}$
Treatments	$SS_{\text{treatments}}$	$ab-1$		
Residual	SS_{residual}	$ab(n-1)$	$MS_{\text{residual}} = \dfrac{SS_{\text{residual}}}{ab(n-1)}$	
Total	SS_{total}	$abn-1$		

Table 7.4.6

ANOVA Table for Example 7.4.1

Source	*SS*	**d. f.**	*MS*	**V. R.**
A	2992.45	3	997.48	67.95
B	1201.05	3	400.35	27.27
AB	608.45	9	67.61	4.61
Treatments	4801.95	15		
Residual	939.60	64	14.68	
Total	5741.55	79		

6. *Decision.* If the assumptions stated earlier hold true, and if each hypothesis is true, it can be shown that each of the variance ratios shown in Table 7.4.5 follows an F distribution with the indicated degrees of freedom. The critical values of F for testing the three hypotheses of our illustrative example are 2.76, 2.76, and 2.04, respectively. Since denominator degrees of freedom equal to 64 are not shown in Table J, 60 was used as the denominator degrees of freedom. We see that each of the three hypotheses would be rejected at the .05 level of significance when tested above. The reader is again cautioned that if all three tests are made simultaneously, the probability of rejecting at least one hypothesis when all are true is something greater than .05. Corresponding to the hypotheses stated in Step 3 above we have $p_1 < .005$, $p_2 < .005$, and $p_3 < .005$.

When $H_0\!:\alpha_1 = \alpha_2 = \alpha_3 = \alpha_4$ is rejected, we conclude that there are differences among the levels of A, that is, differences in the average amount of time spent in home visits with different types of patients. Similarly, when $H_0: \beta_1 = \beta_2 = \beta_3 = \beta_4$ is rejected, we conclude that there are differences among the levels of B, or differences in the average amount of time spent on home visits among the different nurses when grouped by age. When H_0: $(\alpha\beta)_{ij} = 0$ is rejected, we conclude that factors A and B interact, that is, different combinations of levels of the two factors produce different effects. When the hypothesis of no interaction is rejected interest in the levels of factors A and B usually become subordinate to interest in the interaction effects. In other words, we are more interested in learning what combinations of levels are significantly different.

We have treated only the case where the number of observations in each cell is the same. When the number of observations per cell is not the same for every cell the analysis becomes more complex. Many of the references that have been cited cover the analysis appropriate to such a situation, and the reader is referred to them for further information.

Exercises

For each of the following exercises perform the analysis of variance at the indicated level of significance and determine the p-value associated with each tested hypothesis.

7.4.1. In a treatment facility for the mentally retarded an experiment was conducted to compare three different methods for teaching basic self-care skills and three different reward systems. At the end of the experimental period the subjects were given a test designed to measure the degree to which the skills had been learned. The results are shown in the following table.

	Methods		
Rewards	A	B	C
None	52	58	58
	76	56	24
	60	68	32
	58	74	39
Praise	60	60	56
	78	70	66
	75	74	54
	72	77	49
Tangible	98	76	72
	94	80	74
	96	84	76
	98	80	70

(a) Perform an analysis of variance of these data and test the hypotheses that reward effects are zero, method effects are zero, and interaction effects are zero, Let $\alpha' = \alpha'' = \alpha''' = .01$.
(b) What is the magnitude of α, the significance level for the test as a whole?

7.4.2. A mental health team in a local health department conducted a study of mothers' understanding of communicated child-care instructions regarding their children who had been seen in the mental health diagnostic and evaluation clinic. Three methods of consultation were compared, the routine consultation procedure and two experimental procedures. Mothers from three socioeconomic groups were identified. Following the consultations the mothers were interviewed by a second team of professionals who assigned each mother a score designed to measure her level of understanding of the child-care instructions provided by the first team. The following results were obtained.

Socioeconomic Group	Method of Consultation: Routine	A	B
I	56 46 29 33	47 28 28 30	28 42 53 42
II	51 21 36 27	59 47 45 53	68 75 77 84
III	45 41 31 37	55 71 76 85	44 68 77 76

(a) Perform an analysis of variance of these data and test the three possible hypotheses. Let $\alpha' = .01$, $\alpha'' = .05$, and $\alpha''' = .01$.
(b) What is the magnitude of α, the level of significance for the test as a whole?

7.4.3. In a study of the effects of different diets and group therapy in helping overweight persons lose weight, a researcher used 40 overweight women who were carefully matched on as many relevant variables as possible such as age, initial weight, and physical condition. The subjects were randomly assigned to 4 groups of 10 each, and each group of 10 was placed on a different diet. Each group of 10 was further divided at random into two groups. One of these 2 groups participated in a group therapy session twice a week, while the other group did not. At the end of the experimental period the amount of weight lost per person was recorded as shown in the table. Do an analysis of variance of these data and test the three possible hypotheses. Let $\alpha' = \alpha'' = \alpha''' = .05$.

Group Therapy	Diet I	II	III	IV
Yes	15	25	19	22
	12	19	24	22
	18	21	18	18
	16	22	16	19
	13	19	21	15
No	9	13	13	33
	9	15	13	30
	13	12	15	31
	7	15	18	27
	9	12	15	28

7.4.4. A study was conducted to compare the abilities of three drugs to retard reaction time of experimental animals to a certain stimulus. The same strain of animals was trained to respond by three different methods and three animals were used for each training method/drug combination. The following table shows the response time in seconds following administration of the drug.

Training Method	Drug A	B	C
I	5	8	10
	8	8	12
	7	10	10
II	6	10	15
	8	12	14
	6	11	14
III	7	12	16
	8	12	16
	10	14	18

Perform an analysis of variance of these data and test the three possible hypotheses. Let $\alpha' = \alpha'' = \alpha''' = .05$.

7.5 MISCELLANY

A general introductory text cannot begin to cover every aspect of every included topic. Although this chapter, for example, has covered the major concepts of analysis of variance, many topics have not been discussed in the interest of brevity. To provide an awareness of some of the problems that may be encountered, and of some of the additional analyses that are possible in analysis of variance, brief comments on additional topics of importance are given here. For further information refer to the experimental design and analysis of variance texts listed in the references. Most contain a more complete coverage of one or more of these topics.

Missing Data. Even though an experiment may be carried out with the greatest of care, accidents may occur that result in some of the observations being missing when it comes time to do the analysis. Missing observations may result in animal experiments if an animal dies. In experiments involving human beings a subject may be unable to participate in part of the experiment because of illness. In laboratory experiments, cultures and solutions may be destroyed as a result of breakage. An experiment may be completed without mishap, but some of the recorded results may be lost or destroyed.

Generally, one of three procedures may be followed when data are found to be missing:

a. In some instances the analysis may proceed in the usual manner. If in a randomized complete block design, for example, a complete block or a complete treatment is missing the usual analysis may be performed on the remaining data provided that there are, at least, two blocks and two treatments left.

b. The remaining data may be analysed by methods appropriate for the case of unequal subclass numbers. These procedures, which are more complex than the methods presented in this chapter, are discussed in some of the references.

c. It is usually preferable, however, to estimate the missing values. One of two methods is generally employed for this purpose.

One method involves estimating the missing values in such a way that the experimental error sum of squares will be minimized when the usual analysis is performed. A disadvantage of this method is that it results in a biased treatment sum of squares that has to be corrected. Ostle (45) gives a numerical example of this method. Missing values are also frequently estimated by a technique known as *analysis of covariance*. An advantage of the use of covariance analysis is that it gives an unbiased treatment sum of squares as well as a minimum residual sum of squares. This method is illustrated by Steel and Torrie (22). Federer (7) gives an extensive list of references on missing values. References not cited by Federer include the articles by Glenn and Kramer (46), Kramer and Glass (47), and Baird and Kramer (48).

Transformations. Occasionally the assumptions underlying the analysis of variance are not met in the data. An alternative procedure when this happens is to perform a transformation on the data in such a way that the assumptions are more nearly met. By transformation is meant a change in the scale of measurement.

Three frequent objectives in the employment of transformations are to make the variance independent of the mean, to achieve normality, and to achieve additivity of effects (eliminate interaction). Frequently a single transformation will achieve two or more objectives simultaneously. Some of the more commonly used transformations include the following.

1. *The Logarithmic Transformation.* When this transformation is used, the logarithms (usually common logarithms) of the measurements are taken. This transformation is used when the mean is positively correlated with the variance.
2. *The Square Root Transformation.* With this transformation the square roots of the measurements are taken. It is used when the data consist of counts, such as the number of deaths occurring in various groups of experimental animals. If zero counts are encountered, .5 is added to each count before the square root is taken.
3. *The Arcsine Transformation.* This transformation is used when the data are proportions or percentages. The transformation yields $\theta = \arcsin \sqrt{p}$, where θ is the transformed measurement and p is the original measurement.
4. *The Reciprocal Transformation.* When the variance increases as the fourth power of the mean, the reciprocal transformation may be used. Each original observation, θ, is replaced by its reciprocal, $1/\theta$.

In most of the general statistics and experimental design textbooks already mentioned, transformations are discussed. In addition, the subject is covered in more detail in the books by Quenouille (49), Sokal and Rohlf (50), and Pearce (51), and in an article by Bartlett (52). Federer (7) gives additional references.

Nonparametric Alternatives. An alternative procedure that may be followed when the assumptions for analysis of variance are not met is to make use of what is known as a *nonparametric* method of analysis. These methods, in general, are discussed more fully in Chapter 11 where appropriate nonparametric alternatives for some of the experimental designs we have discussed are given.

Efficiency. It is usually of interest to know how much improvement in the experiment as a whole may be expected if one type of design rather than some other type of design is employed. For example, the investigator may wonder if it is worth the effort to use a randomized complete block design instead of a completely randomized design. Even if it is not possible or desirable to choose among designs, the investigator may wish to investigate the merits of increasing sample size or the number of samples. Comparisons like these are judged on the basis of *efficiency* or *relative efficiency*. Basically, efficiency is a ratio of the variances resulting from the use of the designs being compared and is usually expressed as a percentage. Further discussion of this topic may be found in Cochran and Cox (4), Steel and Torrie (22), Scheffé (34), Ostle (45), and Sokal and Rohlf (50).

Other Designs. The two experimental designs considered in this chapter are by no means the only ones employed. The condensation necessary in a general introductory textbook obviates a complete discussion of those that are more frequently encountered. The reader who wishes to investigate the possibilities should refer to the experimental design texts listed in the references. Additional designs discussed in these references include the following.

1. *The Latin Square Design.* When it is possible and desirable to identify and isolate two extraneous sources of variation in an experiment, an extension of the randomized complete block design known as the *Latin square design* may be employed. The term, Latin square, was first used in an analysis of variance context by R. A. Fisher (38) who borrowed it from the Swiss mathematician Leonhard Euler (1707–1783).

In the Latin square design one source of extraneous variation is assigned to the columns of the square, the second source of extraneous variation is assigned to the rows of the square, and the treatments, usually designated by Latin letters, are assigned in such a way that each treatment occurs once and only once in each row and each column. The number of rows, the number of columns, and the number of treatments are all equal.

2. *The Graeco-Latin Square Design.* This is an extension of the Latin square design which allows for the identification and isolation of three extraneous sources of variation. This design gets its name from the fact that another variable, represented by Greek letters, is superimposed on the Latin letters (treatments) of a Latin square in such a way that each Greek letter occurs once in each row, once in each column, and once with each Latin letter.
3. *The Incomplete Block Design.* If a large number of treatments must be included in an experiment, the use of the randomized complete block design may not be feasible. An alternative is to include only a part of the treatments in a block. The blocks that result from this procedure are called *incomplete blocks*.
4. *The Split Plot Design.* The *split plot design* is a special kind of incomplete block design that is frequently used for factorial experiments. Levels of one or more factors are applied to *whole plots* that are divided into *subplots* to which levels of one or more additional factors are applied.

7.6 SUMMARY

The purpose of this chapter is to introduce the student to the basic ideas and techniques of analysis of variance. Two experimental designs, the completely randomized, and the randomized complete block, are discussed in considerable detail. In addition, the concept of a factorial experiment as used with the completely randomized design is introduced. Some additional topics are examined briefly. Individuals who wish to pursue further any aspect of analysis of variance will find the references at the end of the chapter most helpful. The extensive bibliography by Herzberg and Cox (53) indicates further readings.

Review Questions and Exercises

1. Define analysis of variance.
2. For each of the following designs describe a situation in your particular field of interest where the design would be an appropriate experimental design. Use real or realistic data and do the appropriate analysis of variance for each one:
   (a) Completely randomized design.
   (b) Randomized complete block design.
   (c) Completely randomized design with a factorial experiment.
3. Heart rate (beats per minute) was measured in four groups of adult subjects: normal controls (A), angina patients (B), hypertensive subjects (C), and patients with healed myocardial infarction (D). The results were as follows:

A	B	C	D
83	81	75	61
61	65	68	75
80	77	80	78
63	87	80	80
67	95	74	68
89	89	78	65
71	103	69	68
73	89	72	69
70	78	76	70
66	83	75	79
57	91	69	61

Do these data provide sufficient evidence to indicate a difference in the mean heart rate among these four types of subject? Let $\alpha = .05$. Determine the p-value.

4. Random samples were drawn from each of three types of subject: high exposure level employees of a pesticide manufacturing firm, farm laborers exposed to the pesticide for several weeks each year, and persons with no known exposure to the pesticide. Acetylcholinesterase determinations were made on blood samples from each subject with the following results.

Employees	Farm Laborers	Unexposed
6.4	6.5	7.3
6.6	6.8	7.5
6.8	7.0	7.8
6.9	7.1	7.9
9.5	9.7	10.8
6.1	6.2	6.9
7.5	7.7	8.5
8.2	8.4	9.4
4.1	4.2	4.6
5.5	5.6	6.3

Do these data provide sufficient evidence to indicate a difference, on the average, among the three groups? Let $\alpha = .05$. Determine the p-value.

5. Respiratory rate (breaths per minute) was measured in eight experimental animals under three levels of exposure to carbon monoxide. The results were as follows:

	Exposure Level		
Animal	Low	Moderate	High
1	36	43	45
2	33	38	39
3	35	41	33
4	39	34	39
5	41	28	33
6	41	44	26
7	44	30	39
8	45	31	29

Can one conclude on the basis of these data that the three exposure levels, on the average, have a differential effect on respiratory rate? Let $\alpha = .05$. Determine the p-value.

6. An experiment was designed to study the effects of three different drugs and three types of stressful situation in producing anxiety in adolescent subjects. The table below shows the difference between the pre- and post-treatment scores of 18 subjects who participated in the experiment.

Stressful Situation (Factor A)	Drug (Factor B) A	B	C
I	4	1	1
	5	3	0
II	6	6	6
	6	6	3
III	5	7	4
	4	4	5

Perform an analysis of variance of these data and test the three possible hypotheses. Let $\alpha' = \alpha'' = \alpha''' = .05$. Determine the p-values.

7. The following table shows the emotional maturity scores of 27 young adult males cross-classified by age and the extent to which they use marijuana.

Age (Factor A)	Marijuana Usage (Factor B) Never	Occasionally	Daily
15–19	25	18	17
	28	23	24
	22	19	19
20–24	28	16	18
	32	24	22
	30	20	20
25–29	25	14	10
	35	16	8
	30	15	12

Perform an analysis of variance of these data. Let $\alpha' = \alpha'' = \alpha''' = .05$. Compute the p-values.

References

References cited

1. R. A. Fisher, *The Design of Experiments*, Eighth Edition, Oliver and Boyd, Edinburgh, 1966.
2. R. A. Fisher, *Contributions to Mathematical Statistics*, Wiley, New York, 1950.

3. Ronald A. Fisher, *Statistical Methods for Research Workers*, Thirteenth Edition, Hafner, New York, 1958.
4. William G. Cochran and Gertrude M. Cox, *Experimental Designs*, Wiley, New York, 1957.
5. D. R. Cox, *Planning of Experiments*, Wiley, New York, 1958.
6. Owen L. Davies (ed.), *The Design and Analysis of Experiments*, Hafner, New York, 1960.
7. Walter T. Federer, *Experimental Design*, Macmillan, New York, 1955.
8. D. J. Finney, *Experimental Design and its Statistical Basis*, The University of Chicago Press, Chicago, 1955.
9. Peter W. M. John, *Statistical Design and Analysis of Experiments* Macmillan, New York, 1971.
10. Oscar Kempthorne, *The Design and Analysis of Experiments*, Wiley, New York, 1952.
11. C. C. Li, *Introduction to Experimental Statistics*, McGraw-Hill, New York, 1964.
12. William Mendenhall, *Introduction to Linear Models and the Design and Analysis of Experiments*, Wadsworth, Belmont, Cal., 1968.
13. Churchill Eisenhart, "The Assumptions Underlying the Analysis of Variance," *Biometrics*, *21* (1947), 1–21.
14. W. G. Cochran, "Some Consequences When the Assumptions for the Analysis of Variance Are Not Satisfied," *Biometrics*, *3* (1947), 22–38.
15. M. B. Wilk and O. Kempthorne, "Fixed, Mixed and Random Models," *Journal of the American Statistical Association*, *50* (1955), 1144–1167.
16. S. L. Crump, "The Estimation of Variance Components in Analysis of Variance," *Biometrics*, *2* (1946), 7–11.
17. E. P. Cunningham and C. R. Henderson, "An Iterative Procedure for Estimating Fixed Effects and Variance Components in Mixed Model Situations," *Biometrics*, *24* (1968), 13–25.
18. C. R. Henderson, "Estimation of Variance and Covariance Components," *Biometrics*, *9* (1953), 226–252.
19. J. R. Rutherford, "A Note on Variances in the Components of Variance Model," *The American Statistician*, *25* (June 1971), 1, 2.
20. E. F. Schultz, Jr., "Rules of Thumb for Determining Expectations of Mean Squares in Analysis of Variance," *Biometrics*, *11* (1955), 123–135.
21. S. R. Searle, "Topics in Variance Component Estimation," *Biometrics*, *27* (1971), 1–76.
22. Robert G. D. Steel and James H. Torrie, *Principles and Procedures of Statistics*, McGraw-Hill, New York, 1960.

23. David B. Duncan, *Significance Tests for Differences Between Ranked Variates Drawn from Normal Populations*, Ph.D. Thesis (1949), Iowa State College, 117 pp.

24. David B. Duncan, "A Significance Test for Differences Between Ranked Treatments in an Analysis of Variance," *Virginia Journal of Science, 2* (1951), 171–189.

25. David B. Duncan, "On the Properties of the Multiple Comparisons Test," *Virginia Journal of Science, 3* (1952), 50–67.

26. David B. Duncan, "Multiple Range and Multiple-*F* Tests," *Biometrics, 11* (1955), 1–42.

27. C. Y. Kramer, "Extension of Multiple Range Tests to Group Means with Unequal Numbers of Replications," *Biometrics, 12* (1956) 307–310.

28. C. W. Dunnett, "A Multiple Comparisons Procedure for Comparing Several Treatments with a Control," *Journal of the American Statistical Association, 50* (1955), 1096–1121.

29. C. W. Dunnett, "New Tables for Multiple Comparisons with a Control," *Biometrics, 20* (1964), 482–491.

30. J. W. Tukey, "Comparing Individual Means in the Analysis of Variance," *Biometrics, 5* (1949), 99–114.

31. J. W. Tukey, "The Problem of Multiple Comparisons," Ditto, Princeton University, 1953; cited in Roger E. Kirk, *Experimental Design: Procedures for the Behavioral Sciences*, Brooks/Cole, Belmont, California, 1968.

32. D. Newman, "The Distribution of the Range in Samples from a Normal Population in Terms of an Independent Estimate of Standard Deviation," *Biometrika, 31* (1939), 20–30.

33. M. Keuls, "The Use of the Studentized Range in Connection with the Analysis of Variance," *Euphytica, 1* (1952), 112–122.

34. Henry Scheffé, "A Method for Judging All Contrasts in the Analysis of Variance," *Biometrika, 40* (1953), 87–104.

35. Henry Scheffé, *Analysis of Variance*, Wiley, New York (1959).

36. T. A. Bancroft, *Topics in Intermediate Statistical Methods*, Volume I, The Iowa State University Press, Ames, 1968.

37. B. J. Winer, *Statistical Principles in Experimental Design*, McGraw-Hill, New York, 1962.

38. R. A. Fisher, "The Arrangement of Field Experiments," *Journal of Ministry of Agriculture, 33* (1926), 503–513.

39. R. L. Anderson and T. A. Bancroft, *Statistical Theory in Research*, McGraw-Hill, New York, 1952.

40. J. W. Tukey, "One Degree of Freedom for Non-Additivity," *Biometrics*, *5* (1949), 232–242.

41. John Mandel, "A New Analysis of Variance Model for Non-Additive Data," *Technometrics*, *13* (1971), 1–18.

42. A. W. Kimball, "On Dependent Tests of Significance in the Analysis of Variance," *Annals of Mathematical Statistics*, *22* (1951), 600–602.

43. Wilfred J. Dixon and Frank J. Massey, *Introduction to Statistical Analysis*, Third Edition, McGraw-Hill, New York, 1969.

44. William C. Guenther, *Analysis of Variance*, Prentice-Hall, Englewood Cliffs, N.J., 1964.

45. Bernard Ostle, *Statistics in Research*, Second Edition, The Iowa State University Press, Ames, Iowa, 1963.

46. William Alexander Glenn and Clyde Young Kramer, "Analysis of Variance of a Randomized Block Design with Missing Observations," *Applied Statistics*, *7* (1958), 173–185.

47. Clyde Young Kramer and Suzanne Glass, "Analysis of Variance of a Latin Square Design with Missing Observations," *Applied Statistics*, *9* (1960), 43–50.

48. Hugh Robert Baird and Clyde Young Kramer, "Analysis of Variance of a Balanced Incomplete Block Design with Missing Observations," *Applied Statistics*, *9* (1960), 189–198.

49. M. H. Quenoille, *Introductory Statistics*, Pergamon, London, 1950.

50. Robert R. Sokal and F. James Rohlf, *Biometry*, W. H. Freeman, San Francisco, 1969.

51. S. C. Pearce, *Biological Statistics: An Introduction*, McGraw-Hill, New York, 1965.

52. M. S. Bartlett, "The Use of Transformations," *Biometrics*, *3* (1947), 39–52.

53. Agnes M. Herzberg and D. R. Cox, "Recent Work on the Design of Experiments: A Bibliography and a Review," *Journal of the Royal Statistical Society* (Series A), *132* (1969), 29–67.

Other references, books

1. Geoffrey M. Clarke, *Statistics and Experimental Design*, American Elsevier, New York, 1969.

2. D. J. Finney, *An Introduction to the Theory of Experimental Design*, The University of Chicago Press, Chicago, 1960.

3. E. G. Olds, T. B. Mattson, and R. E. Odeh: *Notes on the Use of Transformations in the Analysis of Variance*, WADC Tech Rep 56–308, 1956, Wright Air Development Center.

Other references, journal articles

1. Benjamin A. Barnes, Elinor Pearson, and Eric Reiss, "The Analysis of Variance: A Graphical Representation of a Statistical Concept," *Journal of the American Statistical Association, 50* (1955), 1064–1072.
2. David B. Duncan, "Bayes Rules for a Common Multiple Comparisons Problem and Related Student-*t* Problems," *Annals of Mathematical Statistics, 32* (1961), 1013–1033.
3. David B. Duncan, "A Bayesian Approach to Multiple Comparisons," *Technometrics, 7* (1965), 171–222.
4. Ray A. Waller and David B. Duncan, "A Bayes Rule for the Symmetric Multiple Comparisons Problem," *Journal of the American Statistical Association, 64* (1969) 1484–1503.
5. Alva R. Feinstein, "Clinical Biostatistics II Statistics Versus Science in the Design of Experiments," *Clinical Pharmacology and Therapeutics, 11* (1970), 282–292.
6. B. G. Greenberg, "Why Randomize?" *Biometrics, 7* (1951), 309–322.
7. M. Harris, D. G. Horvitz, and A. M. Mood, "On the Determination of Sample Sizes in Designing Experiments," *Journal of the American Statistical Association, 43* (1948), 391–402.
8. H. Leon Harter, "Multiple Comparison Procedures for Interactions," *The American Statistician, 24* (December 1970), 30–32.
9. Carl E. Hopkins and Alan J. Gross, "Significance Levels in Multiple Comparison Tests," *Health Services Research, 5* (Summer 1970), 132–140.
10. Richard J. Light and Barry H. Margolin, "An Analysis of Variance for Categorical Data," *Journal of the American Statistical Association, 66* (1971), 534–544.
11. Ken Sirotnik, "On the Meaning of the Mean in ANOVA (or the Case of the Missing Degree of Freedom)," *The American Statistician, 25* (October 1971), 36–37.

8

SIMPLE LINEAR REGRESSION AND CORRELATION

8.1 INTRODUCTION

In analyzing data for the health sciences disciplines, we find that it is frequently desirable to learn something about the relationship between two variables. We may, for example, be interested in studying the relationship between blood pressure and age, height and weight, the concentration of an injected drug and heart rate, the consumption level of some nutrient and weight gain, the intensity of a stimulus and reaction time, or total family income and medical care expenditures. The nature and strength of the relationships between variables such as these may be examined by *regression* and *correlation* analysis, two statistical techniques that, although related, serve different purposes.

Regression analysis is helpful in ascertaining the probable form of the relationship between variables, and the ultimate objective when this method of analysis is employed usually is to *predict* or *estimate* the value of one variable corresponding to a given value of another variable. The ideas of regression were first elucidated by the English scientist, Sir Francis Galton (1822–1911) in reports of his research on heredity—first in sweet peas and later in human stature (1–3). He described a tendency of adult offspring, having either short or tall parents, to revert back toward the average height of the general population. He first used the word *reversion*, and later *regression*, to refer to this phenomenon.

Correlation analysis, on the other hand, is concerned with measuring the strength of the relationship between variables. When we compute measures of correlation from a set of data, we are interested in the degree of the *correlation* between variables. Again, the concepts and terminology of correlation analysis originated with Galton, who first used the word *correlation* in 1888 (4).

In this chapter our discussion is limited to the exploration of the relationship between two variables. The concepts and methods of regression are covered first, beginning in the next section. In Section 8.6 the ideas and techniques of correlation are introduced. In the next chapter we consider the case where there is an interest in the relationships among three or more variables.

8.2 THE REGRESSION MODEL

In the typical regression problem, as in most problems in applied statistics, researchers have available for analysis a sample of observations from some real or hypothetical population. Based on the results of their analysis of the sample data, they are interested in reaching decisions about the population from which the sample is presumed to have been drawn. It is important, therefore, that the researchers understand the nature of the population in which they are interested. They should know enough about the population to be able either to construct a mathematical model for its representation or to determine if it reasonably fits some established model. A researcher about to analyze a set of data by the methods of simple linear regression, for example, should be secure in the knowledge that the simple linear regression model is, at least, an approximate representation of the population. It is unlikely that the model will be a perfect portrait of the real situation, since this characteristic is seldom found in models of practical value. A model constructed so that it corresponds precisely with the details of the situation is usually too complicated to yield any information of value. On the other hand, the results obtained from the analysis of data which have been forced into a model that does not fit are also worthless. Fortunately, however, a perfectly fitting model is not a requirement for obtaining useful results. Researchers, then, should be able to distinguish between the occasion when their chosen models and the data are sufficiently compatible for them to proceed, and the case where their chosen model must be abandoned.

Assumptions Underlying Simple Linear Regression. In the simple linear regression model two variables, X and Y, are of interest. The variable X is usually referred to as the *independent variable*, since it is under the control of the investigator, that is, values of X are selected by the investigator and, corresponding to each preselected value of X, one or more values of Y are obtained. The other variable, Y, accordingly, is called the *dependent variable*: and we speak of the regression of Y on X. The following are the assumptions underlying the simple linear regression model.

1. Values of the independent variable X are said to be "fixed." This means that the values of X are preselected by the investigator so that in the collection of the data they are not allowed to vary from these preselected values. In this model, X is referred to by some writers as a *nonrandom* variable and by others as a *mathematical* variable. It should be pointed out at this time that the statement of this assumption classifies our model as the *classical regression model*. Regression analysis also can be carried out on data in which X is a random variable.
2. The variable X is measured without error. Since no measuring procedure is perfect, this means that the magnitude of the measurement error in X is negligible.
3. For each value of X there is a subpopulation of Y values. For the usual inferential procedures of estimation and hypothesis testing to be valid, these subpopulations must be normally distributed. In order that these procedures may be presented it will be assumed that the Y values are normally distributed in the examples and exercises that follow.
4. The variances of the subpopulations of Y are all equal.
5. The means of the subpopulations of Y all lie on the same straight line. This is known as the *assumption of linearity*. This assumption may be expressed symbolically as

$$\mu_{y|x} = \alpha + \beta x \qquad (8.2.1)$$

   where $\mu_{y|x}$ is the mean of the subpopulation of Y values for a particular value of X, and α and β are called population regression coefficients. Geometrically, α and β represent the y-intercept and slope, respectively, of the line on which all the means are assumed to lie.
6. The Y values are statistically independent. In other words, in drawing the sample, it is assumed that the values of Y chosen at one value of X in no way depend on the values of Y chosen at another value of X.

These assumptions may be summarized by means of the following equation which is called the regression model:

$$y = \alpha + \beta x + e \qquad (8.2.2)$$

where y is a typical value from one of the subpopulations of Y, α and β are as defined in Equation 8.2.1, and e is called the error term. If we solve 8.2.2 for e, we have

$$e = y - (\alpha + \beta x) \qquad (8.2.3)$$

and we see that e shows the amount by which y deviates from the mean of the subpopulation of Y values from which it is drawn. As a consequence of the assumption that the subpopulations of Y values are normally distributed with equal variances, the e's for each subpopulation are normally distributed with a variance equal to the common variance of the subpopulations of Y values.

A graphical representation of the regression model is given in Figure 8.2.1.

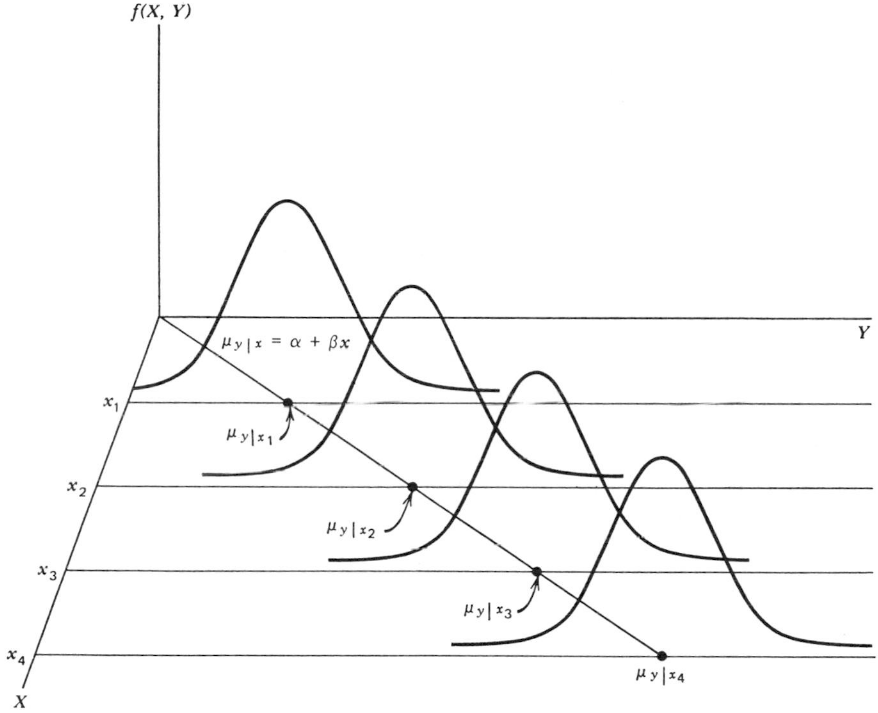

Figure 8.2.1. Representation of the simple linear regression model.

8.3 THE SAMPLE REGRESSION EQUATION

In simple linear regression the object of the researcher's interest is the population regression equation—the equation that describes the true relationship between the dependent variable Y and the independent variable X. In an effort to reach a decision regarding the likely form of this relationship, the researcher draws a sample from the population of interest and, using the resulting data, computes a sample regression equation that forms the basis for reaching conclusions regarding the unknown population regression equation.

Example 8.3.1

A team of professional mental health workers in a long-stay psychiatric hospital wished to measure the level of response of withdrawn patients to a program of remotivation therapy. A standardized test was available for this

Table 8.3.1

Patients' Scores on Standardized Test and New Test, Example 8.3.1

Patient Number	Score on New Test (X)	Score on Standardized Test (Y)
1	50	61
2	55	61
3	60	59
4	65	71
5	70	80
6	75	76
7	80	90
8	85	106
9	90	98
10	95	100
11	100	114

purpose, but it was expensive and time-consuming to administer. To overcome this obstacle the team developed a test that was much easier to administer. To test the usefulness of the new instrument for measuring the level of patient response, the team decided to examine the relationship between scores made on the new test and scores made on the standardized test. The objective was to use the new test if it could be shown that it was a good predictor of a patient's score on the standardized test. The team was interested only in carrying out the analysis for standardized scores between 50 and 100, since a score below 50 did not represent a significant level of response, and scores above 100, although possible, were seldom made by the type of patient under consideration. The team also felt that the use of scores in increments of 5 would give a good coverage of the range of scores between 50 and 100. Accordingly, 11 patients who had made scores on the new test of 50, 55, 60, 65, 70, 75, 80, 85, 90, 95, and 100, respectively, were selected to take the standardized test. The independent and dependent variables, respectively, are scores made on the new test and scores made on the standardized test. The results are shown in Table 8.3.1.

The reader will recognize that the assumption of fixed values of X is satisfied in this example. The values of X were selected in advance and were not allowed to vary as would have been the case had the patients been selected at random before taking the tests.

A first step that is usually useful in studying the relationship between two variables is to prepare a *scatter diagram* of the data such as is shown in Figure 8.3.1. The points are plotted by assigning values of the independent

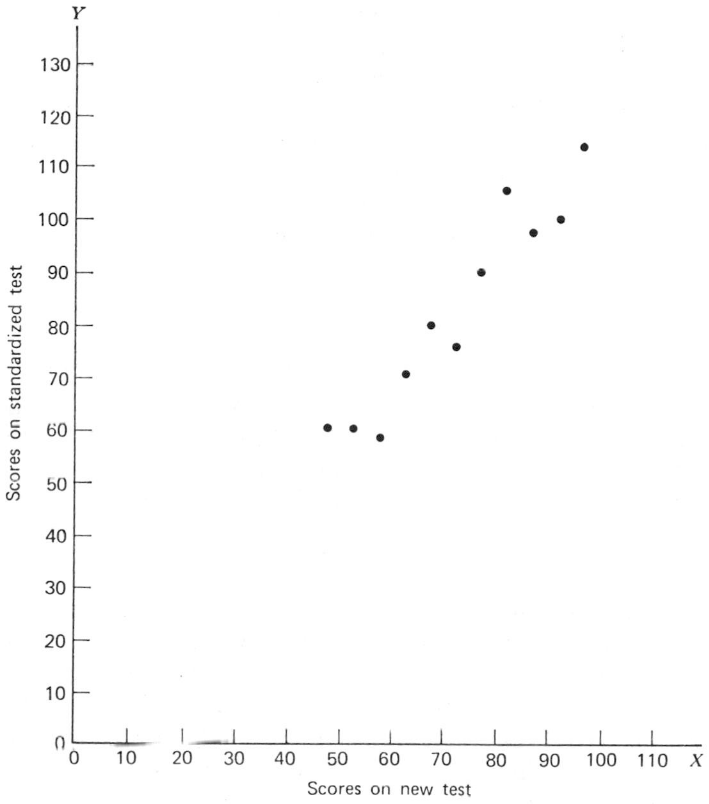

Figure 8.3.1. Scatter diagram of data shown in Table 8.3.1.

variable X to the horizontal axis and values of the dependent variable Y to the vertical axis.

The pattern made by the points plotted on the scatter diagram usually suggests the basic nature of the relationship between two variables. As we look at Figure 8.3.1, for example, the points seem to be scattered around an invisible straight line. The scatter diagram also shows that, in general, patients who score high on the new test also make high scores on the standardized test. These impressions suggest that the relationship between scores on the two tests may be described by a straight line crossing the Y-axis near the origin and making approximately a 45-degree angle with the X-axis. It looks as if it would be simple to draw, freehand, through the data points, the line that describes the relationship between X and Y. It is highly unlikely, however, that the lines drawn by any two people would be exactly the same. In other words, for every person drawing such a line by eye, or freehand, we would expect a slightly different line. The question then arises as to which line best describes the relationship between the variables. We cannot obtain an answer to this question by inspecting the lines. In fact, it is not likely that any freehand line drawn through the data will be the line that best describes the relationship between X and Y, since freehand lines will reflect any defects of vision or judgment that the person drawing the line may possess. Similarly, when judging which of two lines best describes the relationship, subjective evaluation is liable to the same deficiencies.

What is needed is some method for obtaining the desired line that is not fraught with these difficulties.

The Least-Squares Line. The method usually employed for obtaining the desired line is known as the *method of least squares*, and the resulting line is called the *least-squares line*. The reason for calling the method by this name will be explained in the discussion that follows.

We recall from algebra that the general equation for a straight line is given by

$$y = a + bx \tag{8.3.1}$$

where y is a value on the vertical axis, x is a value on the horizontal axis, a is the point where the line crosses the vertical axis, and b shows the amount by which the line rises for each unit increase in x. We refer to a as the y-intercept and b as the *slope* of the line. To draw a line based on Equation 8.3.1, we need the numerical values of the constants a and b. Given these constants, we may substitute various values of x into the equation to obtain corresponding values of y. The resulting points (x_1, y_1), (x_2, y_2), and so on, may be plotted. Since any two such coordinates determine a straight line, we may select any two, locate them on a graph, and connect them to obtain the line corresponding to the equation. It can be shown by mathematics beyond the scope of this book that a and b may be obtained by the simultaneous solution of the following two equations which are known as the *normal equations* for a set of data:

$$\sum y_i = na + b\sum x_i \tag{8.3.2}$$

$$\sum x_i y_i = a\sum x_i + b\sum x_i^2 \tag{8.3.3}$$

In Table 8.3.2 we have the necessary values for substituting into the normal equations.

Substituting appropriate values from Table 8.3.2 into Equations 8.3.2 and 8.3.3 gives

$$916 = 11a + 825b$$

$$71790 = 825a + 64625b$$

We may solve these equations by any familiar method to obtain

$$a = -.9973 \qquad \text{and} \qquad b = 1.1236$$

Table 8.3.2

Intermediate Computations for Normal Equations, Example 8.3.1

Score on New Test	**Score on Standardized Test**			
x	y	x^2	y^2	xy
50	61	2500	3721	3050
55	61	3025	3721	3355
60	59	3600	3481	3540
65	71	4225	5041	4615
70	80	4900	6400	5600
75	76	5625	5776	5700
80	90	6400	8100	7200
85	106	7225	11236	9010
90	98	8100	9604	8820
95	100	9025	10000	9500
100	114	10000	12996	11400
Total 825	916	64625	80076	71790

The linear equation for the least-squares line that describes the relationship between scores on the standardized test and scores on the new test may be written, then, as

$$y_c = -.9973 + 1.1236x \tag{8.3.4}$$

This equation tells us that since a is negative, the line crosses the Y-axis below the origin, and that since b, the slope, is positive, the line extends from the lower left-hand corner of the graph to the upper right-hand corner. We see further that for each unit increase in x, y increases by an amount equal to 1.1236. We have affixed the subscript c to y to indicate that it is a value computed from the equation, rather than an observed value of Y.

By substituting two convenient values of X into Equation 8.3.4, we may obtain the necessary coordinates for drawing the line. Suppose, first, we let $X = 50$ and obtain

$$y_c = -.9973 + 1.1236(50) = 55.1827$$

If we let $X = 100$ we obtain

$$y_c = -.9973 + 1.1236(100) = 111.3627$$

The line, along with the original data, is shown in Figure 8.3.2.

Numerical values for a and b may be obtained by alternative formulas that do not directly involve the normal equations. The formulas are as

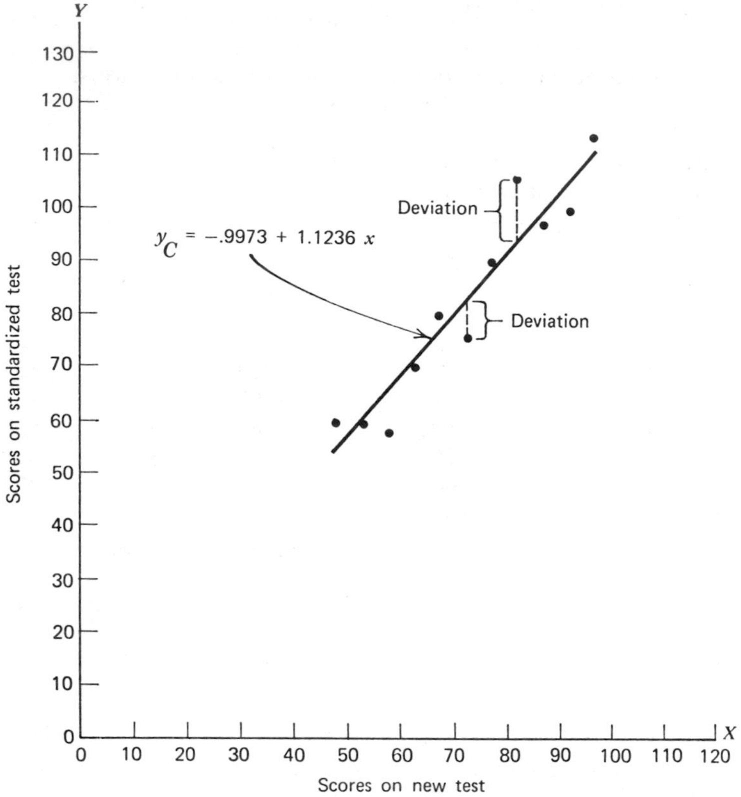

Figure 8.3.2. Original data and least-squares line for Example 8.3.1.

follows:

$$b = \frac{n\sum xy - (\sum x)(\sum y)}{n\sum x^2 - (\sum x)^2} \tag{8.3.5}$$

$$a = \frac{\sum y - b\sum x}{n} \tag{8.3.6}$$

For the present example we have

$$b = \frac{11(71790) - (825)(916)}{11(64625) - (825)^2} = 1.1236$$

$$a = \frac{916 - 1.1236(825)}{11} = -.9973$$

Thus, we see that Equations 8.3.5 and 8.3.6 yield the same results as one obtains by solving the normal equations.

Now that we have obtained what we call the "best" line for describing the relationship between our two variables, we need to determine by what criterion it is considered best. Before the criterion is stated, let us examine Figure 8.3.2. We note that the least-squares line does not pass through any of the observed points that are plotted on the scatter diagram. In other words, the observed points *deviate* from the line by varying amounts.

The line that we have drawn through the points is best in this sense:

The sum of the squared vertical deviations of the observed data points (y_i) *from the least-squares line is smaller than the sum of the squared vertical deviations of the data points from any other line.*

In other words, if we square the vertical distance from each observed point (y_i) to the least-squares line and add these squared values for all points, the resulting total will be smaller than the similarly computed total for any other line that can be drawn through the points. For this reason the line we have drawn is called the least-squares line.

Exercises

For each of the following exercises (a) draw a scatter diagram, and (b) obtain the regression equation and plot it on the scatter diagram.

8.3.1. An experiment was conducted to study the effect of a certain drug in lowering heart rate in adults. The independent variable is dosage in milligrams of the drug, and the dependent variable is the difference between lowest rate following administration of the drug and a predrug control. The following data were collected.

Dose (mg) *X*	Reduction in Heart Rate (Beats/min) *Y*
.5	10
.75	8
1.00	12
1.25	12
1.50	14
1.75	12
2.00	16
2.25	18
2.50	17
2.75	20
3.00	18
3.25	20
3.50	21

8.3.2. The following data show the optical densities of a certain substance at different concentration levels:

Level of Concentration (X)	Optical Density (Y)
80	.08
120	.12
160	.18
200	.21
240	.28
280	.28
320	.38
360	.40
400	.42
440	.50
480	.52
520	.60

8.3.3. A hospital administrator collected the following data on the cost per meal of a standard meal at different volumes of preparation.

Number of Meals Served (X)	Cost per Meal (Y)
30	$1.15
35	1.10
40	.98
45	1.01
50	.97
55	.90
60	.89
70	.85
75	.78
80	.70
65	.80

8.3.4. An experiment was conducted to study the relationship between an objective measurement of anxiety and heart rate in adults. The following data were obtained on 12 normal adults.

Heart Rate per Minute (X)	Objective Measurement of Anxiety (Y)
50	48
55	41
60	45
65	41
70	42
75	36
80	38
85	36
90	30
95	32
100	34
105	25

8.3.5. The following data were collected in a study of the relationship between intelligence and family size.

Number of Children in Family	Average Measured Intelligence Score of All Children in the Family
1	105
2	102
3	104
4	100
5	97
6	101
7	95
8	93
9	97
10	88

8.4 EVALUATING THE REGRESSION EQUATION

Once the regression equation has been obtained it must be evaluated to determine whether it adequately describes the relationship between the two variables and whether it can be used effectively for prediction and estimation purposes.

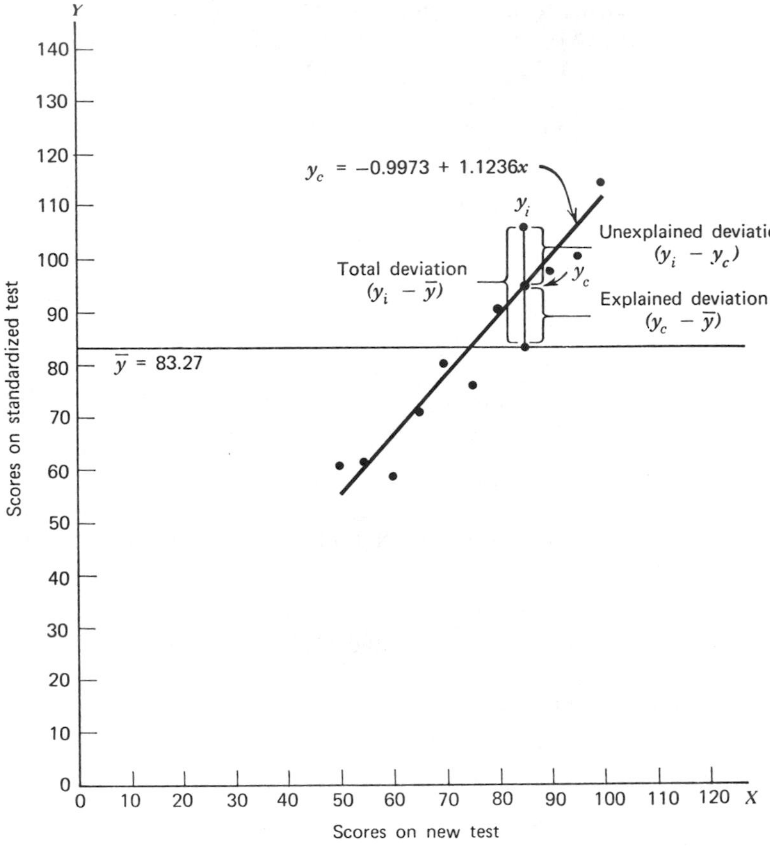

Figure 8.4.1. Scatter diagram showing the total, explained, and unexplained deviations for a selected value of Y, *Example 8.3.1.*

The Coefficient of Determination. One way to evaluate the regression equation is to compare the scatter of the points about the regression line with the scatter about $\bar{y}$, the mean of the sample values of Y. If we take the scatter diagram for Example 8.3.1 and draw through the points a line that intersects the Y-axis at $\bar{y}$ and is parallel to the X-axis, we may obtain a visual impression of the relative magnitudes of the scatter of the points about this line and the regression line. This has been done in Figure 8.4.1.

It appears rather obvious from Figure 8.4.1 that the scatter of the points about the regression line is much less than the scatter about the $\bar{y}$ line. We would not wish, however, to decide on this basis alone that the equation is a useful one. The situation may not be always this clear-cut, so that an objective measure of some sort would be much more desirable. Such an objective measure, called the *coefficient of determination*, is available.

Before defining the coefficient of determination, let us justify its use by examining the logic behind its computation. We begin by considering the point corresponding to any observed value, y_i, and by measuring its vertical distance from the $\bar{y}$ line. We call this the *total deviation* and designate it by $(y_i - \bar{y})$.

If we measure the vertical distance from the regression line to the $\bar{y}$ line, we obtain $(y_c - \bar{y})$ which is called the *explained deviation*, since it shows by how much the total deviation is reduced when the regression line is fitted to the points.

Finally, we measure the vertical distance of the observed point from the regression line to obtain $(y_i - y_c)$ which is called the *unexplained deviation*, since it represents the portion of the total deviation not "explained" or accounted for by the introduction of the regression line. These three quantities are shown for a typical value of Y in Figure 8.4.1.

It is seen, then, that the total deviation for a particular y_i is equal to the sum of the explained and unexplained deviations. We may write this symbolically as

$$\underset{\text{total deviation}}{(y_i - \bar{y})} = \underset{\text{explained deviation}}{(y_c - \bar{y})} + \underset{\text{unexplained deviation}}{(y_i - y_c)} \tag{8.4.1}$$

If we measure these deviations for each value of y_i and y_c, square each deviation, and add up the squared deviations, we have

$$\underset{\substack{\text{total}\\\text{sum}\\\text{of squares}}}{\sum(y_i - y)^2} = \underset{\substack{\text{explained}\\\text{sum}\\\text{of squares}}}{\sum(y_c - \bar{y})^2} + \underset{\substack{\text{unexplained}\\\text{sum}\\\text{of squares}}}{\sum(y_i - y_c)^2} \tag{8.4.2}$$

We may write this relationship in still another way as

$$SS_{\text{total}} = SS_{\text{explained}} + SS_{\text{unexplained}}$$

These quantities may be considered measures of dispersion or variability. The *total sum of squares* for example is a measure of the dispersion of the observed values of Y about their mean $\bar{y}$, that is, this term is a measure of the total variation in the observed values of Y. The reader will recognize this term as the numerator of the familiar formula for the sample variance.

The *explained sum of squares* measures the amount of the total variability in the observed values of Y that is accounted for by the linear relationship between the observed values of X and Y. This quantity is referred to also as the *sum of squares due to linear regression.*

The *unexplained sum of squares* is a measure of the dispersion of the observed Y values about the regression line and sometimes is called the *residual sum of squares.* It is this quantity that is minimized when the least squares line is obtained.

Table 8.4.1

Calculation of Total, Explained, and Unexplained Sums of Squares

Patient Number	**Scores on Standardized Test** (y_i)	$y_c = -.9973 + 1.1236x$	$(y_i - \bar{y})$	$(y_i - \bar{y})^2$	$(y_i - y_c)$	$(y_i - y_c)^2$	$(y_c - \bar{y})$	$(y_c - \bar{y})^2$
1	61	55.1827	−22.2727	496.0732	5.8173	33.8410	−28.0900	789.0481
2	61	60.8007	−22.2727	496.0732	.1993	.0397	−22.4720	504.9908
3	59	66.4187	−24.2727	589.1640	−7.4187	55.0371	−16.8540	284.0573
4	71	72.0367	−12.2727	150.6192	−1.0367	1.0747	−11.2360	126.2477
5	80	77.6547	−3.2727	10.7106	2.3453	5.5004	−5.6180	31.5619
6	76	83.2727	−7.2727	52.8922	−7.2727	52.8922	0.0000	0.0000
7	90	88.8907	6.7273	45.2566	1.1093	1.2305	5.6180	31.5619
8	106	94.5087	22.7273	516.5302	11.4913	132.0500	11.2360	126.2477
9	98	100.1267	14.7273	216.8934	−2.1267	4.5229	16.8540	284.0573
10	100	105.7447	16.7273	279.8026	−5.7447	33.0016	22.4720	504.9908
11	114	111.3627	30.7273	944.1670	2.6373	6.9554	28.0900	789.0481
Total $\bar{y} = 83.2727$	916			3798.1822		326.1455		3471.8116

The necessary calculations for obtaining the total, the explained, and the unexplained sums of squares for our illustrative example are displayed in Table 8.4.1.

For our illustrative example we have

$$SS_{\text{total}} = SS_{\text{explained}} + SS_{\text{unexplained}}$$
$$3798.1822 \approx 3471.8116 + 326.1455$$
$$3798.1822 \approx 3797.9571$$

The failure of the two components on the right of the equality to add to the total on the left is due to rounding.

We may calculate the total sum of squares by the more convenient formula

$$\sum(y_i - \bar{y})^2 = \sum y_i^2 - \frac{(\sum y_i)^2}{n} \tag{8.4.3}$$

and the explained sum of squares may be computed by

$$\sum(y_c - \bar{y})^2 = b^2\sum(x_i - \bar{x})^2 = b^2[\sum x_i^2 - (\sum x_i)^2/n] \tag{8.4.4}$$

The unexplained sum of squares is more conveniently obtained by subtraction. For our illustrative example we have

$$SS_{\text{total}} = 61^2 + 61^2 + \cdots + 114^2 - \frac{(916)^2}{11} = 3798.1818$$

$$SS_{\text{explained}} = (1.1236)^2\left[50^2 + 55^2 + \cdots + 100^2 - \frac{(825)^2}{11}\right]$$
$$= 3471.8116$$

and

$$SS_{\text{unexplained}} = SS_{\text{total}} - SS_{\text{explained}}$$
$$= 3798.1818 - 3471.8116$$
$$= 326.3702$$

The results using the computationally more convenient formulas are the same results as those shown in Table 8.4.1 except for rounding.

It is intuitively appealing to speculate that if a regression equation does a good job of describing the relationship between two variables, the explained sum of squares should constitute a large proportion of the total sum of squares. It would be of interest, then, to determine the magnitude of this proportion by computing the ratio of the explained sum of squares to the total sum of squares. This is exactly what is done in evaluating a regression equation based on sample data, and the result is called the sample *coefficient of determination*, r^2. In other words,

$$r^2 = \frac{\sum(y_c - \bar{y})^2}{\sum(y_i - \bar{y})^2} = \frac{b^2[\sum x_i^2 - (\sum x_i)^2/n]}{\sum y_i^2 - \frac{(\sum y_i)^2}{n}} = SS_{\text{explained}}/SS_{\text{total}}$$

In our present example we have, using the sums of squares values computed by Equations 8.4.3 and 8.4.4,

$$r^2 = \frac{3471.8116}{3798.1818} = .91$$

The sample coefficient of determination measures the closeness of fit of the sample regression equation to the observed values of Y. If we look at Table 8.4.1, we see that when the quantities $(y_i - y_c)$, the vertical distances of the observed values of Y from the equation, are small, the unexplained sum of squares is small. This leads to a large explained sum of squares that leads, in turn, to a large value of r^2. This is illustrated in Figure 8.4.2.

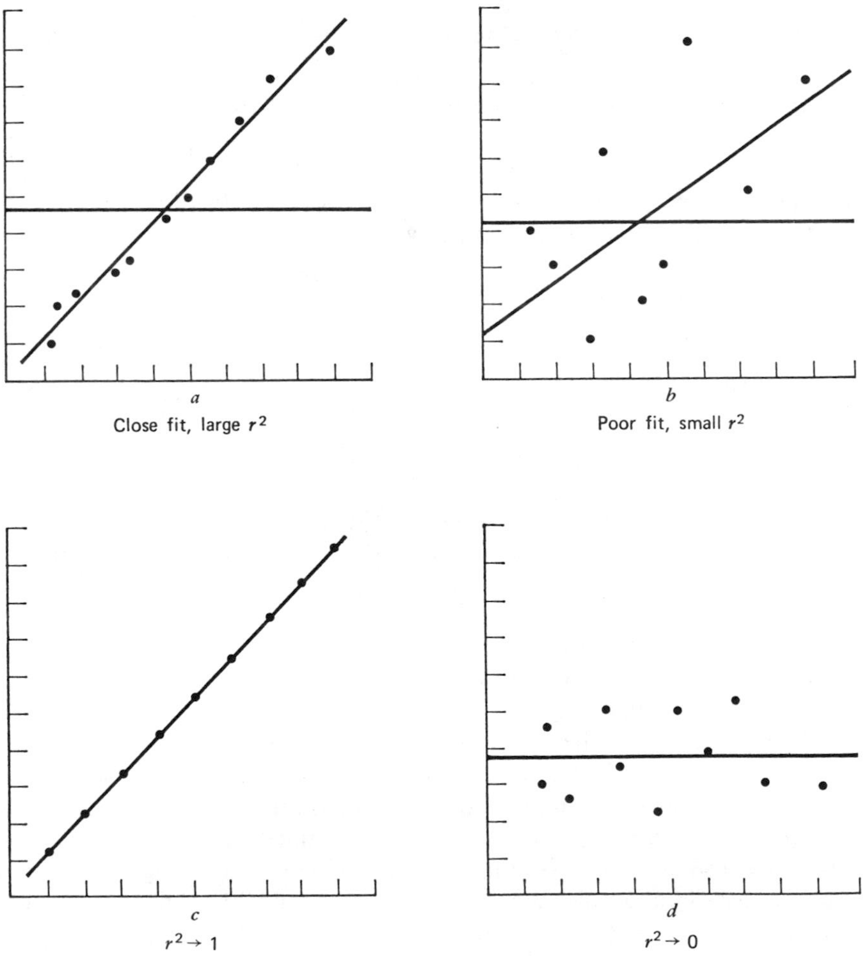

Figure 8.4.2. r^2 *as a measure of closeness-of-fit of the sample regression line to the sample observations.*

In Figure 8.4.2*a* we see that the observations all lie close to the regression line, and we would expect r^2 to be large. In fact, the computed r^2 for these data is .986, indicating that about 99 percent of the total variation in the y_i is explained by the regression.

In Figure 8.4.2*b* we illustrate a case where the y_i are widely scattered about the regression line, and there we suspect that r^2 is small. The computed r^2 for the data is .403, that is, less than 50 percent of the total variation in the y_i is explained by the regression.

The largest value that r^2 can assume is 1, a result that occurs when all of the variation in the y_i is explained by the regression. When $r^2 = 1$ all the observations fall on the regression line. This situation is shown in Figure 8.4.2*c*.

The lower limit of r^2 is 0. This result is obtained when the regression line and the line drawn through $\bar{y}$ coincide. In this situation none of the variation in the y_i is explained by the regression. Figure 8.4.2*d* illustrates a situation in which r^2 is approaching zero.

When r^2 is large, then, the regression has accounted for a large proportion of the total variability in the observed values of Y, and we look with favor on the regression equation. On the other hand, a small r^2, which indicates a failure of the regression to account for a large proportion of the total variation in the observed values of Y, tends to cast doubt on the usefulness of the regression equation. We do not, however, pass final judgment on the equation until it has been subjected to an objective statistical test. Such a test is accomplished by means of analysis of variance which enables us to test the null hypothesis of no linear relationship between X and Y.

From the three sum-of-squares terms and their associated degrees of freedom the analysis of variance table of Table 8.4.2 may be constructed.

In general, the degrees of freedom associated with the sum of squares due to regression is equal to the number of constants in the regression equation minus 1. In the simple linear case we have two constants, a and b, hence, the degrees of freedom for regression are $2 - 1 = 1$. It can be shown that when the hypothesis of no linear relationship between X and Y is true, and when the

Table 8.4.2

ANOVA Table for Simple Linear Regression

Source of Variation	*SS*	**d. f.**	*MS*	**V. R.**
Linear regression	$SS_{\text{explained}}$	1	$SS_{\text{explained}}/1$	$MS_{\text{explained}}/MS_{\text{unexplained}}$
Residual	$SS_{\text{unexplained}}$	$n-2$	$SS_{\text{unexplained}}/(n-2)$	
Total	SS_{total}	$n-1$		

assumptions underlying regression are met, the ratio obtained by dividing the regression mean square by the residual mean square is distributed as F with 1 and $n - 2$ degrees of freedom. The computed V. R., then, is compared with the critical value of F, and if the former exceeds the latter, the null hypothesis that there is no linear relationship between X and Y is rejected.

For our illustrative example suppose that we set up the following hypotheses:

$$H_0\text{: } X \text{ and } Y \text{ are not linearly related}$$

$$H_A\text{: } X \text{ and } Y \text{ are linearly related}$$

$$\alpha = .05$$

Substituting appropriate numerical values into Table 8.4.2 gives Table 8.4.3. Since 95.74 is greater than 5.12, the critical value of F for 1 and 9 degrees of freedom, the null hypothesis of no linear relationship between X and Y is rejected, and we conclude that the two variables are linearly related. For this test, since $95.74 > 13.61$, we have $p < .005$.

The sample coefficient of determination provides a point estimate of ρ^2, the *population coefficient of determination*. The population coefficient of determination, ρ^2, has the same function relative to the population as r^2 has to the sample. It shows what proportion of the total population variation in Y is explained by the regression of Y on X. When the number of degrees of freedom are small, r^2 is positively biased. That is, r^2 tends to be large. An unbiased estimator of ρ^2 is provided by

$$\tilde{r}^2 = 1 - \frac{\sum(y_i - y_c)^2/(n-2)}{\sum(y_i - \bar{y})^2/(n-1)} \tag{8.4.5}$$

Observe that the numerator of the fraction in Equation 8.4.5 is the unexplained mean square and the denominator is the total mean square. These quantities appear in the analysis of variance table. For our illustrative example we have, using the data from Table 8.4.2,

$$\tilde{r}^2 = 1 - \frac{326.3702/9}{3798.1818/10} = 1 - \frac{36.2634}{379.81818} = .9045$$

Table 8.4.3

ANOVA Table for Example 8.3.1

Source of Variation	*SS*	**d. f.**	*MS*	**V. R.**
Linear regression	3471.8116	1	3471.8116	95.74
Residual	326.3702	9	36.2634	
Total	3798.1818	10		

We see that this value is slightly less than

$$r^2 = 1 - \frac{326.3702}{3798.1818} = 1 - .08593 = .91407$$

We see that the difference in r^2 and $\tilde{r}^2$ is due to the factor $(n - 1)/(n - 2)$. When n is large, this factor will approach 1 and the difference between r^2 and $\tilde{r}^2$ will approach zero.

A Hypothesis Test for β. An alternative test of the null hypothesis of no linear relationship between two variables is based on b, the slope of the sample regression equation.

When the assumptions stated in Section 8.2 are met, a and b are unbiased point estimators of the corresponding parameters α and β and since, under these assumptions, the subpopulations of Y values are normally distributed, we may also construct confidence intervals for and test hypotheses about α and β.

When the assumptions of Section 8.2 hold true, the sampling distributions of a and b are each normally distributed with means and variances as follows:

$$\mu_a = \alpha \tag{8.4.6}$$

$$\sigma_a{}^2 = \frac{\sigma_{y|x}^2 \sum x_i{}^2}{n\sum(x_i - \bar{x})^2} \tag{8.4.7}$$

$$\mu_b = \beta \tag{8.4.8}$$

and

$$\sigma_b{}^2 = \frac{\sigma_{y|x}^2}{\sum(x_i - \bar{x})^2} \tag{8.4.9}$$

In Equations 8.4.7 and 8.4.9 $\sigma_{y|x}^2$ is the unexplained variance of the subpopulations of Y values.

With knowledge of the sampling distributions of a and b we may construct confidence intervals and test hypotheses relative to α and β in the usual manner. Inferences regarding α are usually not of interest. On the other hand, a great deal of interest centers on inferential procedures with respect to β. The reason for this is the fact that β tells us so much about the form of the relationship between X and Y. A positive β indicates that, in general, Y increases as X increases, and we say that there is a *direct linear relationship* between X and Y. A negative β indicates that values of Y tend to decrease as values of X increase, and we say that there is an *inverse linear relationship* between X and Y. When there is no linear relationship between X and Y, β is equal to zero. These three situations are illustrated in Figure 8.4.3.

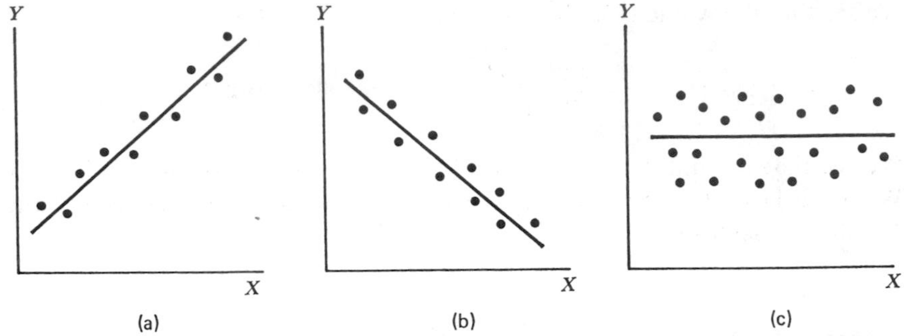

Figure 8.4.3. Scatter diagrams showing direct, inverse, and no linear relationships between X *and* Y. *(a) Direct linear relationship. (b) Inverse linear relationship. (c) No linear relationship.*

In the absence of knowledge of the true value of β, which is the typical situation, we can only draw inferences about it from sample data. Specifically, we may be interested in determining whether the sample data provide sufficient evidence to indicate that β is not equal to zero. We can conclude that β is not equal to zero if we can reject the null hypothesis that $\beta = 0$. If this null hypothesis is rejected we can conclude, with α (note that α as used here refers to a chosen level of significance and not to the *Y*-intercept of the true regression equation) probability of being wrong, that there is evidence of a linear relationship between X and Y. In deciding whether this suggested linear relationship is direct or inverse we will be guided by the sign of b, the estimator of β.

The test statistic when $\sigma^2_{y|x}$ is known is

$$z = \frac{b - \beta_0}{\sigma_b} \tag{8.4.10}$$

where β_0 is the hypothesized value of β. The hypothesized value of β does not have to be zero, but in practice, more often than not, the null hypothesis of interest is that $\beta = 0$.

As a rule $\sigma^2_{y|x}$ is unknown. When this is the case, the test statistic is

$$t = \frac{b - \beta_0}{s_b} \tag{8.4.11}$$

where s_b is an estimate of σ_b, and t is distributed as Student's t with $n - 2$ degrees of freedom. To obtain s_b, we must first estimate $\sigma^2_{y|x}$. An unbiased estimator of this parameter is provided by the unexplained variance computed from the sample data. That is,

$$s^2_{y|x} = \frac{\sum(y_i - y_c)^2}{n - 2} \tag{8.4.12}$$

is an unbiased estimator of $\sigma_{y|x}^2$. This is the unexplained mean square which appears in the analysis of variance table.

When $s_{y|x}^2$ is used to estimate $\sigma_{y|x}^2$ we may obtain the desired and unbiased estimator of $\sigma_b{}^2$,

$$s_b{}^2 = \frac{s_{y|x}^2}{\sum(x_i - \bar{x})^2} \tag{8.4.13}$$

We may write Equation 8.4.13 in the following computationally more convenient form:

$$s_b{}^2 = \frac{s_{y|x}^2}{\sum x_i{}^2 - (\sum x_i)^2/n} \tag{8.4.14}$$

If the probability of observing a value as extreme as the computed value of the test statistic when the null hypothesis is true is less than $\alpha/2$ (since we have a two-sided test), the null hypothesis is rejected.

Let us use our now familiar example to illustrate the procedure of testing the null hypothesis that $\beta = 0$. First we state our hypotheses and decide on a level of significance:

$$H_0: \beta = 0$$
$$H_A: \beta \neq 0$$
$$\alpha = .05$$

We next compute $s_b{}^2$. From Table 8.4.3 we have $s_{y|x}^2 = 36.2634$, so that we may compute

$$s_b{}^2 = \frac{36.2634}{[50^2 + 55^2 + \cdots + 100^2] - \dfrac{(825)^2}{11}} = .013$$

We may compute our test statistic

$$t = \frac{1.1236 - 0}{\sqrt{.013}} = 9.85$$

The probability of getting a value of t this extreme or more extreme when the null hypothesis is true is less than .01, since the probability of getting a value of t as large as or larger than 3.2498 is .005 and the probability of getting a value of t as small as or smaller than -3.2498 is also .005. Since 9.85 is greater than 3.2498, the probability of observing a value of t as large as or larger than 9.85, when the null hypothesis is true, is less than .005. Since the test is two-sided, we must allow for a computed value of t as extreme in the opposite direction, and hence the one-sided p-value is doubled to give $p < 2(.005) = .01$.

Alternatively, we may follow the decision rule approach and note that the critical values of t for a two-sided test, when $\alpha = .05$ and we have $(n - 2) = 9$ degrees of freedom, are ± 2.2622. Since our computed t of 9.85 is larger than

2.2622, we say it is significant, reject H_0, and conclude that the slope of the true regression line is not zero. The practical implication is that we may conclude that there is evidence of a linear relationship between X and Y. The fact that b is positive leads us to believe that β is positive and that the relationship between X and Y is a direct linear relationship. As has already been pointed out, Equation 8.4.11 may be used to test the null hypothesis that β is equal to some value other than 0. The hypothesized value for β, β_0, is substituted into the equation rather than 0. All other quantities, as well as the computations, are the same as in the illustrative example. The degrees of freedom and the method of determining significance are also the same.

A Confidence Interval for β. Once it has been determined that it is unlikely, in light of sample evidence, that β is zero, the researcher may be interested in obtaining an interval estimate of β. The general formula for a confidence interval,

$$\text{estimator} \pm (\text{reliability factor})(\text{standard error of the estimate})$$

may be used. When obtaining a confidence interval for β, the estimator is b, the reliability factor is some value of z or t (depending on whether or not $\sigma^2_{y|x}$ is known), and the standard error of the estimator is

$$\sigma_b = \sqrt{\frac{\sigma^2_{y|x}}{\sum(x_i - \bar{x})^2}}$$

When $\sigma^2_{y|x}$ is unknown, σ_b is estimated by

$$s_b = \sqrt{\frac{s^2_{y|x}}{\sum(x_i - \bar{x})^2}}$$

so that in most practical situations our $100(1 - \alpha)$ percent confidence interval for β is

$$b \pm t_{(1-\alpha/2)} \sqrt{\frac{s^2_{y|x}}{\sum(x_i - \bar{x})^2}} \tag{8.4.15}$$

For our illustrative example we construct the following 95 percent confidence interval for β:

$$1.1236 \pm 2.2622\sqrt{.013}$$
$$1.1236 \pm .2579$$
$$.8657, 1.3815$$

We interpret this interval in the usual manner. From the probabilistic point of view we say that in repeated sampling, 95 percent of the intervals constructed in this way will include β. The practical interpretation is that we are 95 percent confident that the single interval constructed includes β.

It is instructive to note that the confidence interval we constructed does not include zero, so that zero is not a candidate for the parameter being estimated. We feel, then, that it is unlikely that $\beta = 0$. This is compatible with the results of our hypothesis test in which we rejected the null hypothesis that $\beta = 0$. Actually, we can always test $H_0: \beta = 0$ at the α significance level by constructing the $100(1 - \alpha)$ percent confidence interval for β, and we can reject or fail to reject the hypothesis on the basis of whether or not the interval includes zero. If the interval contains zero, the null hypothesis is not rejected; and if zero is not contained in the interval, we reject the null hypothesis.

It must be made clear at this point that failure to reject the null hypothesis that $\beta = 0$ does not mean that X and Y are not related. Not only is it possible that a Type II error may have been committed but it may be true that X and Y are related in some nonlinear manner. On the other hand, when we reject the null hypothesis that $\beta = 0$, we cannot conclude that the *true* relationship between X and Y is linear. Again, it may be that although the data fit the linear regression model fairly well (as evidenced by the fact that the null hypothesis that $\beta = 0$ is rejected), it may be that some nonlinear model would provide an even better fit. Consequently, when we reject H_0 that $\beta = 0$, the best we can say is that more useful results (discussed below) may be obtained by taking into account the regression of Y on X than in ignoring it.

Exercises

8.4.1 to 8.4.5. Refer to Exercises 8.3.1 to 8.3.5 and for each one do the following:

(a) Compute the coefficient of determination.
(b) Prepare an ANOVA table and test the null hypothesis of no linear relationship between the two variables.
(c) Test the null hypothesis that $\beta = 0$ using a .05 level of significance.
(d) Determine the p-value for each hypothesis test.
(e) State your conclusions in terms of the problem.
(f) Construct the 95 percent confidence interval for β.

8.5 USING THE REGRESSION EQUATION

If the results of the evaluation of the sample regression equation indicate that there is a relationship between the two variables of interest, we can put the regression equation to practical use. There are two ways in which the equation can be used. It can be used to *predict* what value Y is likely to assume given a particular value of X. When the assumptions of Section 8.2 are met, a *prediction interval* for this predicted value of Y may be constructed.

We may also use the regression equation to *estimate* the mean of the subpopulation of Y values assumed to exist at any particular value of X. Again, if the previously stated assumptions hold, a confidence interval for this parameter may be constructed. The predicted value of Y and the point estimate of the mean of the subpopulation of Y will be numerically equivalent for any particular value of X but, as we shall see, the prediction interval will be wider than the confidence interval.

Predicting Y for a Given X. Suppose, in our illustrative example, we have a patient who makes a score of 70 on the new test and we want to predict his score on the standardized test. To obtain the predicted value, we substitute 70 for x in the sample regression equation to obtain

$$\begin{aligned} y_c &= -.9973 + 1.1236(70) \\ &= 78 \end{aligned}$$

rounded to the nearest whole number.

If we decide to give the patient the standardized test, we would predict his score to be 78. Since we have no confidence in this prediction, we would prefer an interval with an associated level of confidence. If it is known, or if we are willing to assume that the assumptions of Section 8.2 are met, and when $\sigma^2_{y|x}$ is unknown, the $100(1 - \alpha)$ percent prediction interval for Y is given by

$$y_c \pm t_{(1-\alpha/2)} s_{y|x} \sqrt{1 + \frac{1}{n} + \frac{(x_p - \bar{x})^2}{\sum(x_i - \bar{x})^2}} \tag{8.5.1}$$

where x_p is the particular value of x at which we wish to obtain a prediction interval for Y and the degrees of freedom used in selecting t are $n - 2$. For our illustrative example we may construct the following 95 percent prediction interval:

$$78 \pm 2.2622\sqrt{36.2634}\sqrt{1 + \frac{1}{11} + \frac{(70 - 75)^2}{2750}}$$

$$78 \pm 2.2622(6.02)(1.0488)$$

$$78 \pm 14$$

$$64, 92$$

Our interpretation of a prediction interval is similar to the interpretation of a confidence interval. If we repeatedly draw samples, do a regression analysis, and construct prediction intervals for patients who score 70 on the new test, about 95 percent of them will include the patient's score on the standardized test. This is the probabilistic interpretation. The practical interpretation is that we are 95 percent confident that the single prediction interval constructed includes the patient's score on the standardized test.

Estimating the Mean of Y for a Given X. If, in our illustrative example, we are interested in estimating the mean of the hypothetical subpopulation of scores on the standardized test, made by patients who make a score of 70 on the new test, we would again calculate

$$\begin{aligned} y_c &= -.9973 + 1.1236(70) \\ &= 78 \end{aligned}$$

The $100(1 - \alpha)$ percent confidence interval for $\mu_{y|x}$, when $\sigma^2_{y|x}$ is unknown, is given by

$$y_c \pm t_{(1-\alpha/2)} s_{y|x} \sqrt{\frac{1}{n} + \frac{(x_p - \bar{x})^2}{\sum(x_i - \bar{x})^2}} \tag{8.5.2}$$

We can obtain the following 95 percent confidence interval for $\mu_{y|x=70}$ of our present example by making proper substitutions:

$$78 \pm 2.2622\sqrt{36.2634}\sqrt{\frac{1}{11} + \frac{(70 - 75)^2}{2750}}$$

$$78 \pm 4$$

$$74, 82$$

If we repeatedly drew samples from our population of patients, performed a regression analysis, and estimated $\mu_{y|x=70}$ with a similarly constructed confidence interval, about 95 percent of such intervals would include the true mean. For this reason we are 95 percent confident that the single interval constructed contains the true mean.

If confidence intervals are constructed for several subpopulation means and the upper and lower limits plotted on the same scatter diagram with the regression line, we can obtain a *confidence band* by connecting all the upper limits with one curve and all the lower limits with another curve. Table 8.5.1 contains the 95 percent upper and lower confidence limits for $\mu_{y|x}$ for each value of X in our illustrative example, and Figure 8.5.1 shows the 95 percent confidence band that results when these values are plotted.

Table 8.5.1

95 Percent Confidence Limits for $\mu_{y|x}$ for Each Value of X, Example 8.3.1

x	y_c	**Lower Limit**	**Upper Limit**
50	55.1827	47.5009	62.8645
55	60.8007	54.1798	67.4216
60	66.4187	60.7588	72.0786
65	72.0367	67.1783	76.8951
70	77.6547	73.3482	81.9612
75	83.2727	79.1666	87.3788
80	88.8907	84.5842	93.1972
85	94.5087	89.6503	99.3671
90	100.1267	94.4668	105.7866
95	105.7447	99.1238	112.3656
100	111.3627	103.6809	119.0445

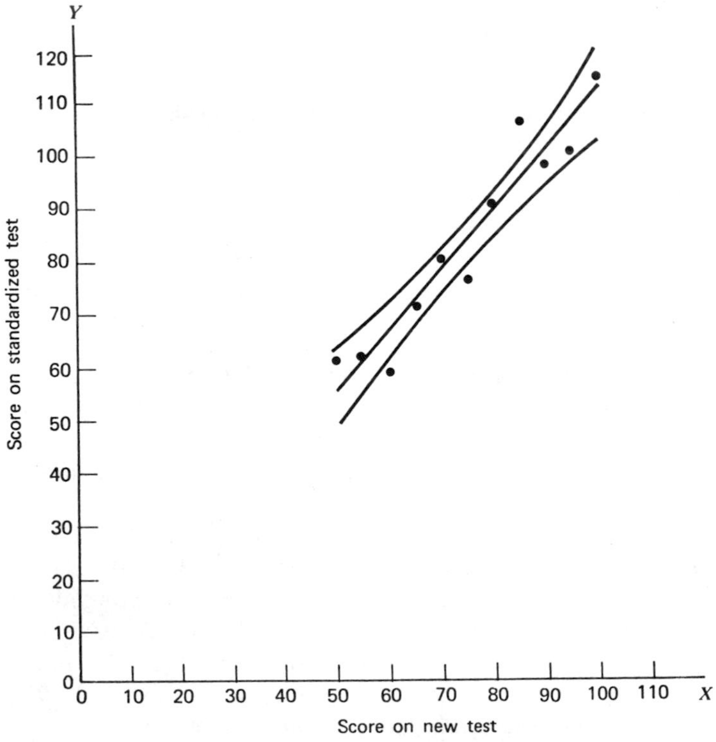

Figure 8.5.1. The 95 percent confidence band for $\mu_{y|x}$, Example 8.3.1.

Notice that the confidence band is wider at the ends than in the middle. In fact, the confidence band is narrowest for $x_p = \bar{x} = 75$. The reason for this is that when $\bar{x} = 75$ is substituted for x_p in Equation 8.5.2, the quantity under the radical is a minimum that results in the narrowest confidence interval. As x_p increases or decreases, the quantity under the radical becomes larger as do the associated confidence intervals.

Graybill and Bowden (5) present a method for constructing confidence bands that are straight lines. They suggest that bands of this type may be preferable to the curvilinear type given above because they are easier to compute and graph, and have a smaller average width.

Dunn (6), who has constructed a confidence band which she states is preferable to that of Graybill and Bowden, suggests that the usual curvilinear confidence band is to be preferred over any of the straight-line variety. This topic is also discussed by Hoel (7), Gafarian (8), Halperin and Gurian (9), and Elston and Grizzle (10).

In a similar manner, prediction bands may be constructed by plotting the prediction intervals at several values of X.

Exercises

In each of the Exercises 8.5.1 to 8.5.5 refer to the appropriate exercise and, for the value of X indicated, (a) construct the 95 percent confidence interval for $\mu_{y|x}$, and (b) construct the 95 percent prediction interval for y_p.

8.5.1. Refer to Exercise 8.3.1 and let $X = 2$.

8.5.2. Refer to Exercise 8.3.2 and let $X = 400$.

8.5.3. Refer to Exercise 8.3.3 and let $X = 50$.

8.5.4. Refer to Exercise 8.3.4 and let $X = 100$.

8.5.5. Refer to Exercise 8.3.5 and let $X = 5$.

8.5.6. Construct the 95 percent confidence band for $\mu_{y|x}$ for Exercise 8.3.5.

8.6 THE CORRELATION MODEL

In the classic regression model, which has been the underlying model in our discussion up to this point, only Y, which has been called the dependent variable, is random. The variable X is defined as a fixed (nonrandom or mathematical) variable, and is referred to as the independent variable. Recall, also, that observations have been described as being obtained by preselecting values of X and determining corresponding values of Y.

When both Y and X are random variables, we have what is called the *correlation model*. Typically, under the correlation model, sample observations are obtained by selecting a random sample of the *units of association* (which may be persons, places, animals, points in time, or any other element on which the two measurements are taken) and by taking on each a measurement of X and a measurement of Y. In this procedure, values of X are not preselected, but occur at random, depending on the unit of association selected in the sample.

Although correlation analysis cannot be carried out meaningfully under the classic regression model, regression analysis can be carried out under the correlation model. Correlation involving two variables implies a co-relationship between variables that puts both on an equal footing, and does not distinguish between them by referring to one as the dependent and the other as the independent variable. In fact, in the basic computational procedures, which are the same as for the regression model, we may fit a straight line to the data either by minimizing $\sum(y_i - y_c)^2$ or by minimizing $\sum(x_i - x_c)^2$. In other words, we may do a regression of X on Y as well as a regression of Y on X. The fitted lines in the two cases in general will be different, and a logical question arises as to which line to fit.

If the objective is solely to obtain a measure of the strength of the relationship between the two variables, it does not matter which line is fitted, since the measure usually computed will be the same in either case. If, however, it is desired to use the equation describing the relationship between the two variables for the purposes discussed in the preceding sections, it does matter which line is fitted. The variable for which we wish to estimate means or to make predictions should be treated as the dependent variable, that is, this variable should be regressed on the other variable.

Under the correlation model, X and Y are assumed to vary together in what is called a *joint distribution*. If the form of this joint distribution is normally distributed, it is referred to as a *bivariate normal distribution*. Inferences regarding this population may be made based on the results of samples properly drawn from it. If, on the other hand, the form of the joint distribution is known to be nonnormal, or if the form is unknown and there is no justification for assuming normality, inferential procedures are invalid, although descriptive measures may be computed.

The following assumptions must hold for inferences about the population to be valid when sampling from a bivariate distribution.

1. For each value of X there is a normally distributed subpopulation of Y values.
2. For each value of Y there is a normally distributed subpopulation of X values.

3. The joint distribution of X and Y is a normal distribution called the *bivariate normal distribution.*
4. The subpopulations of Y values all have the same variance.
5. The subpopulations of X values all have the same variance.

The bivariate normal distribution is represented graphically in Figure 8.6.1. In this illustration we see that if we slice the mound parallel to Y at some value of X, the cutaway reveals the corresponding normal distribution of Y. Similarly, a slice through the mound parallel to X at some value of Y reveals the corresponding normally distributed subpopulation of X.

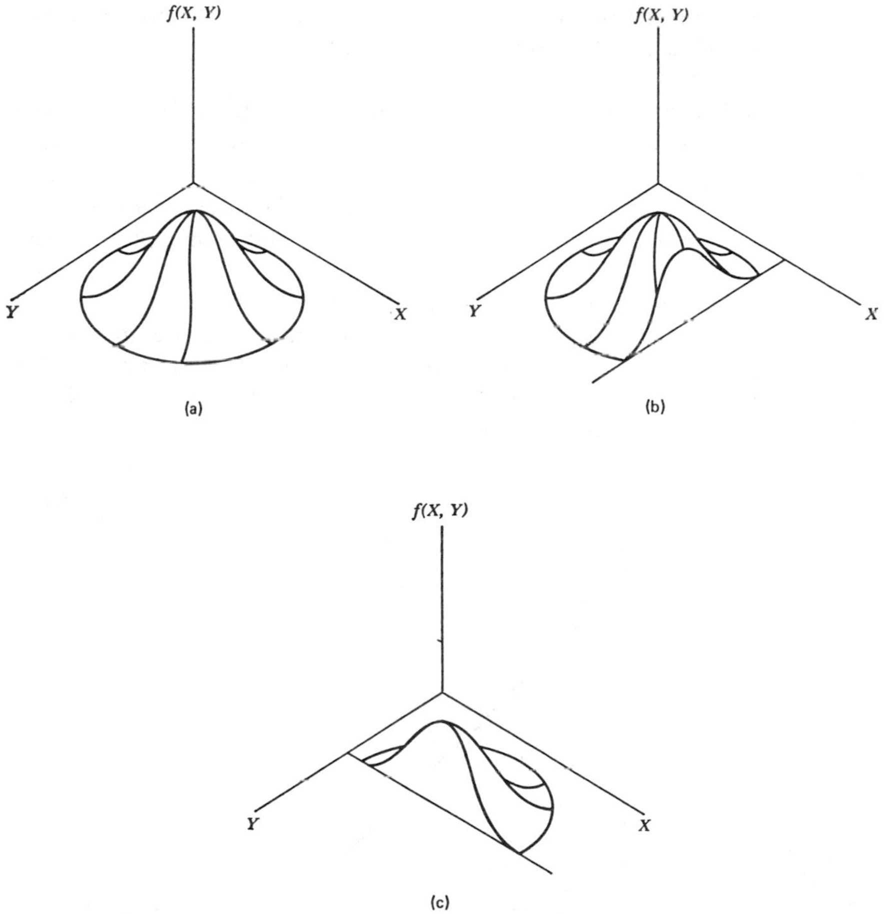

Figure 8.6.1. A bivariate normal distribution. (a) A bivariate normal distribution. (b) A cutaway showing normally distributed subpopulation of Y *for given* X. *(c) A cutaway showing normally distributed subpopulation of* X *for given* Y.

8.7 THE CORRELATION COEFFICIENT

The bivariate normal distribution discussed in Section 8.6 has five parameters σ_x, σ_y, μ_x, μ_y, and ρ. The first four are, respectively, the standard deviations and means associated with the individual distributions. The other parameter, ρ, is called the population *correlation coefficient* and measures the strength of the linear relationship between X and Y.

The population correlation coefficient is the square root of ρ^2, the population coefficient of determination previously discussed, and since the coefficient of determination takes on values between 0 and 1 inclusive, ρ may assume any value between -1 and $+1$. If $\rho = 1$ there is perfect direct linear correlation between the two variables, while $\rho = -1$ indicates perfect inverse linear correlation. If $\rho = 0$ the two variables are not correlated. The sign of ρ will always be the same as the sign of β, the slope of the regression line for X and Y.

The sample correlation coefficient, r, describes the relationship between the sample observations on two variables in the same way that ρ describes the relationship in a population.

Figure 8.4.2*d*, and 8.4.2*c*, respectively, show typical scatter diagrams where $r \to 0$ ($r^2 \to 0$) and $r = +1$ ($r^2 = 1$). Figure 8.7.1 shows a typical scatter diagram where $r = -1$.

We are usually interested in knowing if we may conclude that $\rho \neq 0$, that is, that X and Y are correlated. Since ρ is usually unknown, we draw a random sample from the population of interest, compute r, the estimator of ρ, and test $H_0: \rho = 0$ against the alternative $\rho \neq 0$. The procedure will be illustrated in the following example.

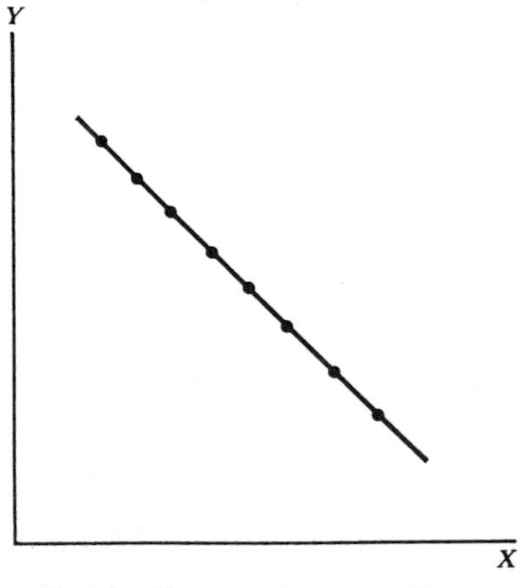

Figure 8.7.1. Scatter diagram for r = *− 1.*

Table 8.7.1

Systolic Blood Pressure Readings (mm Hg) by Two Methods in 25 Patients with Essential Hypertension

Patient Number	**Method I**	**Method II**
1	132	130
2	138	134
3	144	132
4	146	140
5	148	150
6	152	144
7	158	150
8	130	122
9	162	160
10	168	150
11	172	160
12	174	178
13	180	168
14	180	174
15	188	186
16	194	172
17	194	182
18	200	178
19	200	196
20	204	188
21	210	180
22	210	196
23	216	210
24	220	190
25	220	202

Example 8.7.1

Blood pressure readings by two different methods were made on 25 patients with essential hypertension. The systolic readings by the two methods are shown in Table 8.7.1.

The clinician wished to investigate the strength of the relationship between the two measurements. The scatter diagram and least-squares regression line are shown in Figure 8.7.2.

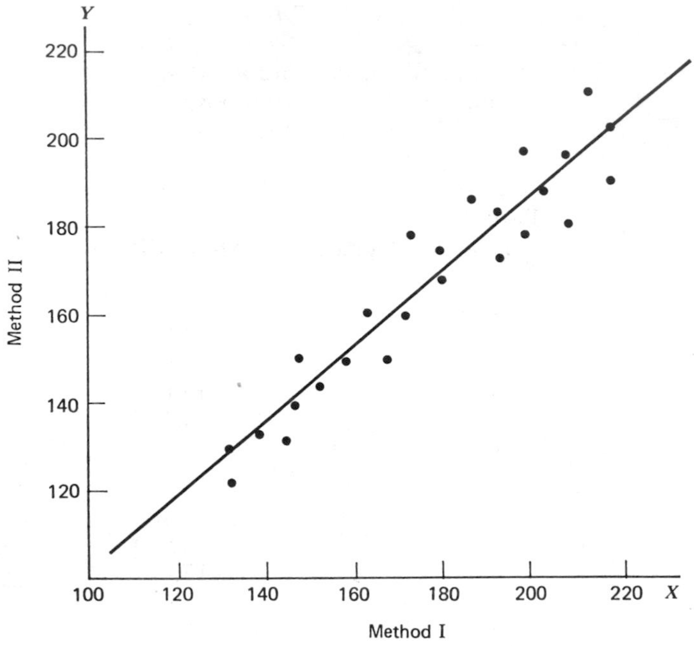

Figure 8.7.2. Systolic blood pressure readings (mm Hg), 25 patients with essential hypertension.

The preliminary calculations necessary for obtaining the least-squares regression line are shown in Table 8.7.2. Since the investigator wishes to obtain a regression equation to use for estimating and predicting purposes, the sample correlation coefficient will be obtained by the methods discussed under the regression model.

Method I readings were treated as the independent variable, since the clinician anticipated that he might want to predict a Method II reading given a Method I reading.

By substituting from Table 8.7.2 into Equations 8.3.2 and 8.3.3, the following normal equations are obtained:

$$4172 = 25a + 4440b$$
$$757{,}276 = 4440a + 808408b$$

When these equations are solved we have

$$a = 20.8928$$
$$b = .8220$$

The least-squares equation is

$$y_c = 20.8928 + .8220x$$

Table 8.7.2

Preliminary Calculations for Obtaining Least-Squares Regression Line, Example 8.7.1

Method I (x)	**Method II** (y)	x^2	y^2	xy
132	130	17424	16900	17160
138	134	19044	17956	18492
144	132	20736	17424	19008
146	140	21316	19600	20440
148	150	21904	22500	22200
152	144	23104	20736	21888
158	150	24964	22500	23700
130	122	16900	14884	15860
162	160	26244	25600	25920
168	150	28224	22500	25200
172	160	29584	25600	27520
174	178	30276	31684	30972
180	168	32400	28224	30240
180	174	32400	30276	31320
188	186	35344	34596	34968
194	172	37636	29584	33368
194	182	37636	33124	35308
200	178	40000	31684	35600
200	196	40000	38416	39200
204	188	41616	35344	38352
210	180	44100	32400	37800
210	196	44100	38416	41160
216	210	46656	44100	45360
220	190	48400	36100	41800
220	202	48400	40804	44440
Total 4440	4172	808408	710952	757276

The coefficient of determination, which is equal to the explained sum of squares divided by the total sum of squares, is (using Equations 8.4.3 and 8.4.4)

$$r^2 = \frac{b^2[\sum x_i^2 - (\sum x_i)^2/n]}{\sum y_i^2 - (\sum y_i)^2/n} \tag{8.7.1}$$

Substituting values from Table 8.7.2 and the regression equation into Equation 8.7.1 gives

$$r^2 = \frac{(.8220)^2[808{,}408 - (4440)^2/25]}{710{,}952 - (4172)^2/25}$$

$$= .911$$

Finally, the correlation coefficient is

$$r = \sqrt{r^2} = \sqrt{.911} = .95$$

An alternative formula for computing r is given by

$$r = \frac{n\sum x_i y_i - (\sum x_i)(\sum y_i)}{\sqrt{n\sum x_i^2 - (\sum x_i)^2}\sqrt{n\sum y_i^2 - (\sum y_i)^2}} \tag{8.7.2}$$

An advantage of this formula is that r may be computed without first computing b. This is the desirable procedure when it is not anticipated that the regression equation will be used. Substituting from Table 8.7.2 in Equation 8.7.2 gives

$$r = \frac{25(757{,}276) - (4440)(4172)}{\sqrt{25(808{,}408) - (4440)^2}\sqrt{25(710{,}952) - (4172)^2}}$$

$$= .95$$

To see if this value of r is of sufficient magnitude to indicate that the two variables of interest are correlated, we test the hypothesis

$$H_0 : \rho = 0$$

against the alternative

$$H_A : \rho \neq 0$$

When $\rho = 0$, it can be shown that

$$t = r\sqrt{\frac{n-2}{1-r^2}} \tag{8.7.3}$$

is distributed as Student's t distribution with $n - 2$ degrees of freedom.

If we let $\alpha = .05$, the critical values of t in the present example are ± 2.0687. If, from our data, we compute a value of t greater than or equal to $+2.0687$ or less than or equal to -2.0687, we will reject the null hypothesis. Our calculated value of t is

$$t = .95\sqrt{\frac{23}{1 - .9025}}$$

$$= 14.59$$

and since it does exceed the critical value of t, we reject the null hypothesis and conclude that the two variables are correlated. Since $14.59 > 2.8073$, we have for this test, $p < .01$.

The use of the t statistic computed in the above test is appropriate only for testing $H_0 : \rho = 0$. If it is desired to test $H_0 : \rho = \rho_0$, where ρ_0 is some value other than zero, we must use another approach. Fisher (11) suggests that r be transformed to z_r as follows

$$z_r = \frac{1}{2} \ln \frac{1+r}{1-r} \tag{8.7.4}$$

where ln is a natural logarithm. It can be shown that z_r is approximately normally distributed with a mean of $z_\rho = \frac{1}{2}\ln\{(1 + \rho)/(1 - \rho)\}$ and estimated standard deviation of

$$\frac{1}{\sqrt{n - 3}} \tag{8.7.5}$$

To test the null hypothesis that ρ is equal to some value other than zero the test statistic is

$$Z = \frac{z_r - z_\rho}{1/\sqrt{n - 3}} \tag{8.7.6}$$

which follows approximately the unit normal distribution.

To determine z_r for an observed r and z_ρ for a hypothesized ρ, we consult Table L, thereby avoiding the direct use of natural logarithms.

Suppose in our present example we wish to test

$$H_0: \rho = .98$$

against the alternative

$$H_A: \rho \neq .98$$

at the .05 level of significance. By consulting Table L we find that for

$$r = .95, \qquad z_r = 1.83178$$

and for

$$\rho = .98, \qquad z_\rho = 2.29756$$

Our test statistic, then, is

$$\begin{aligned} Z &= \frac{1.83178 - 2.29756}{1/\sqrt{25 - 3}} \\ &= -2.18 \end{aligned}$$

Since -2.18 is less than the critical value of $z = -1.96$, we must reject H_0 and conclude that the population correlation coefficient is not .98.

For sample sizes less than 25, Fisher's Z transformation should be used with caution, if at all. An alternative procedure due to Hotelling (12) may be used for sample sizes equal to or greater than 10. In this procedure the following transformation of r is employed

$$z^* = z_r - \frac{3z_r + r}{4n} \tag{8.7.7}$$

The standard deviation of z^* is

$$\sigma_{z^*} = \frac{1}{\sqrt{n - 1}} \tag{8.7.8}$$

The test statistic is

$$Z^* = \frac{z^* - \zeta^*}{1/\sqrt{n - 1}} = (z^* - \zeta^*)\sqrt{n - 1} \tag{8.7.9}$$

where

$$\zeta^* \text{ (pronounced zeta)} = z_\rho - \frac{(3z_\rho + \rho)}{4n}$$

Critical values for comparison purposes are obtained from the unit normal distribution.

In our present example, to test $H_0: \rho = .98$ against $H_A: \rho \neq .98 (\alpha = .05)$, using the Hotelling transformation we have

$$z^* = 1.83178 - \frac{3(1.83178) + .95}{4(25)} = 1.76733$$

$$\zeta^* = 2.29756 - \frac{3(2.29756) + .98}{4(25)} = 2.21883$$

$$Z^* = (1.76733 - 2.21883)\sqrt{25 - 1}$$
$$= -2.21$$

Since -2.21 is smaller than -1.96, the null hypothesis is rejected and the same conclusion is reached as when the Fisher transformation is used.

Confidence Interval for ρ**.** Fisher's transformation may be used to construct $100(1 - \alpha)$ percent confidence intervals for ρ. The general formula for a confidence interval

estimator ± (reliability factor)(standard error)

is employed. We first convert our estimator, r, to z_r, construct a confidence interval about z_ρ, and then reconvert the limits to obtain a $100(1 - \alpha)$ percent confidence interval about ρ. The general formula then becomes

$$z_r \pm z(1/\sqrt{n - 3}) \tag{8.7.10}$$

For our present example the 95 percent confidence interval for z_ρ is given by

$$1.83178 \pm 1.96(1/\sqrt{25 - 3})$$
$$1.83178 \pm .41787$$
$$1.41391, 2.24965$$

Converting these limits, which are values of z_r, into values of r gives

z_r	r
1.41391	.890
2.24965	.975

We are 95 percent confident, then, that ρ is contained in the interval .890 to .975. Because of the limited entries in the table, these limits must be considered as only approximate.

An alternative method of constructing confidence intervals for ρ is to use the special charts prepared by David (13).

Exercises

In each of the following exercises:

(a) Prepare a scatter diagram.
(b) Compute the sample correlation coefficient.
(c) Test $H_0: \rho = 0$ at the .05 level of significance and state your conclusions.
(d) Determine the p-value for the test.
(e) Construct the 95 percent confidence interval for ρ.

8.7.1. A random sample of the records of a certain hospital yielded the following information on the length of hospital stay in days and the annual family income (rounded to the nearest $500) of 15 discharged patients.

Annual Family Income (X)	Length of Stay (Y)
$2000	11
2500	12
3000	9
3500	8
4000	9
4500	10
5000	7
5500	8
6000	4
6500	7
7000	5
7500	6
8000	3
8500	4
9000	4

$$\sum x_i = 82{,}500$$
$$\sum x_i^2 = 523{,}750{,}000$$
$$\sum y_i = 107$$
$$\sum y_i^2 = 871$$
$$\sum x_i y_i = 510{,}500$$

8.7.2. The following table shows the systolic blood pressures of each of 25 pairs of identical twins.

First Twin (X)	Second Twin (Y)
118	115
116	119
118	116
120	119
122	118
122	138
122	124
120	128
124	126
125	130
138	130
140	125
142	164
144	160
145	158
162	145
180	184
180	190
182	188
185	180
170	174
172	170
150	160
152	155
155	160

$\sum x_i = 3{,}604 \qquad \sum x_i^2 = 532{,}832$

$\sum y_i = 3{,}676 \qquad \sum y_i^2 = 555{,}618$

$\sum x_i y_i = 543{,}120$

8.7.3. Two methods of measuring cardiac output were compared in 10 experimental animals with the following results

Cardiac Output (l./min) Method I (X)	Method II (Y)
.8	.5
1.0	1.2
1.3	1.1
1.4	1.3
1.5	1.1
1.4	1.8
2.0	1.6
2.4	2.0
2.7	2.4
3.0	2.8

8.7.4. The following are 15 readings on traffic volume and carbon monoxide concentration taken at a metropolitan air quality sampling site.

Traffic Volume (Cars per Hour) (X)	CO (ppm) (Y)
100	8.8
110	9.0
125	9.5
150	10.0
175	10.5
190	10.5
200	10.5
225	10.6
250	11.0
275	12.1
300	12.1
325	12.5
350	13.0
375	13.2
400	14.5

$\sum x_i = 3{,}550 \qquad \sum y_i = 167.8$

$\sum x_i^2 = 974{,}450 \qquad \sum y_i^2 = 1{,}915.36$

$\sum x_i y_i = 41{,}945$

8.7.5. A random sample of 25 nurses selected from a state registry of nurses yielded the following information on each nurse's score on the state board examination and his or her final score in school. Both scores relate to the nurse's area of affiliation.

Final Score (X)	State Board Score (Y)
87	440
87	480
87	535
88	460
88	525
89	480
89	510
89	530
89	545
89	600
90	495
90	545

Final Score (X)	State Board Score (Y)
90	575
91	525
91	575
91	600
92	490
92	510
92	575
93	540
93	595
94	525
94	545
94	600
94	625

$$\sum x_i = 2{,}263 \qquad \sum y_i = 13{,}425$$
$$\sum x_i^2 = 204{,}977 \qquad \sum y_i^2 = 7{,}264{,}525$$
$$\sum x_i y_i = 1{,}216{,}685$$

8.8 SOME PRECAUTIONS

Regression and correlation analysis are very powerful statistical tools when they are properly employed. Their inappropriate use, however, can lead only to meaningless results. To aid in the proper use of these techniques, we make the following suggestions,

1. The assumptions underlying regression and correlation analysis should be carefully reviewed before the data are collected. Although it is rare to find that assumptions are met to perfection, practitioners should have some idea about the magnitude of the gap that exists between the data to be analyzed and the assumptions of the proposed model, so that they may decide whether they should choose another model; proceed with the analysis, but use caution in the interpretation of the results; or use the chosen model with confidence.
2. In simple linear regression and correlation analysis, the two variables of interest are measured on the same entity, called the unit of association. If we are interested in the relationship between height and weight, for example, these two measurements are taken on the same individual. It usually does not make sense to speak of the correlation, say, between the heights of one group of individuals and the weights of another group.
3. No matter how strong is the indication of a relationship between two variables, it should not be interpreted as one of cause and effect. If, for example, a significant sample correlation coefficient between two variables

X and Y is observed, it can mean one of several things:

(a) X causes Y.
(b) Y causes X.
(c) Some third factor, either directly or indirectly, causes both X and Y.
(d) An unlikely event has occurred and a large sample correlation coefficient has been generated by chance from a population in which X and Y are, in fact, not correlated.
(e) The correlation is purely nonsensical, a situation that may arise when measurements of X and Y are not taken on a common unit of association.

4. The sample regression equation should not be used to predict or estimate outside the range of values of the independent variable represented in the sample. This practice, called *extrapolation*, is risky. The true relationship between two variables, although linear over an interval of the independent variable, sometimes may be described best as a curve outside this interval. If our sample by chance is drawn only from the interval where the relationship is linear, we have only a limited representation of the population, and to project the sample results beyond the interval represented by the sample may lead to false conclusions. Figure 8.8.1 illustrates one of the possible pitfalls of extrapolation.

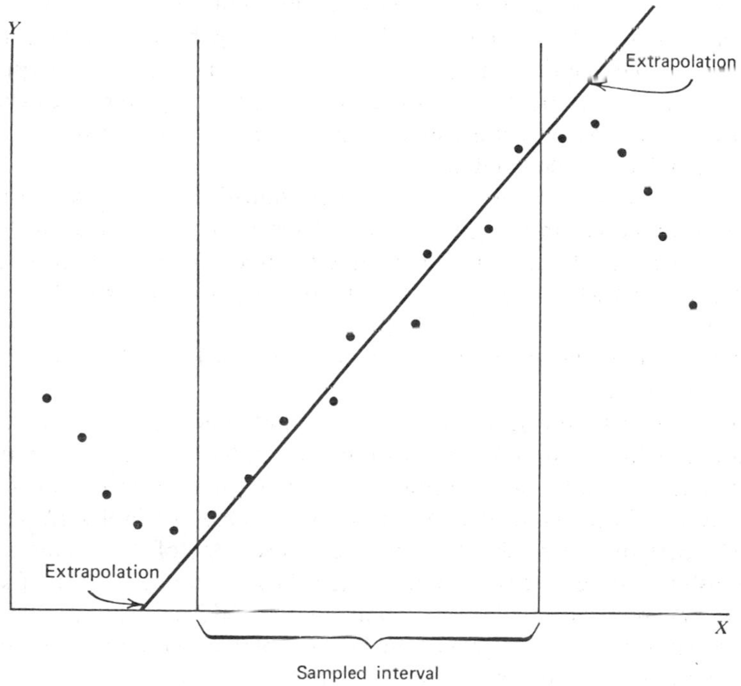

Figure 8.8.1. Example of extrapolation.

8.9 SUMMARY

In this chapter two important tools of statistical analysis, simple linear regression and correlation, are examined. The following outline for the application of these techniques has been suggested.

1. *Identify the model.* The practitioner must know whether the regression model or the correlation model is the appropriate one for answering his questions.
2. *Review assumptions.* It has been pointed out several times that the validity of the conclusions depends on how well the data analyzed fit the chosen model.
3. *Obtain the regression equation.* We have seen how the regression equation is obtained by the method of least squares. Although the computations, when done by hand, are rather lengthy, involved, and subject to error; this is not the problem today that it has been in the past. Electronic computers are now in such widespread use that one is tempted to say that the researcher or statistician without access to one is the exception rather than the rule. No apology for lengthy computations is necessary to the researcher who has a computer available.
4. *Evaluate the equation.* We have seen that the usefulness of the regression equation for estimating and predicting purposes is determined by means of the analysis of variance, which tests the significance of the regression mean square. The strength of the relationship between two variables under the correlation model is assessed by testing the null hypothesis that there is no correlation in the population. If this hypothesis can be rejected we may conclude, at the chosen level of significance, that the two variables are correlated.
5. *Use the equation.* Once it has been determined that it is likely that the regression equation provides a good description of the relationship between two variables, X and Y, it may be used for one of two purposes:
   (a) to predict what value Y is likely to assume, given a particular value of X, or
   (b) to estimate the mean of the subpopulation of Y values for a particular value of X.

This necessarily abridged treatment of simple linear regression and correlation may have raised more questions than it has answered. It may have occurred to the reader, for example, that a dependent variable can be more precisely predicted using two or more independent variables rather than one. Or, perhaps, he or she may feel that knowledge of the strength of the relationship among several variables might be of more interest than knowledge of the relationship between only two variables. The exploration of these possibilities is the subject of the next chapter, and the reader's curiosity along these lines should be, at least, partially relieved.

For those who would like to pursue the topic further, a number of excellent references, in addition to those already cited, follow at the end of this chapter.

Review Questions and Exercises

1. What are the assumptions underlying simple linear regression analysis when one of the objectives is to make inferences about the population from which the sample data were drawn?
2. Why is the regression equation called the least-squares equation?
3. Explain the meaning of a in the sample regression equation.
4. Explain the meaning of b in the sample regression equation.
5. Explain the following terms:
   (a) Total sum of squares
   (b) Explained sum of squares
   (c) Unexplained sum of squares
6. Explain the meaning of, and the method of computing, the coefficient of determination.
7. What is the function of the analysis of variance in regression analysis?
8. Describe two ways in which one may test the null hypothesis that $\beta = 0$.
9. For what two purposes can a regression equation be used?
10. What are the assumptions underlying simple correlation analysis when inference is an objective?
11. What is meant by the unit of association in regression and correlation analysis?
12. What are the possible explanations for a significant sample correlation coefficient?
13. Explain why it is risky to use a sample regression equation to predict or to estimate outside the range of values of the independent variable represented in the sample.
14. Describe a situation in your particular area of interest where simple regression analysis would be useful. Use real or realistic data and do a complete regression analysis.
15. Describe a situation in your particular area of interest where simple correlation analysis would be useful. Use real or realistic data and do a complete correlation analysis.

In each of the following exercises carry out the required analysis and test hypotheses at the indicated significance levels. Compute the p-value for each test.

16. The following are the plasma testosterone levels and age at first conviction for violent and aggressive crimes collected on a sample of young male prisoners.

Testosterone Level	Age at 1st Conviction	Testosterone Level	Age at 1st Conviction
1305	11	710	17
1000	12	1150	18
1175	13	605	20
1495	14	690	21
1060	15	700	23
800	16	625	24
1005	16	610	27
		450	30

Do these data provide sufficient evidence, at the .05 level of significance, to indicate that the two variables are correlated?

17. Some health researchers have reported an inverse relationship between central nervous system malformations and the hardness of the related water supplies. Suppose data were collected on a sample of 20 geographic areas with the following results.

C.N.S. Malformation Rate (per 1000 Births)	Water Hardness (ppm.)	C.N.S. Malformation Rate (per 1000 Births)	Water Hardness (ppm.)
7.2	50	6.3	160
8.1	25	12.5	50
11.2	15	15.0	45
9.3	75	6.5	60
9.4	100	8.0	100
5.0	150	10.0	155
5.8	180	5.3	200
3.3	250	4.9	240
3.6	275	7.2	40
4.8	220	11.9	65

Construct a scatter diagram and compute r. What are your conclusions? ($\alpha = .05$)

18. The mean systolic blood pressure during surgery and amount of blood loss were recorded for 16 patients.

Mean Systolic BP During Surgery (mmHg)	Blood Loss (ml)	Mean Systolic BP During Surgery (mmHg)	Blood Loss (ml)
95	274	80	190
90	170	110	288
125	352	90	205
105	317	105	150
110	171	90	175
105	150	110	64
90	245	110	276
90	120	140	318

Prepare a scatter diagram, compute r, and test for significance at the .05 level.

19. In a study of the effect of a dietary component on plasma lipid composition, the following data were obtained on a sample of 15 experimental animals:

n=15

Measure of Dietary Component (X)	Measure of Plasma Lipid Level (Y)
18	38
21	40
28	47
35	54
47	66
33	52
40	59
41	60
28	47
21	40
30	49
46	65
44	63
38	57
19	38

$\Sigma x_i = 489$ $\bar{x} = 32.6$ 775 $\bar{y} = 51.67$

Obtain the regression equation for these data, compute r^2, and test $H_0: \beta = 0$ by both the F test and the t test.

20. The following are the pulmonary blood flow (PBF) and pulmonary blood volume (PBV) values recorded for 16 infants and children with congential heart disease.

Y PBV (ml/sqM)	*X* PBF (L/min/sqM)
168	4.31
280	3.40
391	6.20
420	17.30
303	12.30
429	13.99
605	8.73
522	8.90
224	5.87
291	5.00
233	3.51
370	4.24
531	19.41
516	16.61
211	7.21
439	11.60

Find the regression equation describing the linear relationship between the two variables, compute r^2, and test $H_0: \beta = 0$ by both the F test and the t test. Let $\alpha = .05$.

21. Fifteen specimens of human sera were tested comparatively for tuberculin antibody by two methods. The logarithms of the titers obtained by the two methods were as follows:

Method $A(X)$	Method $B(Y)$
3.31	4.09
2.41	3.84
2.72	3.65
2.41	3.20
2.11	2.97
2.11	3.22
3.01	3.96
2.13	2.76
2.41	3.42
2.10	3.38
2.41	3.28
2.09	2.93
3.00	3.54
2.08	3.14
2.11	2.76

Find the regression equation describing the relationship between the two variables, compute r^2, and test $H_0: \beta = 0$ by both the F test and the t test.

22. The following table shows the methyl mercury intake and whole blood mercury values in 12 subjects exposed to methyl mercury through consumption of contaminated fish.

X Methyl Mercury Intake (μg Hg/day)	Y Mercury in Whole Blood (ng/g)
180	90
200	120
230	125
410	290
600	310
550	290
275	170
580	375
105	70
250	105
460	205
650	480

Find the regression equation describing the linear relationship between the two variables, compute r^2, and test $H_0: \beta = 0$ by both the F and t tests. Let $\alpha = .05$. Construct a 95 percent confidence interval for β.

References

References cited

1. Francis Galton, *Natural Inheritance*, Macmillan, London (1899).
2. Francis Galton, *Memories of My Life*, Methuen, London, 1908.
3. Karl Pearson, *The Life, Letters and Labours of Francis Galton*, Volume III A, Cambridge at the University Press, 1930.
4. Francis Galton, "Co-relations and Their Measurement, Chiefly from Anthropometric Data," *Proceedings of the Royal Society*, *XLV* (1888), 135–145.
5. F. A. Graybill and D. C. Bowden, "Linear Segment Confidence Bands for Simple Linear Models," *Journal of the American Statistical Association*, *62* (1967), 403–408.

6. Olive Jean Dunn, "A Note on Confidence Bands for a Regression Line Over a Finite Range," *Journal of the American Statistical Association*, *63* (1968), 1028–1033.
7. P. G. Hoel, "Confidence Regions for Linear Regression," *Proceedings of the Second Berkeley Symposium on Mathematical Statistics and Probability*, University of California Press, Berkeley, 1951, pp. 75–81.
8. A. V. Gafarian, "Confidence Bands in Straight Line Regression," *Journal of the American Statistical Association*, *59* (1964), 182–213.
9. M. Halperin and J. Gurian, "Confidence Bands in Linear Regression with Constraints in the Independent Variables," *Journal of the American Statistical Association*, *63* (1968), 1020–1027.
10. R. C. Elston and J. E. Grizzle, "Estimation of Time Response Curves and their Confidence Bands," *Biometrics*, *18* (1962), 148–159.
11. R. A. Fisher, "On the Probable Error of a Coefficient of Correlation Deduced from a Small Sample," *Metron*, *1* (1921), 3–21.
12. H. Hotelling, "New Light on the Correlation Coefficient and its Transforms," *Journal of the Royal Statistical Society*, Ser B, *15* (1953), 193–232.
13. F. N. David, *Tables of the Ordinates and Probability Integral of the Distribution of the Correlation Coefficient in Small Samples*, Cambridge University Press, Cambridge, 1938.

Other references, books

1. F. S. Acton, *Analysis of Straight Line Data*, Wiley, New York, 1959.
2. Andrew R. Baggaley, *Intermediate Correlational Methods*, Wiley, New York, 1964.
3. Cuthbert Daniel and Fred S. Wood, *Fitting Equations to Data*, Wiley-Interscience, New York, 1971.
4. N. R. Draper and H. Smith, *Applied Regression Analysis*, Wiley, New York, 1966.
5. Mordecai Ezekiel and Karl A. Fox, *Methods of Correlation and Regression Analysis*, Third Edition, Wiley, New York, 1959.
6. Arthur S. Goldberger, *Topics in Regression Analysis*, Macmillan, Toronto, 1968.
7. R. L. Plackett, *Principles of Regression Analysis*, Oxford University Press, London, 1960.
8. K. W. Smillie, *An Introduction to Regression and Correlation*, Academic Press, New York, 1966.
9. Peter Sprent, *Models in Regression*, Methuen, London, 1969.
10. E. J. Williams, *Regression Analysis*, Wiley, New York, 1959.

11. Stephen Wiseman, *Correlation Methods*, Manchester University Press, Manchester, 1966.

Other references, journal articles

1. R. G. D. Allen, "The Assumptions of Linear Regression," *Economica, 6 N.S.* (1939), 191–204.
2. M. S. Bartlett, "The Fitting of Straight Lines if Both Variables Are Subject to Error," *Biometrics, 5* (1949), 207–212.
3. J. Berkson, "Are There Two Regressions?" *Journal of the American Statistical Association, 45* (1950), 164–180.
4. Dudley J. Cowden, "A Procedure for Computing Regression Coefficients," *Journal of the American Statistical Association, 53* (1958), 144–150.
5. A. S. C. Ehrenberg, "Bivariate Regression Is Useless," *Applied Statistics, 12* (1963), 161–179.
6. M. G. Kendall, "Regression, Structure, and Functional Relationship, Part I," *Biometrika, 28* (1951), 11–25.
7. M. G. Kendall, "Regression, Structure and Functional Relationship II," *Biometrika, 39* (1952), 96–108.
8. D. V. Lindley, "Regression Lines and the Linear Functional Relationship," *Journal of the Royal Statistical Society* (Supplement), *IX* (1947), 218–244.
9. A. Madansky, "The Fitting of Straight Lines When Both Variables Are Subject to Error," *Journal of the American Statistical Association, 54* (1959), 173–205.
10. A. Wald, "The Fitting of Straight Lines if Both Variables Are Subject to Error," *Annals of Mathematical Statistics, 11* (1940), 284–300.
11. W. G. Warren, "Correlation or Regression: Bias or Precision," *Applied Statistics, 20* (1971), 148–164.
12. Charles P. Winsor, "Which Regression?" *Biometrics, 2* (1946), 101–109.

9

MULTIPLE REGRESSION AND CORRELATION

9.1 INTRODUCTION

In Chapter 8 we explore the concepts and techniques for analyzing and making use of the relationship between two variables. We see that this analysis may lead to an equation that can be used to predict the value of some dependent variable given the value of an associated independent variable.

Intuition tells us that, in general, we ought to be able to improve our predicting ability by including more independent variables in such an equation.

For example, a researcher may find that intelligence scores of individuals may be predicted from physical factors such as birth order, birth weight, and length of gestation along with certain hereditary and external environmental factors. Length of stay in a chronic disease hospital may be related to the patient's age, marital status, sex, and income, not to mention the obvious factor of diagnosis. The response of an experimental animal to some drug may depend on the size of the dose, and the age and weight of the animal. A nursing supervisor may be interested in the strength of the relationship between a nurse's performance on the job, score on the state board examination, scholastic record, and score on some achievement or aptitude test. Or a hospital administrator studying admissions from various communities served by the hospital may be interested in determining what factors seem to be responsible for differences in admission rates.

The concepts and techniques for analyzing the association among several variables are natural extensions of those explored in the previous chapters. The computations, as one would expect, are more complex and tedious. However, as is pointed out in Chapter 8, this presents no real problem whenever an electronic computer is available. It is not unusual to find researchers investigating the relationships among a dozen or more variables. For those who have access to a computer, the decision as to how many variables to include in an analysis is based not on the complexity and length of the computations, but on such considerations as their meaningfulness, the cost of their inclusion, and the importance of their contribution.

In this chapter we follow closely the sequence of the previous chapter. The regression model is considered first, followed by a discussion of the correlation model. In considering the regression model, the following points are covered: a description of the model, methods for obtaining the regression equation, evaluation of the equation, and the uses that may be made of the equation. In both models the possible inferential procedures and their underlying assumptions are discussed.

9.2 THE MULTIPLE REGRESSION MODEL

In the multiple regression model we assume that a linear relationship exists between some variable Y, which we call the dependent variable, and k independent variables, $X_1, X_2, \ldots, X_k$. The independent variables are sometimes referred to as *explanatory variables*, because of their use in explaining the variation in Y, and *predictor variables*, because of their use in predicting Y.

The accompanying assumptions are as follows.

1. The X_i are nonrandom (fixed) variables. This assumption distinguishes the multiple regression model from the multiple correlation model, which will be presented in Section 9.6. This condition indicates that any inferences which are drawn from sample data apply only to the set of X values observed and not to some larger collection of X's. Under the regression model, correlation analysis is not meaningful. Under the correlation model to be presented later, the regression techniques that follow may be applied.
2. For each set of X_i values there is a subpopulation of Y values. To construct certain confidence intervals and test hypotheses, it must be known, or the researcher must be willing to assume that these subpopulations of Y values are normally distributed. Since we will want to demonstrate these inferential procedures, the assumption of normality will be made in the examples and exercises in this chapter.
3. The variances of the subpopulations of Y are all equal.
4. The Y values are independent. That is, the values of Y selected for one set of X values do not depend on the values of Y selected at another set of X values.

These assumptions may be stated in more compact fashion as

$$y_j = \beta_0 + \beta_1 x_{1j} + \beta_2 x_{2j} + \cdots + \beta_k x_{kj} + e_j \tag{9.2.1}$$

where y_j is a typical value from one of the subpopulations of Y values, the β_i are called the regression coefficients, $x_{1j}, x_{2j}, \ldots, x_{kj}$ are, respectively, particular values of the independent variables $X_1, X_2, \ldots, X_k$, and e_j is a random variable with mean 0 and variance σ^2, the common variance of the subpopulations of Y values. To construct confidence intervals for and test hypotheses about the regression coefficients, we assume that the e_j are normally and independently distributed. The statements regarding e_j are a consequence of the assumptions regarding the distributions of Y values. We will refer to Equation 9.2.1 as the *multiple regression model.*

When Equation 9.2.1 consists of one dependent variable and two independent variables, that is, when the model is written

$$y_j = \beta_0 + \beta_1 x_{1j} + \beta_2 x_{2j} + e_j \tag{9.2.2}$$

a *plane* in three-dimensional space may be fitted to the data points as illustrated in Figure 9.2.1. When the model contains more than two independent variables, it is described geometrically as a *hyperplane.*

In Figure 9.2.1 the observer should visualize some of the points as being located above the plane and some as being located below the plane. The deviation of a point from the plane is represented by

$$e_j = y_j - \beta_0 - \beta_1 x_{1j} - \beta_2 x_{2j} \tag{9.2.3}$$

In Equation 9.2.2, β_0 represents the point where the plane cuts the Y-axis, that is, it represents the Y-intercept of the plane. β_1 measures the average change in Y for a unit increase in X_1 when X_2 remains unchanged, and β_2 measures the average change in Y for a unit increase in X_2 when X_1 remains unchanged. For this reason β_1 and β_2 are referred to as *partial regression coefficients.*

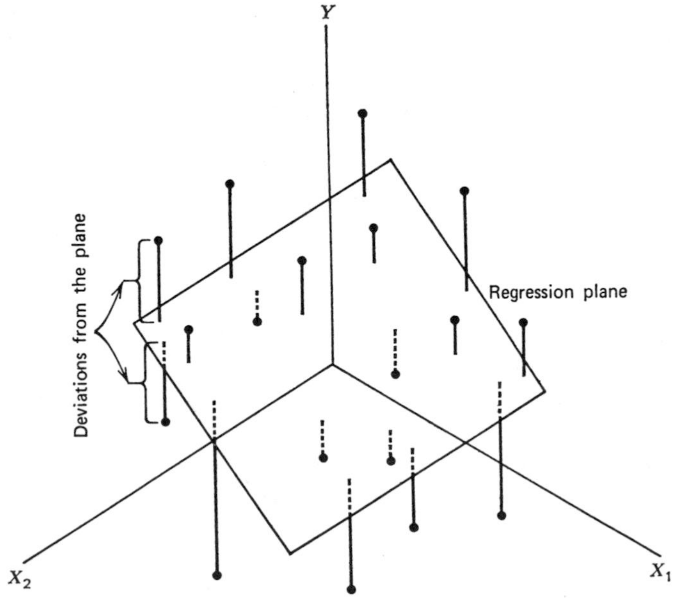

Figure 9.2.1 Multiple regression plane and scatter of points.

9.3 OBTAINING THE MULTIPLE REGRESSION EQUATION

Unbiased estimates of the parameters, $\beta_0, \beta_1, \ldots, \beta_k$ of the model specified in Equation 9.2.1 are obtained by the method of least squares. This means that the sum of the squared deviations of the observed values of Y from the resulting regression surface is minimized. In the three-variable case, as illustrated in Figure 9.2.1, the sum of the squared deviations of the observations from the plane are a minimum when β_0, β_1, and β_2 are estimated by the method of least squares. In other words, by the method of least squares, sample estimates of $\beta_0, \beta_1, \ldots, \beta_k$ are selected in such a way that the quantity

$$\sum e_j^2 = \sum (y_j - \beta_0 x_{1j} - \beta_1 x_{2j} - \cdots - \beta x_{kj})$$

is minimized. This quantity, referred to as the sum of squares of the residuals may also be written as

$$\sum (y_j - y_c)^2 \tag{9.3.1}$$

indicating the fact that the sum of squares of deviations of the observed values of Y from the values of Y calculated from the estimated equation is minimized.

Estimates, $b_0, b_1, b_2, \ldots, b_k$, of the regression coefficients are obtained by solving the following set of normal equations:

$$\left.\begin{array}{l}
nb_0 + b_1\sum x_{1j} + b_2\sum x_{2j} + \cdots + b_k\sum x_{kj} = \sum y_j \\
b_0\sum x_{1j} + b_1\sum x_{1j}^2 + b_2\sum x_{1j}x_{2j} + \cdots + b_k\sum x_{1j}x_{kj} = \sum x_{1j}y_j \\
b_0\sum x_{2j} + b_1\sum x_{2j}x_{1j} + b_2\sum x_{2j}^2 + \cdots + b_k\sum x_{2j}x_{kj} = \sum x_{2j}y_j \\
\cdots \quad \cdots \quad \cdots \quad \cdots \quad \cdots \quad \cdots \quad \cdots \quad \cdots \quad \cdots \\
b_0\sum x_{kj} + b_1\sum x_{kj}x_{1j} + b_2\sum x_{kj}x_{2j} + \cdots + b_k\sum x_{kj}^2 = \sum x_{kj}y_j
\end{array}\right\} \tag{9.3.2}$$

Let us illustrate the calculation of the estimated regression equation and its uses for the case where we have one dependent variable and two independent variables.

When the model contains only two independent variables, the sample regression equation is

$$y_{cj} = b_0 + b_1 x_{1j} + b_2 x_{2j} \tag{9.3.3}$$

Example 9.3.1

In a study of length of stay of patients in a chronic disease hospital researchers wished to see how well they could predict length of stay (Y) given the independent variables number of previous admissions (X_1) and age (X_2). The data shown in Table 9.3.1 were obtained for a sample of $n = 15$ patients.

To obtain the least-squares equation, the following normal equations must be solved for the sample regression coefficients:

$$\left.\begin{array}{l}
nb_0 + b_1\sum x_{1j} + b_2\sum x_{2j} = \sum y_j \\
b_0\sum x_{1j} + b_1\sum x_{1j}^2 + b_2\sum x_{1j}x_{2j} = \sum x_{1j}y_j \\
b_0\sum x_{2j} + b_1\sum x_{1j}x_{2j} + b_2\sum x_{2j}^2 = \sum x_{2j}y_j
\end{array}\right\} \tag{9.3.4}$$

Table 9.3.1

Length of Stay in Days, Age in Years, and Number of Previous Admissions, 15 Patients Admitted to a Chronic Disease Hospital

Length of Stay (Y)	**Number of Previous Admissions** (X_1)	**Age** (X_2)
15	0	21
15	0	18
21	0	22
28	1	24
30	1	25
35	1	25
40	1	26
35	2	34
30	2	25
45	2	38
50	3	44
60	3	51
45	4	39
60	4	54
50	5	55

Note that the number of equations is equal to the number of parameters to be estimated. We may solve the three equations as they stand or we may reduce them to a set of two equations by transforming each value into a deviation from its mean. If we designate these deviations by y'_j, x'_{1j}, and x'_{2j}, we have

$$\left.\begin{aligned} y'_j &= y_j - \bar{y} \\ x'_{1j} &= x_{1j} - \bar{x}_1 \\ x'_{2j} &= x_{2j} - \bar{x}_2 \end{aligned}\right\} \tag{9.3.5}$$

If we restate the original sample regression equation (Equation 9.3.3) in terms of these transformations, we have

$$y'_{cj} = b'_0 + b'_1 x'_{1j} + b'_2 x'_{2j} \tag{9.3.6}$$

where b'_0, b'_1, and b'_2 are appropriate coefficients for the transformed variables. The relationship between the two sets of coefficients can be determined by substituting the deviations from the means of the original variables into Equation 9.3.6 and then simplifying. Thus,

$$y_{cj} - \bar{y} = b'_0 + b'_1(x_{1j} - \bar{x}_1) + b'_2(x_{2j} - \bar{x}_2)$$

$$y_{cj} = \bar{y} + b'_0 + b'_1 x_{1j} - b'_1\bar{x}_1 + b'_2 x_{2j} - b'_2\bar{x}_2$$

$$y_{cj} = b'_0 + \bar{y} - b'_1\bar{x}_1 - b'_2\bar{x}_2 + b'_1 x_{1j} + b'_2 x_{2j} \tag{9.3.7}$$

When we set the coefficients of like terms in Equation 9.3.3 and 9.3.7, equal to each other, we obtain

$$b_1 = b'_1$$
$$b_2 = b'_2$$

and, therefore,

$$b_0 = b'_0 + \bar{y} - b'_1\bar{x}_1 - b'_2\bar{x}_2 = b'_0 + \bar{y} - b_1\bar{x}_1 - b_2\bar{x}_2 \qquad (9.3.8)$$

A new set of normal equations based on Equation 9.3.6 is

$$nb'_0 + b'_1\sum x'_{1j} + b'_2\sum x'_{2j} = \sum y'_j$$
$$b'_0\sum x'_{1j} + b'_1\sum x'^2_{1j} + b'_2\sum x'_{1j}x'_{2j} = \sum x'_{1j}y_j$$
$$b'_0\sum x'_{2j} + b'_1\sum x'_{1j}x'_{2j} + b'_2\sum x'^2_{2j} = \sum x'_{2j}y_j$$

Using the transformations from Equation 9.3.5, and the property that $\sum(x_i - \bar{x}) = 0$, we obtain

$$nb'_0 + b'_1(0) + b'_2(0) = 0$$
$$b'_0(0) + b'_1\sum(x_{1j} - \bar{x}_1)^2 + b'_2\sum(x_{1j} - \bar{x}_1)(x_{2j} - \bar{x}_2) = \sum(x_{1j} - \bar{x}_1)(y_j - \bar{y})$$
$$b'_0(0) + b'_1\sum(x_{1j} - \bar{x}_1)(x_{2j} - \bar{x}_2) + b'_2\sum(x_{2j} - \bar{x}_2)^2 = \sum(x_{2j} - \bar{x}_2)(y_j - \bar{y})$$

Note that $b'_0 = 0$. Thus by Equation 9.3.8

$$b_0 = \bar{y} - b_1\bar{x}_1 - b_2\bar{x}_2$$

and when we substitute b_1 and b_2 for b'_1 and b'_2, respectively, our normal equations collapse to the following.

$$\left.\begin{aligned} b_1\sum x'^2_{1j} + b_2\sum x'_{1j}x'_{2j} &= \sum x'_{1j}y'_j \\ b_1\sum x'_{1j}x'_{2j} + b_2\sum x'^2_{2j} &= \sum x'_{2j}y'_j \end{aligned}\right\} \qquad (9.3.9)$$

Table 9.3.2 contains the sums of squares and cross products of the original values necessary for computing the sums of squares and cross products of y'_j, x'_{1j}, and x'_{2j}.

Using the data in Table 9.3.2, we compute

$$\sum x'^2_{1j} = \sum(x_{1j} - \bar{x}_1)^2 = \sum x_{1j}{}^2 - (\sum x_{1j})^2/n$$
$$= 91 - (29)^2/15 = 34.93$$

$$\sum x'^2_{2j} = \sum(x_{2j} - \bar{x}_2)^2 = \sum x_{2j}{}^2 - (\sum x_{2j})^2/n$$
$$= 18{,}975 - (501)^2/15 = 2241.60$$

$$\sum x'_{1j}x'_{2j} = \sum(x_{1j} - \bar{x}_1)(x_{2j} - \bar{x}_2) = \sum x_{1j}x_{2j} - \sum x_{1j}\sum x_{2j}/n$$
$$= 1226 - (29)(501)/15 = 257.40$$

$$\sum x'_{1j}y'_j = \sum(x_{1j} - \bar{x}_1)(y_j - \bar{y}) = \sum x_{1j}y_j - \sum x_{1j}\sum y_j/n$$
$$= 1353 - (29)(559)/15 = 272.27$$

$$\sum x'_{2j}y'_j = \sum(x_{2j} - \bar{x}_2)(y_j - \bar{y}) = \sum x_{2j}y_j - \sum x_{2j}\sum y_j/n$$
$$= 21{,}039 - (501)(559)/15 = 2368.40$$

Table 9.3.2

Sums of Squares and Sums of Cross Products for Example 9.3.1

	y_j	x_{1j}	x_{2j}	$x_{1j}x_{2j}$	$x_{1j}y_j$	$x_{2j}y_j$	x_{1j}^2	x_{2j}^2	y_j^2
	15	0	21	0	0	315	0	441	225
	15	0	18	0	0	270	0	324	225
	21	0	22	0	0	462	0	484	441
	28	1	24	24	28	672	1	576	784
	30	1	25	25	30	750	1	625	900
	35	1	25	25	35	875	1	625	1225
	40	1	26	26	40	1040	1	676	1600
	35	2	34	68	70	1190	4	1156	1225
	30	2	25	50	60	750	4	625	900
	45	2	38	76	90	1710	4	1444	2025
	50	3	44	132	150	2200	9	1936	2500
	60	3	51	153	180	3060	9	2601	3600
	45	4	39	156	180	1755	16	1521	2025
	60	4	54	216	240	3240	16	2916	3600
	50	5	55	275	250	2750	25	3025	2500
Totals	559	29	501	1,226	1,353	21,039	91	18,975	23,775
Means	37.27	1.93	33.40						

When we substitute these values into Equations 9.3.9, we have

$$\left.\begin{aligned} 34.93b_1 + 257.40b_2 &= 272.27 \\ 257.40b_1 + 2241.60b_2 &= 2368.40 \end{aligned}\right\} \qquad (9.3.10)$$

These equations may be solved by any standard method to obtain

$$b_1 = .06$$
$$b_2 = 1.05$$

We obtain b_0 from the relationship:

$$b_0 = \bar{y} - b_1\bar{x}_1 - b_2\bar{x}_2 \qquad (9.3.11)$$

For our example, we have

$$\begin{aligned} b_0 &= 37.27 - (.06)(1.93) - (1.05)(33.40) \\ &= 2.08 \end{aligned}$$

Our sample multiple regression equation, then, is

$$y_c = 2.08 + .06x_{1j} + 1.05x_{2j} \qquad (9.3.12)$$

We have used an example containing only three variables for simplicity. As the number of variables increases, the algebraic manipulations and arithmetic calculations become more tedious and subject to error, although they are natural extensions of the procedures given in the present example.

Snedecor and Cochran (1) and Steel and Torrie (2) give numerical examples for four variables, and Anderson and Bancroft (3) illustrate the calculations involved when there are five variables. The techniques used by these authors are applicable for any number of variables.

Fortunate are researchers who, finding it necessary to employ the techniques of multiple regression analysis, have access to an electronic computer and ready-made programs that will handle a large number of variables. They can forget about the algebraic and arithmetic complexities of their problems and concentrate on the evaluation of the adequacy of their models and the interpretation of their results.

After the multiple regression equation has been obtained, the next step involves its evaluation and interpretation. It is this facet of the analysis that is covered in the next section.

Exercises

Obtain the regression equation for each of the following sets of data.

9.3.1. In a study designed to discover what factors might be related to birth weight, the following data were obtained on 10 new born babies.

Birth Weight in Grams (Y)	Socioeconomic Status Score (X_1)	Birth Order (X_2)
1361	8	4
1588	7	3
1815	4	4
2087	5	3
2268	5	2
2404	4	2
3402	3	2
3629	3	1
3765	2	1
4083	1	1
26402	42	23

$\sum x_{1j}^2 = 218$ $\quad \sum x_{2j}^2 = 65$ $\quad \sum y_j^2 = 78{,}536{,}258$

$\sum x_{1j}x_{2j} = 114$ $\quad \sum x_{1j}y_j = 93{,}361$ $\quad \sum x_{2j}y_j = 51{,}354$

9.3.2. A researcher collected the following data on 15 children.

Intelligence Score (Y)	Birth Order (X_1)	Mother's Age at Birth of Child (X_2)
110	1	25
115	1	24
120	1	22
118	1	24
110	2	20
108	2	20
105	2	20
104	3	24
98	3	25
99	4	30
98	4	24
100	5	29
90	5	30
93	5	30
90	6	28
Totals 1558	45	375

$\sum x_{1j}^2 = 177$ $\quad\sum x_{2j}^2 = 9563$ $\quad\sum y_j^2 = 163{,}112$

$\sum x_{1j}x_{2j} = 1191$ $\quad\sum x_{1j}y_j = 4458$ $\quad\sum x_{2j}y_j = 38{,}620$

9.3.3. In a study of factors thought to be related to admission patterns to a large general hospital, a hospital administrator obtained these data on ten communities in the hospital's catchment area:

Community	Persons per 1000 Population Admitted During Study Period (Y)	Index of Availability of Other Health Services (X_1)	Index of Indigency (X_2)
1	61.6	6.0	6.3
2	53.2	4.4	5.5
3	65.5	9.1	3.6
4	64.9	8.1	5.8
5	72.7	9.7	6.8
6	52.2	4.8	7.9
7	50.2	7.6	4.2
8	44.0	4.4	6.0
9	53.8	9.1	2.8
10	53.5	6.7	6.7
Total	571.6	69.9	55.6

$\sum x_{1j}^2 = 525.73$ $\sum x_{2j}^2 = 331.56$ $\sum y_j^2 = 33{,}349.92$

$\sum x_{1j}x_{2j} = 374.31$ $\sum x_{1j}y_j = 4104.32$ $\sum x_{2j}y_j = 3183.57$

9.3.4. The administrator of a general hospital obtained the following data on 20 surgery patients during a study to determine what factors appear to be related to length of stay.

	Postoperative Length of Stay in Days (Y)	Number of Current Medical Problems (X_1)	Preoperative Length of Stay in Days (X_2)
	6	1	1
	6	2	1
	11	2	2
	9	1	3
	16	3	3
	16	1	5
	4	1	1
	8	3	1
	11	2	2
	13	3	2
	13	1	4
	9	1	2
	17	3	3
	17	2	4
	12	4	1
	6	1	1
	5	1	1
	12	3	2
	8	1	2
	9	2	2
Total	208	38	43

$\sum x_{1j}^2 = 90$ $\sum x_{2j}^2 = 119$ $\sum y_j^2 = 2478$

$\sum x_{1j}x_{2j} = 79$ $\sum x_{1j}y_j = 430$ $\sum x_{2j}y_j = 519$

9.3.5. Refer to Exercise 8.7.5. Additional information on the score made by each nurse on an aptitude test, taken at the time of entering nursing school, was made available to the researcher. The complete data are as follows.

State Board Score (Y)	Final Score (X_1)	Aptitude Test Score (X_2)
440	87	92
480	87	79
535	87	99
460	88	91
525	88	84
480	89	71
510	89	78
530	89	78
545	89	71
600	89	76
495	90	89
545	90	90
575	90	73
525	91	71
575	91	81
600	91	84
490	92	70
510	92	85
575	92	71
540	93	76
595	93	90
525	94	94
545	94	94
600	94	93
625	94	73
Total 13,425	2263	2053
$\sum x_{1j}^2 = 204{,}977$	$\sum x_{2j}^2 = 170{,}569$	$\sum y_j^2 = 7{,}264{,}525$
$\sum x_{1j}x_{2j} = 185{,}838$	$\sum x_{1j}y_j = 1{,}216{,}685$	$\sum x_{2j}y_j = 1{,}101{,}220$

9.4 EVALUATING THE MULTIPLE REGRESSION EQUATION

Before one makes use of a multiple regression equation, it is desirable to determine first whether it is, in fact, worth using. In our study of simple linear regression we have learned that the usefulness of a regression equation may be evaluated by a consideration of the sample coefficient of determination and estimated slope. In evaluating our multiple regression equation we focus our attention on the *coefficient of multiple determination* and the partial regression coefficients.

The Coefficient of Multiple Determination. In Chapter 8 the coefficient of determination is discussed in considerable detail. The concept extends logically to the multiple regression case. The total variation present in the Y values may be partitioned into two components—the explained variation, which measures the amount of the total variation that is explained by the fitted regression surface, and the unexplained variation, which is that part of the total variation not explained by fitting the regression surface. The measure of variation in each case is a sum of squared deviations. The total variation is the sum of squared deviations of each observation of Y from the mean of the observations and is designated by $\sum(y_j - \bar{y})^2$. The explained variation, designated by $\sum(y_c - \bar{y})^2$, is the sum of squared deviations of the calculated values from the mean of the observed Y values. This sum of squared deviations is sometimes called the *sum of squares due to regression.* The unexplained variation, written as $\sum(y_j - y_c)^2$, is the sum of squared deviations of the original observations from the calculated values. This quantity is sometimes referred to as the *sum of squares about regression.* We may summarize the relationship among the three sums of squares with the following equation:

$$\sum(y_j - \bar{y})^2 = \sum(y_c - \bar{y})^2 + \sum(y_j - y_c)^2 \qquad (9.4.1)$$

$$SS_{\text{total}} = SS_{\text{explained}} + SS_{\text{unexplained}}$$

total sum of squares = explained sum of squares
+ unexplained sum of squares

The total, explained, and unexplained sum of squares are computed as follows:

$$SS_{\text{total}} = \sum(y_j - \bar{y})^2 = \sum y_j^2 - (\sum y_j)^2/n \qquad (9.4.2)$$

$$\begin{aligned} SS_{\text{explained}} &= \sum(y_c - \bar{y})^2 \\ &= b_1\sum x'_{1j}y'_j + b_2\sum x'_{2j}y'_j + \cdots + b_k\sum x'_{kj}y'_j \end{aligned} \qquad (9.4.3)$$

$$SS_{\text{unexplained}} = SS_{\text{total}} - SS_{\text{explained}} \qquad (9.4.4)$$

For our illustrative example we have (using data from Table 9.3.2 and some previous calculations)

$$SS_{\text{total}} = 23{,}775 - (559)^2/15 = 2942.93$$

$$SS_{\text{explained}} = (.06)(272.27) + (1.05)(2368.40) = 2503.16$$

$$SS_{\text{unexplained}} = 2942.93 - 2503.16 = 439.77$$

The coefficient of multiple determination, $R^2_{y.12\ldots k}$, is obtained by dividing the explained sum of squares by the total sum of squares. That is,

$$R^2_{y.12\ldots k} = \frac{\sum(y_c - \bar{y})^2}{\sum(y_j - \bar{y})^2} \tag{9.4.5}$$

The subscript $y.12\ldots k$ indicates that in the analysis Y is treated as the dependent variable and the X variables from X_1 through X_k are treated as the independent variables. The value of $R^2_{y.12\ldots k}$ indicates what proportion of the total variation in the observed Y values is explained by the regression of Y on $X_1, X_2, \ldots, X_k$. In other words, we may say that $R^2_{y.12\ldots k}$ is a measure of the goodness of fit of the regression surface. This quantity is analogous to r^2, which was computed in Chapter 8.

For our present example we have

$$R^2_{y.12} = \frac{2503.16}{2942.93} = .85$$

We say that 85 percent of the total variation in the Y values is explained by the fitted regression plane.

To determine whether the overall regression is significant, we may perform an analysis of variance. In doing this we are testing the null hypothesis that $\beta_1 = \beta_2 = \cdots = \beta_k = 0$, that is, that all the independent variables are of no value in explaining the variation in the Y values. The general ANOVA table is shown as Table 9.4.1. In Table 9.4.1, MSR stands for mean square due to regression and MSE stands for mean square about regression or, as it is sometimes called, the error mean square.

For our illustrative example the analysis of variance is shown in Table 9.4.2.

When we consult Table J with 2 and 12 degrees of freedom we find that our computed V. R. of 34.15 is significant at the .005 level (that is, $p < .005$). We conclude, therefore, that the regression explains a significant proportion

Table 9.4.1

ANOVA Table for Multiple Regression

Source	*SS*	**d. f.**	*MS*	**V. R.**
Due to regression	$SS_{\text{explained}}$	k	$MSR = SS_{\text{explained}}/k$	MSR/MSE
About regression	$SS_{\text{unexplained}}$	$n - k - 1$	$MSE = SS_{\text{unexplained}}/(n - k - 1)$	
Total	SS_{total}	$n - 1$		

Table 9.4.2

ANOVA Table, Example 9.3.1

Source	*SS*	d. f.	*MS*	V. R.
Due to regression	2503.16	2	1251.58	34.15
About regression	439.77	12	36.65	
Total	2942.93	14		

of the total variation in Y. In other words, we conclude that the fitted plane provides a good fit to the data.

Inferences Regarding Individual β's. An alternative procedure for evaluating the strength of the linear relationship between Y and the independent variables is to test the null hypothesis that $\beta_i = 0$ against the alternative $\beta_i \neq 0$ $(i = 1, 2, \ldots, k)$. The validity of this procedure rests on the assumptions stated earlier: that for each combination of X_i values there is a normally distributed subpopulation of Y values with variance σ^2. When these assumptions hold true, it can be shown that each of the sample estimates, b_i, are normally distributed with mean β_i and variance $c_{ii}\sigma^2$. Since σ^2 is unknown, it will have to be estimated. An estimate is provided by the mean square about regression which is shown in the ANOVA table. We may designate this quantity generally as $s^2_{y.12\ldots k}$. For our particular example we have, from Table 9.4.2, $s^2_{y.12} = 36.65$, and $s_{y.12} = 6.05$. We must digress briefly at this point, however, to explain the computation of c_{ii}.

Computation of the c_{ii}. The c_{ii} values are called *Gauss multipliers*. For those familiar with matrix algebra it may be enlightening to point out that they may be obtained by inverting the matrix of sums of squares and cross products that can be constructed by using the left-hand terms of the normal equations given in Equation 9.3.5. The c's may be found without the use of matrix algebra by solving the following two sets of equations:

$$\left.\begin{aligned} c_{11}\sum x'^2_{1j} + c_{12}\sum x'_{1j}x'_{2j} &= 1 \\ c_{11}\sum x'_{1j}x'_{2j} + c_{12}\sum x'^2_{2j} &= 0 \end{aligned}\right\} \qquad (9.4.6)$$

$$\left.\begin{aligned} c_{21}\sum x'^2_{1j} + c_{22}\sum x'_{1j}x'_{2j} &= 0 \\ c_{21}\sum x'_{1j}x'_{2j} + c_{22}\sum x'^2_{2j} &= 1 \end{aligned}\right\} \qquad (9.4.7)$$

In the above equations $c_{12} = c_{21}$. Note also that the sums of squares and cross products are the same as those in the normal equations (Equation 9.3.5).

When the analysis involves more than two independent variables, the c's are obtained by expanding Equations 9.4.6 and 9.4.7 so that there is one set of equations for each independent variable. Each set of equations also contains as many individual equations as there are independent variables. The 1 is placed to the right of the equal sign in all equations containing a term of the form $c_{ii}\sum x_i'^2$. For example, in Equation 9.4.6, a 1 is to the right of the equal sign in the equation containing $c_{11}\sum x_{1j}'^2$. Ezekiel and Fox (4) have written out the equations for the case of three independent variables, and they, as well as Snedecor and Cochran (1), Steel and Torrie (2), and Anderson and Bancroft (3) demonstrate the use of the abbreviated Doolittle Method (5) of obtaining the c's as well as the regression coefficients. Anderson and Bancroft (3) give a numerical example for four independent variables.

When we substitute data from our illustrative example into Equations 9.4.6 and 9.4.7, we have

$$\left.\begin{aligned} 34.93c_{11} + 257.40c_{12} &= 1 \\ 257.40c_{11} + 2241.60c_{12} &= 0 \end{aligned}\right\}$$

$$\left.\begin{aligned} 34.93c_{21} + 257.40c_{22} &= 0 \\ 257.40c_{21} + 2241.60c_{22} &= 1 \end{aligned}\right\}$$

The solution of these equations yields

$$c_{11} = .1861$$

$$c_{12} = c_{21} = -.0213711$$

$$c_{22} = .0029001$$

We may now return to the problem of inference procedures regarding the individual partial regression coefficients. To test the null hypothesis that β_i is equal to some particular value, say β_{i0}, the following t statistic may be computed:

$$t = \frac{b_i - \beta_{i0}}{s_{bi}} \tag{9.4.8}$$

where the degrees of freedom are equal to $n - k - 1$, and

$$s_{bi} = s_{y.12\ldots k}\sqrt{c_{ii}} \tag{9.4.9}$$

The standard error of the difference between two partial regression coefficients is given by

$$s_{(bi-bj)} = \sqrt{s_{y.12\ldots k}^2(c_{ii} + c_{jj} - 2c_{ij})} \tag{9.4.10}$$

so that we may test $H_0: \beta_i = \beta_j$ by computing

$$t = \frac{b_i - b_j}{s_{(bi-bj)}} \tag{9.4.11}$$

which has $n - k - 1$ degrees of freedom. Confidence intervals for β_i and $\beta_i - \beta_j$ may be constructed in the usual way by using a value from the t distribution for the reliability factor and standard errors given above.

For our hospital length of stay example let us test the null hypothesis that number of previous admissions is irrelevant in predicting length of hospital stay. We proceed as follows:

$$H_0\colon \beta_1 = 0$$
$$H_A\colon \beta_1 \neq 0$$
$$\text{Let } \alpha = .05$$

$$t = \frac{b_1 - 0}{s_{b_1}} = \frac{.06}{6.05\sqrt{.1861}} = \frac{.06}{2.609928} = .023$$

The null hypothesis is not rejected, since the computed value of t, .023, is between -2.1788 and $+2.1788$, the critical values of t for a two-sided test when $\alpha = .05$ and the degrees of freedom are 12. We conclude, then, that there may not be a significant linear relationship between Y and X_1 when X_2 is held constant. At least these data do not provide evidence for such a relationship. In other words, the data of the present sample do not provide sufficient evidence to indicate that number of previous admissions, when used in a regression equation along with age, is a useful variable in predicting length of hospital stay. [For this test, $p > 2(.10) = .20$.]

Now, let us perform a similar test for the second partial regression coefficient, β_2.

$$H_0\colon \beta_2 = 0$$
$$H_A\colon \beta_2 \neq 0$$
$$\alpha = .05$$

$$t = \frac{b_2 - 0}{s_{b_2}} = \frac{1.05}{6.05\sqrt{.0029001}} = \frac{1.05}{.325808} = 3.223$$

In this case the null hypothesis is rejected, since 3.223 is greater than 2.1788. We conclude that there is a linear relationship between X_2 and Y when X_1 is held constant, and that age, used in this manner, is a useful variable for predicting length of hospital stay. [For this test, $p < 2(.005) = .01$.]

When the researcher has been led to conclude that a partial regression coefficient is not 0, he or she may be interested in obtaining an interval for this β_i. A $100(1 - \alpha)$ percent confidence interval for a β_i is given by

$$b_i \pm t_{(1-\alpha/2,\, n-k-1)} s_{y.12\ldots k}\sqrt{c_{ii}}$$

For our illustrative example we may compute the following 95 percent confidence interval for β_2:

$$1.05 \pm (2.1788)(6.05)\sqrt{.0029001}$$
$$1.05 \pm .71$$
$$.34,\ 1.76$$

We may give this interval the usual probabilistic and practical interpretations. We are 95 percent confident that β_2 is contained in the interval from .34 to

1.76 since, in repeated sampling, 95 percent of the intervals that may be constructed in this manner will include the true parameter.

One should be aware of the problems involved in carrying out multiple hypothesis tests and constructing multiple confidence intervals from the same sample data. The effect on α of performing multiple hypothesis tests from the same data is discussed in Section 7.6. A similar problem arises when one wishes to construct confidence intervals for two or more partial regression coefficients. The intervals will not be independent, so that the tabulated confidence coefficient does not, in general apply. In other words, all such intervals would not be $100(1 - \alpha)$ percent confidence intervals. Durand (6) gives a procedure that may be followed when confidence intervals for more than one partial regression coefficient are desired.

Another problem sometimes encountered in the application of multiple regression is an apparent incompatibility in the results of the various tests of significance that one may perform. In a given problem for a given level of significance, one or the other of the following situations may be observed.

1. R^2 and all b_i significant.
2. R^2 and some but not all b_i significant.
3. R^2 but none of the b_i significant.
4. All b_i significant but not R^2.
5. Some b_i significant, but not all nor R^2.
6. Neither R^2 nor any b_i significant.

Geary and Leser (7) identify these six situations, and after pointing out that situations 1 and 6 present no problem (since they both imply compatible results), discuss each of the other situations in some detail.

Notice that situation 2 exists in our illustrative example where we have a significant R^2 but only one out of two significant regression coefficients. Geary and Leser (7) point out that this situation is very common, especially when a large number of independent variables have been included in the regression equation, and that the only problem is to decide whether or not to eliminate from the analysis one or more of the variables associated with nonsignificant coefficients.

Exercises

9.4.1. Refer to Exercise 9.3.1. (a) Calculate the coefficient of multiple determination; (b) perform an analysis of variance; (c) test the significance of each b_i $(i > 0)$. Let $\alpha = .05$ for all tests of significance. Determine the p-value for all tests.

9.4.2. Refer to Exercise 9.3.2. Do the analysis suggested in 9.4.1.

9.4.3. Refer to Exercise 9.3.3. Do the analysis suggested in 9.4.1.

9.4.4. Refer to Exercise 9.3.4. Do the analysis suggested in 9.4.1.

9.4.5. Refer to Exercise 9.3.5. Do the analysis suggested in 9.4.1.

9.5 USING THE MULTIPLE REGRESSION EQUATION

As we learned in the previous chapter, a regression equation may be used to compute a particular value of Y, y_c, when given a particular value of X. Similarly we may use our multiple regression equation to obtain a y_c value when we are given particular values of the two or more X variables present in the equation.

Just as was the case in simple linear regression, we may, in multiple regression, interpret a y_c value in one of two ways. First we may interpret y_c as an estimate of the mean of the subpopulation of Y values assumed to exist for particular combinations of X_i values. Under this interpretation y_c is called an *estimate*, and when it is used for this purpose, the equation is thought of as an *estimating equation*. The second interpretation of y_c is that it is the value Y is most likely to assume for given values of the X_i. In this case y_c is called the *predicted value* of Y, and the equation is called a *prediction equation*. In both cases, intervals may be constructed about the y_c value when the assumptions of Section 9.2 hold true. When y_c is interpreted as an estimate of a population mean, the interval is called a *confidence interval*, and when y_c is interpreted as a predicted value of Y, the interval is called a *prediction interval*. Now let us see how each of these intervals is constructed.

The Confidence Interval for the Mean of a Subpopulation of Y Values Given Particular Values of the X_i**.** We have seen that a $100(1-\alpha)$ percent confidence interval for a parameter may be constructed by the general procedure of adding to and subtracting from the estimator, a quantity equal to the reliability factor corresponding to $1-\alpha$ multiplied by the standard error of the estimator. We have also seen that in the present situation our estimator is

$$y_c = b_0 + b_1 x_{1j} + b_2 x_{2j} + \cdots + b_k x_{kj} \tag{9.5.1}$$

The standard error of this estimator for the case of two independent variables, is given by

$$s_{y.12}\sqrt{\frac{1}{n} + c_{11}x_{1j}'^2 + c_{22}x_{2j}'^2 + 2c_{12}x_{1j}'x_{2j}'} \tag{9.5.2}$$

where x_{ij}' values are particular values of the X_i expressed as deviations from their mean. Expression 9.5.2. is easily generalized to any number of independent variables. See for example, Anderson and Bancroft (3). The $100(1-\alpha)$

percent confidence interval for the three-variable case, then, is as follows:

$$y_c \pm t_{(1-\alpha/2,n-k-1)}s_{y.12}\sqrt{\frac{1}{n}+c_{11}x_{1j}'^2+c_{22}x_{2j}'^2+2c_{12}x_{1j}'x_{2j}'} \qquad (9.5.3)$$

For our illustrative example, suppose we wish to estimate the mean length of stay for all 25-year-old patients with two previous admissions. In other words, given $x_{1j}=2$ and $x_{2j}=25$ what is our estimate of the mean of the corresponding subpopulation of Y values? To obtain a point estimate, we substitute $x_{1j}=2$ and $x_{2j}=25$ into Equation 9.3.8:

$$\begin{aligned} y_c &= 2.08 + .06(2) + 1.05(25) \\ &= 28.45 \end{aligned}$$

To compute the standard error we first obtain $x'_{1j}=(x_{1j}-\bar{x}_1)=(2-1.93)=.07$, and $x'_{2j}=(x_{2j}-\bar{x}_2)=(25-33.40)=-8.40$. Substituting these and other appropriate values into Expression 9.5.3 gives

$$28.45 \pm (2.1788)(6.05) \times \sqrt{\tfrac{1}{15}+(.1861)(.07)^2+(.0029001)(-8.40)^2+2(-.0213711)(.07)(-8.40)}$$

$$28.45 \pm 7.19$$

$$21.26,\ 35.64$$

We interpret this interval in the usual ways. We are 95 percent confident that the interval from 21.26 to 35.64 includes the mean of the subpopulation of Y values for the specified combination of X_i values, since this parameter would be included in about 95 percent of the intervals that can be constructed in the manner shown.

The Prediction Interval for a Particular Value of Y Given Particular Values of the X_i. When we interpret y_c as the value Y is most likely to assume when particular values of the X_i are observed, we may construct a prediction interval in the same way in which the confidence interval was constructed. The only difference in the two is the standard error. The standard error of the prediction is slightly larger than the standard error of the estimate, which causes the prediction interval to be wider than the confidence interval.

The standard error of the prediction for the three-variable case is given by

$$s_{y.12}\sqrt{1+\frac{1}{n}+c_{11}x_{1j}'^2+c_{22}x_{2j}'^2+2c_{12}x_{1j}'x_{2j}'} \qquad (9.5.3)$$

so that the $100(1-\alpha)$ percent prediction interval is

$$y_c \pm t_{(1-\alpha/2,n-k-1)}s_{y.12}\sqrt{1+\frac{1}{n}+c_{11}x_{1j}'^2+c_{22}x_{2j}'^2+2c_{12}x_{1j}'x_{2j}'} \qquad (9.5.4)$$

Suppose, for our illustrative example, a 25-year-old patient with two previous admissions is admitted. How long is that patient likely to stay? Our best point prediction is found by computing y_c. That is,

$$\begin{aligned} y_c &= 2.08 + .06(2) + 1.05(25) \\ &= 28.45 \end{aligned}$$

the same value obtained previously when we interpreted y_c as a point estimate of the subpopulation mean.

We may obtain the following 95 percent prediction interval by using Expression 9.5.4:

$$28.45 \pm (2.1788)(6.05)$$
$$\times \sqrt{1 + \tfrac{1}{15} + (.1861)(.07)^2 + (.0029001)(-8.40)^2 + 2(-.0213711)(.07)(-8.40)}$$
$$28.45 \pm 15.01$$
$$13.44, 43.46$$

We are 95 percent confident that this patient would remain in the hospital somewhere between 13.44 and 43.46 days.

Exercises

For each of the following exercises compute the y_c value and construct (a) 95 percent confidence, and (b) 95 percent prediction intervals for the specified values of X_i.

9.5.1. Refer to Exercise 9.3.1 and let $x_{1j} = 5$ and $x_{2j} = 3$.

9.5.2. Refer to Exercise 9.3.2 and let $x_{1j} = 2$ and $x_{2j} = 20$.

9.5.3. Refer to Exercise 9.3.3 and let $x_{1j} = 5$ and $x_{2j} = 6$.

9.5.4. Refer to Exercise 9.3.4 and let $x_{1j} = 1$ and $x_{2j} = 2$.

9.5.5. Refer to Exercise 9.3.5 and let $x_{1j} = 90$ and $x_{2j} = 80$.

9.6 THE CORRELATION MODEL

We pointed out in the preceding chapter that while regression analysis is concerned with the form of the relationship between variables, the objective of correlation analysis is to gain insight into the strength of the relationship. This is also true in the multivariable case, and in this section we investigate methods for measuring the strength of the relationship among several variables. First, however, let us define the model and assumptions on which our analysis rests.

We may write the correlation model as

$$y_j = \beta_0 + \beta_1 x_{1j} + \beta_2 x_{2j} + \cdots + \beta_k x_{kj} + e_j \tag{9.6.1}$$

Where y_j is a typical value from the population of values of the variable, Y, the β's are the regression coefficients defined in Section 9.2, the x_{ij} are particular (known) values of the random variables X_i. This model is similar to the multiple regression model, but there is one important distinction. In the multiple regression model, given in Equation 9.2.1, the X_i are nonrandom variables, but in the multiple correlation model the X_i are random variables. In other words, in the correlation model there is a joint distribution of Y and the X_i that we call a *multivariate distribution.* Under this model, the variables are no longer thought of as being dependent or independent, since logically they are interchangeable and either of the X_i may play the role of Y.

Typically random samples of units of association are drawn from a population of interest, and measurements of Y and the X_i are made.

A least-squares plane or hyperplane is fitted to the sample data by methods described in Section 9.3, and the same uses may be made of the resulting equation. Inferences may be made about the population from which the sample was drawn if it can be assumed that the underlying distribution is normal, that is, if it can be assumed that the joint distribution of Y and the X_i is a *multivariate normal distribution.* In addition, sample measures of the degree of the relationship among the variables may be computed and, under the assumption that sampling is from a multivariate normal distribution, the corresponding parameters may be estimated by means of confidence intervals, and hypothesis tests may be carried out. Specifically, we may compute an estimate of the *multiple correlation coefficient* that measures the dependence between Y and the X_i. This is a straightforward extension of the concept of correlation between two variables that we discuss in Chapter 8. We may also compute *partial correlation coefficients* that measure the intensity of the relationship between any two variables when the influence of all other variables has been removed.

To illustrate the concepts and techniques of correlation analysis, let us consider an example.

Example 9.6.1

The measurements shown in Table 9.6.1 were taken on 11 apparently normal males between the ages of 14 and 24 years. The researcher who gathered the data wished to investigate the nature and strength of the relationships among the three variables.

Table 9.6.1

Measurements Taken on 11 Apparently Normal Males Between the Ages of 14 and 24 Years

Serum Cholesterol, mg/100 cc (Y)	**Weight in Kilograms** (X_1)	**Systolic Blood Pressure** (X_2)
162.2	51.0	108
158.0	52.9	111
157.0	56.0	115
155.0	56.5	116
156.0	58.0	117
154.1	60.1	120
169.1	58.0	124
181.0	61.0	127
174.9	59.4	122
180.2	56.1	121
174.0	61.2	125

The Multiple Correlation Coefficient. As a first step in analyzing the relationships among the variables, we look at the multiple correlation coefficient.

The multiple correlation coefficient is the square root of the coefficient of determination and, consequently, the sample value may be computed by taking the square root of Equation 9.4.5. That is,

$$R_{y.12\ldots k} = \sqrt{R^2_{y.12\ldots k}} = \sqrt{\frac{\sum(y_c - \bar{y})^2}{\sum(y_j - \bar{y})^2}} \tag{9.6.2}$$

The numerator of the term under the radical in Equation 9.6.2, which is the explained sum of squares, is given by Equation 9.4.3, which we recall, contains b_1 and b_2, the sample partial regression coefficients. We compute these by the methods of Section 9.3.

First, the various sums, sums of squares, and sums of cross products must be computed. They are as follows:

$$\sum x_{1j} = 630.20 \qquad \sum x_{2j} = 1306.00 \qquad \sum y_j = 1821.50$$
$$\sum x_{1j}{}^2 = 36{,}209.68 \qquad \sum x_{2j}{}^2 = 155{,}410.00 \qquad \sum y_j{}^2 = 302{,}723.51$$
$$\sum x_{1j}x_{2j} = 74{,}995.80 \qquad \sum x_{1j}y_j = 104{,}485.19 \qquad \sum x_{2j}y_j = 216{,}682.00$$

When we compute the sums of squares and cross products of

$$y'_j = (y_j - \bar{y})$$
$$x'_{1j} = (x_{1j} - \bar{x}_1) \qquad \text{and} \qquad x'_{2j} = (x_{2j} - \bar{x}_2)$$

we have

$$\sum x'^2_{1j} = 36{,}209.68 - (630.20)^2/11 = 104.95$$
$$\sum x'^2_{2j} = 155{,}410.00 - (1306.00)^2/11 = 352.18$$
$$\sum y'^2_j = 302{,}723.51 - (1821.5)^2/11 = 1099.67$$
$$\sum x'_{1j}x'_{2j} = 74{,}995.8 - (630.20)(1306.00)/11 = 173.87$$
$$\sum x'_{1j}y'_j = 104{,}485.19 - (630.20)(1821.50)/11 = 129.80$$
$$\sum x'_{2j}y'_j = 216{,}682.00 - (1306.00)(1821.50)/11 = 420.27$$

The normal equations, by Equations 9.3.9, are

$$104.95b_1 + 173.87b_2 = 129.80$$
$$173.87b_1 + 352.18b_2 = 420.27$$

The simultaneous solution of these equations gives $b_1 = -4.06$, $b_2 = 3.20$. We obtain b_0 by substituting appropriate values into Equation 9.3.11:

$$b_0 = 165.59 - (-4.06)(57.29) - (3.20)(118.73) = 18.25$$

The least-squares equation, then, is

$$y_c = 18.25 - 4.06x_{1j} + 3.20x_{2j}$$

This equation may be used for estimation and prediction purposes and may be evaluated by the methods discussed in Section 9.4.

We now have the necessary quantities for computing the multiple correlation coefficient. We first compute the explained sum of squares by Equation 9.4.3:

$$SS_{\text{explained}} = (-4.06)(129.80) + (3.20)(420.27)$$
$$= 817.876$$

The total sum of squares by Equation 9.4.2 is

$$SS_{\text{total}} = 302{,}723.51 - (1821.5)^2/11$$
$$= 1{,}099.669$$

The coefficient of multiple determination, then, is

$$R^2_{y.12} = \frac{817.876}{1099.669} = .7437$$

and the multiple correlation coefficient is

$$R_{y.12} = \sqrt{.7437} = .86$$

We interpret $R_{y.12}$ as a measure of the correlation between serum cholesterol level, weight, and systolic blood pressure in our sample of apparently normal males between 14 and 24 years of age. If our data constitute a random sample from the population of such persons we may use $R_{y.12}$ as an estimate of $\rho_{y.12}$ the true population multiple correlation coefficient. We may also interpret $R_{y.12}$ as the simple correlation coefficient between y_i and y_c, respectively, the observed and calculated values of the "dependent" variable. Perfect correspondence between the observed and calculated values of Y will result in a correlation coefficient of 1, while a complete lack of a linear relationship between observed and calculated values yields a correlation coefficient of 0. The multiple correlation coefficient is always given a positive sign.

We may test the null hypothesis that $\rho_{y.12\ldots k} = 0$ by computing

$$F = \frac{R^2_{y.12\ldots k}}{1 - R^2_{y.12\ldots k}} \cdot \frac{n - k - 1}{k} \tag{9.6.3}$$

The numerical value obtained from Equation 9.6.3 is compared with the tabulated value of F with k and $n - k - 1$ degrees of freedom. The reader will recall that this is identical to the test of $H_0: \beta_1 = \beta_2 = \cdots = \beta_k = 0$ described in Section 9.4.

For our present example let us test the null hypothesis that $\rho_{y.12} = 0$ against the alternative that $\rho_{y.12} \neq 0$. We compute

$$F = \frac{.7437}{(1 - .7437)} \cdot \frac{(11 - 2 - 1)}{2} = 11.61$$

Since 11.61 is greater than 11.04, $p < .005$, so that we may reject the null hypothesis at the .005 level of significance and conclude that serum cholesterol level is linearly correlated with weight and systolic blood pressure in the sampled population.

Further comments on the significance of observed multiple correlation coefficients may be found in Ezekiel and Fox (4) who discuss a paper on the subject by R. A. Fisher (8) and present graphs for constructing confidence intervals when the number of variables is eight or less. Kramer (9) presents tables for constructing confidence limits when the number of variables is greater than eight.

Partial Correlation. The researcher may wish to have a measure of the strength of the linear relationship between two variables when the effect of the remaining variables has been removed. Such a measure is provided by the *partial correlation* coefficient. For example, the partial correlation coefficient $\rho_{y1.2}$ is a measure of the correlation between Y and X_1 when X_2 is held constant. By this we mean that only Y and X_1 are involved in the correlation.

The partial correlation coefficients may be computed from the *simple correlation coefficients.* The simple correlation coefficients measure the correlation between two variables when no effort has been made to control other variables. In other words, they are the coefficients for any pair of variables that would be obtained by the methods of simple correlation discussed in Chapter 8.

For three variables these simple correlation coefficients may be obtained:
r_{y1}, the simple correlation between Y and X_1
r_{y2}, the simple correlation between Y and X_2
r_{12}, the simple correlation between X_1 and X_2
These may be computed as follows:

$$r_{y1} = \sum x'_{1j}y'_j/\sqrt{\sum x'^2_{1j}\sum y'^2_j} \tag{9.6.4}$$

$$r_{y2} = \sum x'_{2j}y'_j/\sqrt{\sum x'^2_{2j}\sum y'^2_j} \tag{9.6.5}$$

$$r_{12} = \sum x'_{1j}x'_{2j}/\sqrt{\sum x'^2_{1j}\sum x'^2_{2j}} \tag{9.6.6}$$

For our illustrative example we may use previously computed quantities to obtain

$$r_{y1} = 129.80/\sqrt{(104.95)(1099.67)} = .382$$
$$r_{y2} = 420.27/\sqrt{(352.18)(1099.67)} = .675$$
$$r_{12} = 173.87/\sqrt{(104.95)(352.18)} = .904$$

The sample partial correlation coefficients that may be computed in the three-variable case are

1. The partial correlation between Y and X_1 when X_2 is held constant:

$$r_{y1.2} = (r_{y1} - r_{y2}r_{12})/\sqrt{(1 - r_{y2}^2)(1 - r_{12}^2)} \tag{9.6.7}$$

2. The partial correlation between Y and X_2 when X_1 is held constant:

$$r_{y2.1} = (r_{y2} - r_{y1}r_{12})/\sqrt{(1 - r_{y1}^2)(1 - r_{12}^2)} \tag{9.6.8}$$

3. The partial correlation between X_1 and X_2 when Y is held constant:

$$r_{12.y} = (r_{12} - r_{y1}r_{y2})/\sqrt{(1 - r_{y1}^2)(1 - r_{y2}^2)} \tag{9.6.9}$$

If we use the simple correlation coefficients already computed, we obtain the following partial correlation coefficients for our illustrative example:

$$r_{y1.2} = [.382 - (.675)(.904)]/\sqrt{(1 - .675^2)(1 - .904^2)} = -.723$$
$$r_{y2.1} = [.675 - (.382)(.904)]/\sqrt{(1 - .382^2)(1 - .904^2)} = .834$$
$$r_{12.y} = [.904 - (.382)(.675)]/\sqrt{(1 - .382^2)(1 - .675^2)} = .948$$

We may test the null hypothesis that the population partial correlation coefficient corresponding to any one of the above is 0 by means of the t test. For example, to test $H_0: \rho_{y1.2\ldots k} = 0$, we compute

$$t = r_{y1.2\ldots k}\sqrt{\frac{n - k - 1}{1 - r^2_{y1.2\ldots k}}} \tag{9.6.10}$$

which is distributed as Student's t with $n - k - 1$ degrees of freedom.

Let us illustrate the procedure for our current example by testing $H_0: \rho_{12.y} = 0$ against the alternative, $H_A: \rho_{12.y} \neq 0$. The computed t is

$$t = .948\sqrt{\frac{11 - 2 - 1}{1 - .948^2}}$$
$$= 8.425$$

Since the computed t of 8.425 is larger than the tabulated t of 3.5554 for 8 degrees of freedom and $\alpha = .01$, (two-sided test), we may reject H_0 at the .01 level of significance and conclude that there is a significant correlation between systolic blood pressure and weight when serum cholesterol level is held constant. Significance tests for the other two partial correlation coefficients will be left as an exercise for the reader.

Although our illustration of correlation analysis is limited to the three-variable case, the concepts and techniques extend logically to the case of four or more variables. The number and complexity of the calculations increases rapidly as the number of variables increases.

Exercises

9.6.1. The following data were obtained on 12 males between the ages of 12 and 18 years (all measurements are in centimeters):

	Height (Y)	Radius Length (X_1)	Femur Length (X_2)
	149.0	21.00	42.50
	152.0	21.79	43.70
	155.7	22.40	44.75
	159.0	23.00	46.00
	163.3	23.70	47.00
	166.0	24.30	47.90
	169.0	24.92	48.95
	172.0	25.50	49.90
	174.5	25.80	50.30
	176.1	26.01	50.90
	176.5	26.15	50.85
	179.0	26.30	51.10
Total	1992.1	290.87	573.85

$\sum x_{1j}^2 = 7087.6731$ $\quad \sum x_{2j}^2 = 27541.8575$ $\quad \sum y_j^2 = 331851.09$

$\sum x_{1j}x_{2j} = 13970.5835$ $\quad \sum x_{1j}y_j = 48492.886$ $\quad \sum x_{2j}y_j = 95601.09$

(a) Find the sample multiple correlation coefficient and test the null hypothesis that $\rho_{y.12} = 0$

(b) Find each of the partial correlation coefficients and test each for significance. Let $\alpha = .05$ for all tests.

(c) Determine the p-value for each test.

(d) State your conclusions.

9.6.2. The following data were collected on 15 obese girls.

Weight in Kilograms (Y)	Lean Body Weight (X_1)	Mean Daily Caloric Intake (X_2)
79.2	54.3	2670
64.0	44.3	820
67.0	47.8	1210
78.4	53.9	2678
66.0	47.5	1205
63.0	43.0	815
65.9	47.1	1200
63.1	44.0	1180
73.2	44.1	1850
66.5	48.3	1260
61.9	43.5	1170
72.5	43.3	1852
101.1	66.4	1790
66.2	47.5	1250
99.9	66.1	1789
Total 1087.9	741.1	22739

$\sum x_{1j}^2 = 37{,}439.95$ $\quad$ $\sum x_{2j}^2 = 39{,}161{,}759$ $\quad$ $\sum y_j^2 = 81{,}105.63$

$\sum x_{1j}x_{2j} = 1{,}154{,}225.2$ $\quad$ $\sum x_{1j}y_j = 55{,}021.31$ $\quad$ $\sum x_{2j}y_j = 1{,}707{,}725.3$

(a) Find the multiple correlation coefficient and test it for significance.
(b) Find each of the partial correlation coefficients and test each for significance. Let $\alpha = .05$ for all tests.
(c) Determine the p-value for each test.
(d) State your conclusions.

9.6.3. Refer to Exercise 9.3.5. Assume that the data fit the correlation model.
(a) Compute the multiple correlation coefficient and test it for significance.
(b) Compute each of the partial correlation coefficients and test each for significance. Let $\alpha = .05$ for all tests.
(c) Determine the p-value for each test.
(d) What are your conclusions?

9.6.4. Refer to Example 9.6.1. Test $r_{y1.2}$ and $r_{y2.1}$ for significance at the .05 level. Determine the p-value for each test.

9.7 CHOOSING THE INDEPENDENT VARIABLES FOR THE MULTIPLE REGRESSION EQUATION

One of the more troublesome problems in the use of multiple regression analysis is deciding what independent variables should be included in the equation. A final decision in most cases is the result of both statistical and nonstatistical considerations.

In the intial stages of determining the regression equation, the investigator will be guided by his knowledge of relevant variables and which ones are likely to be useful for prediction and estimation purposes. He or she will also take into account the relative costs and ease of obtaining measurements.

In this computer era the volume and complexity of calculations associated with a large number of variables do not pose the problem they once did. Even so, it is usually desirable (particularly from the point of view of cost and convenience of obtaining measurements) to include in the final equation fewer independent variables than are available. It is at this point that the investigator may employ statistical analysis as an aid to arriving at a decision. There are several procedures that can be followed. The most thorough, but also the most tedious and time-consuming method, even with the aid of a computer, is to regress Y on every subset of the X_i, that is, Y is regressed on each X, then on each pair of X's, then on each group of three X's, and so on. The best, according to some statistical criterion, of these regression equations will be the one selected unless some nonstatistical consideration such as cost necessitates a compromise. Because of the magnitude of the computations this method is not widely used.

A second approach, called the step-up or forward method, consists of introducing independent variables, one at a time, into the regression and at each stage statistically evaluating the "goodness" of the equation. The procedure continues until, according to some statistical criterion, a satisfactory equation is obtained.

A third method, called the step-down or backward method, is the reverse of the forward method. By this method the regression of Y on all X_i is carried out, and then independent variables are eliminated one at a time until a satisfactory equation has been obtained.

For a discussion of these and other methods for determining what independent variables to include in the analysis, refer to books and articles by Allen (10), Beale et al. (11), Draper and Smith (12), Garside (13), Gorman and Toman (14), Hocking and Leslie (15), Larson and Bancroft (16), Lindley (17), Schultz and Goggans (18), Smillie (19), Sprent (20), and Summerfield and Lubin (21).

9.8 SUMMARY

In this chapter we examine how the concepts and techniques of simple linear regression and correlation analysis are extended to the multiple-variable case. The least-squares method of obtaining the regression equation is presented and illustrated. This chapter also is concerned with the calculation of descriptive measures, tests of significance, and the uses to be made of the multiple regression equation. In addition, the methods and concepts of correlation analysis, including partial correlation, are discussed For those who wish to extend their knowledge of multiple regression and correlation analysis, the references at the end of the chapter provide a good beginning.

Review Questions and Exercises

1. What are the assumptions underlying multiple regression analysis when one wishes to infer about the population from which the sample data have been drawn?
2. What are the assumptions underlying the correlation model when inference is an objective?
3. Explain fully the following terms:
   (a) Coefficient of multiple determination
   (b) The multiple correlation coefficient
   (c) Simple correlation coefficient
   (d) Partial correlation coefficient
4. Describe a situation in your particular area of interest where multiple regression analysis would be useful. Use real or realistic data and do a complete regression analysis.
5. Describe a situation in your particular area of interest where multiple correlation analysis would be useful. Use real or realistic data and do a complete correlation analysis.

In the exercises that follow carry out the indicated analysis and test hypotheses at the indicated significance levels. Compute the p-value for each test.

6. The following table shows certain pulmonary function values observed in 10 hospitalized patients.

X_1 Vital Capacity (liters)	X_2 Total Lung Capacity (liters)	Y Forced Expiratory Volume (liters) per Second
2.2	2.5	1.6
1.5	3.2	1.0
1.6	5.0	1.4
3.4	4.4	2.6
2.0	4.4	1.2
1.9	3.3	1.5
2.2	3.2	1.6
3.3	3.3	2.3
2.4	3.7	2.1
.9	3.6	.7

Compute the multiple correlation coefficient and test for significance at the .05 level.

7. The following table shows the weight and total cholesterol and triglyceride levels in 15 patients with primary type II hyperlipoproteinemia just prior to initiation of treatment.

Y Weight (kg)	X_1 Total Cholesterol (mg/100 ml)	X_2 Triglyceride (mg/100 ml)
76	302	139
97	336	101
83	220	57
52	300	56
70	382	113
67	379	42
75	331	84
78	332	186
70	426	164
99	399	205
75	279	230
78	332	186
70	410	160
77	389	153
76	302	139

Compute the multiple correlation coefficient and test for significance at the .05 level.

8. In a study of the relationship between creatinine excretion, height, and weight the data shown in the following table were collected on 20 infant males.

Infant	Creatinine Excretion (mg/day) Y	Weight (kg) X_1	Height (cm) X_2
1	100	9	72
2	115	10	76
3	52	6	59
4	85	8	68
5	135	10	60
6	58	5	58
7	90	8	70
8	60	7	65
9	45	4	54
10	125	11	83

Infant	Creatinine Excretion (mg/day) Y	Weight (kg) X_1	Height (cm) X_2
11	86	7	64
12	80	7	66
13	65	6	61
14	95	8	66
15	25	5	57
16	125	11	81
17	40	5	59
18	95	9	71
19	70	6	62
20	120	10	75

(a) Find the multiple regression equation describing the relationship among these variables.
(b) Compute R^2 and do an analysis of variance.
(c) Let $X_1 = 10$ and $X_2 = 60$ and find the predicted value of Y.

9. A study was conducted to examine those variables thought to be related to the job satisfaction of nonprofessional hospital employees. A random sample of 15 employees gave the following results:

Score on Job Satisfaction Test (Y)	Coded Intelligence Score (X_1)	Index of Personal Adjustment (X_2)
54	15	8
37	13	1
30	15	1
48	15	7
37	10	4
37	14	2
31	8	3
49	12	7
43	1	9
12	3	1
30	15	1
37	14	2
61	14	10
31	9	1
31	4	5

(a) Find the multiple regression equation describing the relationship among these variables.

(b) Compute the coefficient of multiple determination and do an analysis of variance.

(c) Let $X_1 = 10$ and $X_2 = 5$ and find the predicted value of Y.

10. A medical research team obtained the index of adiposity, basal insulin, and basal glucose values on 21 normal subjects. The results are shown in the following table. The researchers wished to investigate the strength of the association among these variables.

Index of Adiposity Y	Basal Insulin (μU/ml) X_1	Basal Glucose (mg/100ml) X_2
90	12	98
112	10	103
127	14	101
137	11	102
103	10	90
140	38	108
105	9	100
92	6	101
92	8	92
96	6	91
114	9	95
108	9	95
160	41	117
91	7	101
115	9	86
167	40	106
108	9	84
156	43	117
167	17	99
165	40	104
168	22	85

Compute the multiple correlation coefficient and test for significance at the .05 level.

References

References cited

1. George W. Snedecor and William G. Cochran, *Statistical Methods*, Sixth Edition, The Iowa State University Press, Ames, Iowa, 1967.
2. Robert G. D. Steel and James H. Torrie, *Principles and Procedures of Statistics*, McGraw-Hill, New York, 1960.
3. R. L. Anderson and T. A. Bancroft, *Statistical Theory in Research*, McGraw-Hill, New York, 1952.

4. Mordecai Ezekiel and Karl A. Fox, *Methods of Correlation and Regression Analysis*, Third Edition, Wiley, New York, 1959.

5. M. H. Doolittle, "Method Employed in the Solution of Normal Equation and the Adjustment of a Triangulation," *U.S. Coast and Geodetic Survey Report*, 1878.

6. David Durand, "Joint Confidence Region for Multiple Regression Coefficients," *Journal of the American Statistical Association*, *49* (1954), 130–146.

7. R. C. Geary and C. E. V. Leser, "Significance Tests in Multiple Regression," *The American Statistician*, *22* (February 1968), 20–21.

8. R. A. Fisher, "The General Sampling Distribution of the Multiple Correlation Coefficient," *Proceedings of the Royal Society* A, *121* (1928), 654–673.

9. K. H. Kramer, "Tables for Constructing Confidence Limits on the Multiple Correlation Coefficient," *Journal of the American Statistical Association*, *58* (1963), 1082–1085.

10. David M. Allen, "Mean Square Error of Prediction as a Criterion for Selecting Variables," *Technometrics*, *13* (1971), 469–475.

11. E. M. L. Beale, M. G. Kendall, and D. W. Mann, "The Discarding of Variables in Multivariate Analysis," *Biometrika*, *54* (1967), 357–366.

12. N. R. Draper and H. Smith, *Applied Regression Analysis*, Wiley, New York, 1966.

13. M. J. Garside, "The Best Sub-Set in Multiple Regression Analysis," *Applied Statistics*, *14* (1965), 196–200.

14. J. W. Gorman and R. J. Toman, "Selection of Variables for Fitting Equations to Data," *Technometrics*, *8* (1966), 27–52.

15. R. R. Hocking and R. N. Leslie, "Selection of the Best Sub-Set in Regression Analysis," *Technometrics*, *9* (1967), 531–540.

16. H. J. Larson and T. A. Bancroft, "Sequential Model Building for Prediction in Regression Analysis I," *Annals of Mathematical Statistics*, *34* (1963), 462–479.

17. D. V. Lindley, "The Choice of Variables in Multiple Regression," *Journal of the Royal Statistical Society* B, *30* (1968), 31–66.

18. E. F. Schultz, Jr. and J. F. Goggans, "A Systematic Procedure for Determining Potent Independent Variables in Multiple Regression and Discriminant Analysis," Agri. Exp. Sta. Bull. 336, Auburn University, 1961.

19. K. W. Smillie, *An Introduction to Regression and Correlation*, Academic Press, New York, 1966.

20. Peter Sprent, *Models in Regression*, Methuen, London, 1969.

21. A. Summerfield and A. Lubin, "A Square Root Method of Selecting a Minimum Set of Variables in Multiple Regression: I, The Method," *Psychometrika, 16* (3):271 (1951).

Other references, books

1. Frank Andrews, James Morgan, and John Sonquist, *Multiple Classification Analysis*, Ann Arbor, Survey Research Center, 1967.
2. T. W. Anderson, *Introduction to Multivariate Statistical Analysis*, Wiley, New York, 1958.
3. Cuthbert Daniel and Fred S. Wood, *Fitting Equations to Data*, Wiley-Interscience, New York, 1971.
4. Alan E. Treloar, *Correlation Analysis*, Burgess, Minneapolis, 1949.

Other references, journal articles

1. R. G. Newton and D. J. Spurrell, "A Development of Multiple Regression for the Analysis of Routine Data," *Applied Statistics, 16* (1967), 51–64.
2. Potluri Rao, "Some Notes on Misspecification in Multiple Regression," *The American Statistician, 25* (December 1971), 37–39.
3. Neil S. Weiss, "A Graphical Representation of the Relationships Between Multiple Regression and Multiple Correlation," *The American Statistician, 24* (April 1970), 25–29.
4. E. J. Williams, "The Analysis of Association Among Many Variates," *Journal of the Royal Statistical Society, 29* (1967), 199–242.

Other references, other publications

1. R. L. Bottenbery and Y. H. Ward, Jr., *Applied Multiple Linear Regression*, U.S. Department of Commerce, Office of Technical Services, AD 413128, 1963.
2. Jean Draper, *Interpretation of Multiple Regression Analysis Part I, Problems of Interpreting Large Samples of Data*, The University of Arizona, College of Business and Public Administration, Division of Economics and Business Research, 1968.

10

THE CHI-SQUARE DISTRIBUTION AND THE ANALYSIS OF FREQUENCIES

10.1 INTRODUCTION

In the chapters on estimation and hypothesis testing brief mention is made of the chi-square distribution in the construction of confidence intervals for and the testing of hypotheses concerning a population variance. This distribution, which is one of the most widely used distributions in statistical applications, has many other uses. Some of the more common ones are presented in this chapter along with a more complete description of the distribution itself, which follows in the next section.

10.2 THE MATHEMATICAL PROPERTIES OF THE CHI-SQUARE DISTRIBUTION

The chi-square distribution may be derived from normal distributions. Suppose that from a normally distributed random variable Y with mean μ and variance σ^2 we randomly and independently select samples of size $n = 1$. Each value selected may be transformed to the unit normal variable z by the familiar formula:

$$z = \frac{y_i - \mu}{\sigma} \qquad (10.2.1)$$

Each value of z may be squared to obtain z^2. When we investigate the sampling distribution of z^2, we find that it follows a chi-square distribution with 1 degree of freedom. That is,

$$\chi^2_{(1)} = \left(\frac{y - \mu}{\sigma}\right)^2 = z^2$$

Now suppose that we randomly and independently select samples of size $n = 2$ from the normally distributed population of Y values. Within each sample we may transform each value of y to the unit normal variable z and square as before. If the resulting values of z^2 for each sample are added, we may designate this sum by

$$\chi^2_{(2)} = \left(\frac{y_1 - \mu}{\sigma}\right)^2 + \left(\frac{y_2 - \mu}{\sigma}\right)^2 = z_1{}^2 + z_2{}^2$$

since it follows the chi-square distribution with 2 degrees of freedom, the number of independent squared terms that are added together.

The procedure may be repeated for any sample size n. The sum of the resulting z^2 values in each case will be distributed as chi-square with n degrees of freedom. In general, then,

$$\chi^2_{(n)} = z_1{}^2 + z_2{}^2 + \cdots + z_n{}^2 \tag{10.2.2}$$

follows the χ^2 distribution with n degrees of freedom. The mathematical form of the chi-square distribution is as follows:

$$f(u) = \frac{1}{\left(\frac{k}{2} - 1\right)!} \frac{1}{2^{k/2}} u^{(k/2)-1} e^{-(u/2)}, \qquad u > 0 \tag{10.2.3}$$

where e is the irrational number 2.71828 · · · and k is the number of degrees of freedom. The variate u is usually designated by the Greek letter chi (χ) and, hence, the distribution is called the χ^2-distribution. As we pointed out in Chapter 5, the χ^2 distribution has been tabulated in Table I. Further use of the table is demonstrated as the need arises in succeeding sections.

The mean and variance of the χ^2 distribution are k and $2k$, respectively. The modal value of the distribution is $k - 2$ for values of k greater than or equal to 2 and is zero for $k = 1$.

The shapes of the χ^2 distributions for several values of k are shown in Figure 5.9.1. We observe in this figure that the shapes for $k = 1$ and $k = 2$ are quite different from the general shape of the distribution for $k > 2$. We also see from this figure that χ^2 assumes values between 0 and infinity. It cannot take on negative values, since it is the sum of values that have been squared.

A final characteristic of the χ^2 distribution worth noting is that the sum of two or more independent χ^2 variables also follows a χ^2 distribution. We make use of the χ^2 distribution in this chapter in testing hypotheses where the data available for analysis are in the form of frequencies. These hypothesis testing procedures are discussed under the topics of *tests of goodness-of-fit*, *test of independence*, and *test of homogeneity*. We shall discover that, in a sense, all of the χ^2 tests that we employ may be thought of as goodness-of-fit tests, in that they test the goodness-of-fit of observed frequencies to frequencies that one would expect if the data were generated under some particular theory or hypothesis. We, however, reserve the phrase "goodness-of-fit" for use in a more restricted sense. We use the phrase "goodness-of-fit" to refer to a comparison of a sample distribution to some theoretical distribution that it is assumed describes the population from which the sample came. The justification of our use of the distribution in these situations is due to Karl Pearson (1) who showed that the χ^2 distribution may be used as a test of the agreement between observation and hypothesis whenever the data are in the form of frequencies.

An extensive treatment of the χ^2 distribution is to be found in the book by Lancaster (2).

10.3 TESTS OF GOODNESS-OF-FIT

As we have pointed out, a goodness-of-fit test is appropriate when one wishes to decide if an observed distribution of frequencies is incompatible with some preconceived or hypothesized distribution.

We may, for example, wish to determine whether or not a sample of observed values of some random variable is compatible with the hypothesis that it was drawn from a population of values that is normally distributed. The procedure for reaching a decision consists of placing the values into mutually exclusive categories or class intervals and noting the frequency of occurrence of values in each category. We then make use of our knowledge of normal distributions to determine the frequencies for each category that one could expect if the sample had come from a normal distribution. If the discrepancy between what was observed and what one would expect, given that sampling was from a normal distribution, is too great to be attributed to chance, we conclude that the sample did not come from a normal distribution. If the discrepancy is of such magnitude that it could have come about due to chance, we conclude that the sample may have come from a normal distribution. In a similar manner, tests of goodness-of-fit may be carried out in cases where the hypothesized distribution is the binomial, the Poisson, or any other distribution. Let us illustrate in more detail with some examples.

Example 10.3.1. The Normal Distribution

Suppose that a research team making a study of hospitals in the United States collects data on a sample of 250 hospitals which enables the team to compute for each the inpatient occupancy ratio, a variable that shows, for a 12-month period, the ratio of average daily census to the average number of beds maintained. Suppose the sample yielded the distribution of ratios (expressed as percents), shown in Table 10.3.1.

Table 10.3.1

Results of Study Described in Example 10.3.1

Inpatient Occupancy Ratio	Number of Hospitals
0.0 to 39.9	16
40.0 to 49.9	18
50.0 to 59.9	22
60.0 to 69.9	51
70.0 to 79.9	62
80.0 to 89.9	55
90.0 to 99.9	22
100.0 to 109.9	4
Total	250

Do these data provide sufficient evidence to indicate that the sample did not come from a normally distributed population? The question suggests a test of the null hypothesis, H_0, that the data were drawn from a normally distributed population against the alternative, H_A, that the data did not come from a normally distributed population.

Since the mean and variance of the hypothesized distribution are not specified, the sample data must be used to estimate them. These parameters, or their estimates, will be needed to compute the frequency that would be expected in each class interval when the null hypothesis is true. The mean and standard deviation computed from the sample data are

$$\bar{x} = 69.91$$

$$s = 19.02$$

As the next step in the analysis we must obtain for each class interval the frequency of occurrence of values that we would expect when the null hypothesis is true, that is, if the sample were, in fact, drawn from a normally distributed population of values. To do this, we first determine the expected relative frequency of occurrence of values for each class interval and then multiply these expected relative frequencies by the total number of values to obtain the expected number of values for each interval.

It will be recalled from our study of the normal distribution that the relative frequency of occurrence of values equal to or greater than some specified value, say x_0, of the normally distributed random variable X, is equivalent to the area under the curve and to the right of x_0 as represented

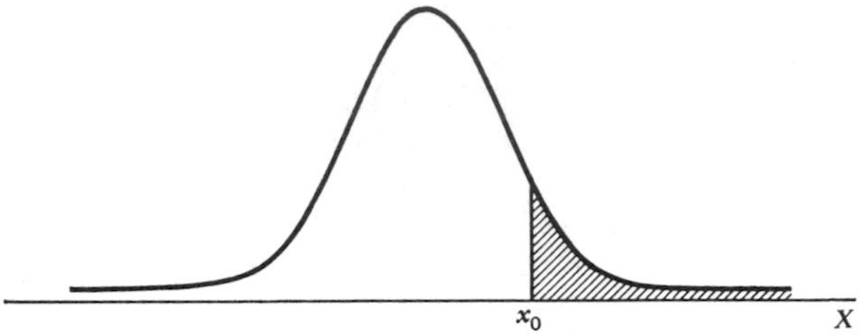

Figure 10.3.1. A normal distribution showing the relative frequency of occurrence of values greater than or equal to X_0. *The shaded area represents the relative frequency of occurrence of values equal to or greater than* X_0.

by the shaded area in Figure 10.3.1. We obtain the numerical value of this area by converting x_0 to a standard normal deviate by the formula $z_0 = (x_0 - \mu)/\sigma$, and finding the appropriate value in Table F. We use this procedure to obtain the expected relative frequencies corresponding to each of the class intervals in Table 10.3.1. We estimate μ and σ with $\bar{x}$ and s as computed from the sample. The first step consists of obtaining z values corresponding to the lower limit of each class interval. The area between two successive z values will give the expected relative frequency of occurrence of values for the corresponding class interval.

For example, to obtain the expected relative frequency of occurrence of values in the interval 40.0 to 49.9 we proceed as follows:

$$\text{The } z \text{ value corresponding to } X = 40.0 \text{ is } z = \frac{40.0 - 69.91}{19.02} = -1.57$$

$$\text{The } z \text{ value corresponding to } X = 50.0 \text{ is } z = \frac{50.0 - 69.91}{19.02} = -1.05$$

In Table F we find that the area to the left of -1.05 is $.5 - .3531 = .1469$, and the area to the left of -1.57 is $.5 - .4418 = .0582$. The area between -1.05 and -1.57 is equal to $.1469 - .0582 = .0887$, which is equal to the expected relative frequency of occurrence of values of occupancy ratios between the interval 40.0 to 49.9. This tells us that if the null hypothesis is true, that is, if the occupancy ratio values are normally distributed, we should expect 8.9 percent of the values in our sample to be between 40.0 and 49.9. When we multiply our total sample size, 250, by .0887 we find the expected frequency for the interval to be 22.18. Similar calculations will give the expected frequencies for the other intervals as shown in Table 10.3.2.

We are now interested in examining the magnitudes of the discrepancies between the observed frequencies and the expected frequencies, since we note that the two sets of frequencies do not agree. We know that even if our sample were drawn from a normal distribution of values, sampling variability alone would make it highly unlikely that the observed and expected

Table 10.3.2

Class Intervals, and Expected Frequencies for Example 10.3.1

Class Interval	$z = (x_i - \bar{x})/s$ at Lower Limit of Interval	Expected Relative Frequency	Expected Frequency
<40.0		.0582	14.55
40.0 to 49.9	−1.57	.0887	22.18
50.0 to 59.9	−1.05	.1546	38.65
60.0 to 69.9	−.52	.1985	49.62
70.0 to 79.9	.00	.2019	50.48
80.0 to 89.9	.53	.1535	38.38
90.0 to 99.9	1.06	.0875	21.88
100.0 to 109.9	1.58	.0397	9.92
110.0 and greater	2.11	.0174	4.35
Total		1.0000	250.00

frequencies would agree perfectly. We wonder, then, if the discrepancies between the observed and expected frequencies are small enough that we feel it reasonable that they could have occurred by chance alone, when the null hypothesis is true. If they are of this magnitude, we will be unwilling to reject the null hypothesis that the sample came from a normally distributed population.

If the discrepancies are so large that it does not seem reasonable that they could have occurred by chance alone when the null hypothesis is true, we will want to reject the null hypothesis. The criterion against which we judge whether the discrepancies are "large" or "small" is provided by the χ^2 distribution.

It can be shown that when the null hypothesis is true, the statistic

$$X^2 = \sum_{i=1}^{k} \frac{(O_i - E_i)^2}{E_i} \tag{10.3.1}$$

is distributed approximately as χ^2 with $k - r$ degrees of freedom.

In Equation 10.3.1 O_i refers to the ith observed frequency and E_i refers to the ith expected frequency. In determining the degrees of freedom, k is equal to the number of groups for which observed and expected frequencies are available, and r is the number of restrictions or constraints imposed on the given comparison. A restriction is imposed when we force the sum of the expected frequencies to equal the sum of the observed frequencies, and an additional restriction is imposed for each parameter that is estimated from the sample. For a full discussion of the theoretical justification for subtracting one degree of freedom for each estimated parameter, see Cramer (3).

Table 10.3.3

Observed and Expected Frequencies and $(O_i - E_i)^2/E_i$ for Example 10.3.1

Class Interval	**Observed Frequency (O_i)**	**Expected Frequency (E_i)**	$(O_i - E_i)^2/E_i$
<40.0	16	14.55	.145
40.0 to 49.9	18	22.18	.788
50.0 to 59.9	22	38.65	7.173
60.0 to 69.9	51	49.62	.038
70.0 to 79.9	62	50.48	2.629
80.0 to 89.9	55	38.38	7.197
90.0 to 99.9	22	21.88	.001
100.0 to 109.9	4	9.92	3.533
110.0 and greater	0	4.35	4.350
Total	250	250.00	25.854

The quantity $\sum[(O_i - E_i)^2/E_i]$ will be small if the observed and expected frequencies are close together, and will be large if the differences are large.

The computed value of X^2 is compared with the tabulated value of χ^2 with $k - r$ degrees of freedom. If X^2 is greater than the tabulated χ^2 for any value of α, the null hypothesis may be rejected at that level of significance.

Let us illustrate the procedure with the data from our current example. The observed and expected frequencies along with each value of $(O_i - E_i)^2/E_i$ are shown in Table 10.3.3. The first entry in the last column, for example, is computed from $(16 - 14.55)^2/14.55 = .145$. The other values of $(O_i - E_i)^2/E_i$ are computed in a similar manner.

From Table 10.3.3 we see that $X^2 = \sum[(O_i - E_i)^2/E_i] = 25.854$. The appropriate degrees of freedom are 9 (the number of groups or class intervals) $- 3$ (for the three restrictions: making $\sum E_i = \sum O_i$, and estimating μ and σ from the sample data) $= 6$. When we compare $X^2 = 25.854$ with values of χ^2 in Table I, we see that it is larger than $\chi^2_{.995} = 18.548$, so that we can reject the null hypothesis that the sample came from a normally distributed population at the .005 level of significance. In other words, the probability of obtaining a value of X^2 as large as 25.854, when the null hypothesis is true, is less than 5 in 1000 ($p < .005$). We say that such a rare event did not occur due to chance alone (when H_0 is true), so we look for another explanation. The other explanation is that the null hypothesis is false.

Sometimes the parameters are known or may be estimated from information external to the sample so that they may be specified in the null hypothesis. It should be noted that had the mean and variance of the population been specified as part of the null hypothesis, we would not have had to estimate them from the sample and our degrees of freedom would have been $9 - 1 = 8$.

Small Expected Frequencies. Frequently in applications of the chi-square test the expected frequency for one or more categories will be small, perhaps much less than 1. In the literature the point is frequently made that the approximation of X^2 to χ^2 is not strictly valid when some of the expected frequencies are small. There is disagreement among writers, however, over what size expected frequencies are allowable before making some adjustment or abandoning χ^2 in favor of some alternative test. Some writers, especially the earlier ones, suggest lower limits of 10 while others suggest that all expected frequencies should be no less than 5. Cochran (4, 5), writing in the early 1950s, suggests that for goodness-of-fit tests of unimodal distributions (such as the normal) the minimum expected frequency can be as low as 1. If, in practice, one encounters one or more expected frequencies less than 1, adjacent categories may be combined to achieve the suggested minimum. Combining reduces the number of categories and, therefore, the number of degrees of freedom. Cochran's suggestions appear to have been followed extensively by practitioners in recent years. More recent research on the subject of small expected frequencies includes that of Roscoe and Byars (6), Yarnold (7), Tate and Hyer (8), Slakter (9, 10), and Lewontin and Felsenstein (11).

Although one frequently encounters in the literature, the use of chi-square to test for normality, it is not the most appropriate test to use when the hypothesized distribution is continuous. The Kolmogorov-Smirnov test, described in Chapter 11, was especially designed for goodness-of-fit tests involving continuous distributions.

Example 10.3.2. The Binomial Distribution

In a study designed to determine patient acceptance of a new pain reliever, 100 physicians each selected a sample of 25 patients to participate in the study. Each patient, after trying the new pain reliever for a specified period of time, was asked whether it was preferable to the pain reliever used regularly in the past.

The results of the study are shown in Table 10.3.4.

We are interested in determining whether or not these data are compatible with the hypothesis that they were drawn from a population that follows a binomial distribution. Again, we employ a chi-square goodness-of-fit test.

Since the binomial parameter, p, is not specified, it must be estimated from the sample data. A total of 500 patients out of the 2500 patients participating in the study said they preferred the new pain reliever, so that our point estimate of p is $\tilde{p} = 500/2500 = .20$. The expected relative frequencies can be

Table 10.3.4

Results of Study Described in Example 10.3.2

Number of Patients Out of 25 Preferring New Pain Reliever	**Number of Doctors Reporting This Number**	**Total Number of Patients Preferring New Pain Reliever by Doctor**
0	5	0
1	6	6
2	8	16
3	10	30
4	10	40
5	15	75
6	17	102
7	10	70
8	10	80
9	9	81
10 or more	0	0
Total	100	500

obtained by evaluating the binomial function

$$f(x) = \binom{25}{x} .2^x .8^{25-x}$$

for $x = 0, 1, \ldots, 25$. For example, to find the probability that out of a sample of 25 patients none would prefer the new pain reliever, when, in the total population the true proportion preferring the new pain reliever is .2, we would evaluate

$$f(0) = \binom{25}{0} .2^0 .8^{25-0}$$

This can be done most easily by consulting Table C where we see that $P(X = 0) = 1 - P(X \geq 1) = 1 - .9962 = .0038$. The relative frequency of occurrence of samples of size 25 in which no patients prefer the new pain reliever is .0038. To obtain the corresponding expected frequency we multiply .0038 by 100 to get .38. Similar calculations yield the remaining expected frequencies which, along with the observed frequencies, are shown in Table 10.3.5. We see in this table that the first expected frequency is less than 1, so that we follow Cochran's suggestion and combine this group with the second group. When we do this, all of the expected frequencies are greater than 1.

Table 10.3.5

Number of Patients Out of 25 Preferring New Pain Reliever	Number of Doctors Reporting This Number (Observed Frequency, O_i)	Expected Relative Frequency	Expected Frequency, E_i
0	5 } 11	.0038	.38 } 2.74
1	6 }	.0236	2.36 }
2	8	.0708	7.08
3	10	.1358	13.58
4	10	.1867	18.67
5	15	.1960	19.60
6	17	.1633	16.33
7	10	.1109	11.09
8	10	.0623	6.23
9	9	.0295	2.95
10 or more	0	.0173	1.73
Total	100	1.0000	100.00

From the data we compute

$$X^2 = \frac{(11 - 2.74)^2}{2.74} + \frac{(8 - 7.08)^2}{7.08} + \cdots + \frac{(0 - 1.73)^2}{1.73} = 47.624$$

The appropriate degrees of freedom are 10 (the number of groups left after combining the first two) less 2, or 8. One degree of freedom is lost because we force the total of the expected (frequencies to equal the total observed frequencies, and one degree of freedom is sacrificed because we estimate p from the sample data.

We compare our computed X^2 with the tabulated χ^2 with 8 degrees of freedom and find that it is significant at the .005 level of significance. We reject the null hypothesis that the data came from a binomial distribution.

Example 10.3.3. The Poisson Distribution

Our final example of a chi-square goodness-of-fit test illustrates the procedure when the Poisson is the hypothesized distribution.

Let us refer to Example 3.4.1 and test the null hypothesis that emergency admissions follow a Poisson distribution with $\lambda = 3$. Suppose that over a period of 90 days the numbers of emergency admissions were as shown in Table 10.3.6.

Table 10.3.6

Number of Emergency Admissions to a Hospital During a 90-Day Period

Day	Emergency Admissions	Day	Emergency Admissions	Day	Emergency Admissions	Day	Emergency Admissions
1.	2	24.	5	47.	4	70.	3
2.	3	25.	3	48.	2	71.	5
3.	4	26.	2	49.	2	72.	4
4.	5	27.	4	50.	3	73.	1
5.	3	28.	4	51.	4	74.	1
6.	2	29.	3	52.	2	75.	6
7.	3	30.	5	53.	3	76.	3
8.	0	31.	1	54.	1	77.	3
9.	1	32.	3	55.	2	78.	5
10.	0	33.	2	56.	3	79.	2
11.	1	34.	4	57.	2	80.	1
12.	0	35.	2	58.	5	81.	7
13.	6	36.	5	59.	2	82.	7
14.	4	37.	0	60.	7	83.	1
15.	4	38.	6	61.	8	84.	5
16.	4	39.	4	62.	3	85.	1
17.	3	40.	4	63.	1	86.	4
18.	4	41.	5	64.	3	87.	4
19.	3	42.	1	65.	1	88.	9
20.	3	43.	3	66.	0	89.	2
21.	3	44.	1	67.	3	90.	3
22.	4	45.	2	68.	2		
23.	3	46.	3	69.	1		

The data of Table 10.3.6 are summarized in Table 10.3.7.

To obtain the expected frequencies we first obtain the expected relative frequencies by evaluating the Poisson function given by Equation 3.4.1 for each entry in the left-hand column of Table 10.3.7. For example, the first expected relative frequency is obtained by evaluating

$$f(0) = \frac{e^{-3}3^0}{0!}$$

We may use Table E of the Appendix to find this and all the other expected relative frequencies that we need. Each of the expected relative frequencies is multiplied by 90 to obtain the corresponding expected frequencies. These values along with the observed and expected frequencies and the components of X^2, $(O_i - E_i)^2/E_i$, are displayed in Table 10.3.8.

Table 10.3.7

Summary of Data Presented in Table 10.3.6

Number of Emergency Admissions in a Day	Number of Days This Number of Emergency Admissions Occurred
0	5
1	14
2	15
3	23
4	16
5	9
6	3
7	3
8	1
9	1
10 or more	0
Total	90

Table 10.3.8

Observed and Expected Frequencies and Components of X^2 for Example 10.3.3

Number of Emergency Admissions	Number of Days This Number Occurred, O_i	Expected Relative Frequency	Expected Frequency	$\frac{(O_i - E_i)^2}{E_i}$
0	5	.050	4.50	.056
1	14	.149	13.41	.026
2	15	.224	20.16	1.321
3	23	.224	20.16	.400
4	16	.168	15.12	.051
5	9	.101	9.09	.001
6	3	.050	4.50	.500
7	3	.022	1.98	.525
8	1 } 2	.008	.72 } 1.08	.784
9	1	.003	.27	
10 or more	0	.001	.09	
Total	90	1.000	90.00	3.664

In Table 10.3.8 we see that

$$X^2 = \sum \frac{(O_i - E_i)^2}{E_i} = \frac{(5 - 4.50)^2}{4.50} + \cdots + \frac{(2 - 1.08)^2}{1.08} = 3.664$$

We also note that the last three expected frequencies are less than 1, so that they must be combined to avoid having any expected frequencies less than 1. This means that we have only nine effective categories for computing degrees of freedom. Since the parameter, λ, was specified in the null hypothesis, we do not lose a degree of freedom for reasons of estimation, so that the appropriate degrees of freedom are $9 - 1 = 8$. By consulting Table I of the Appendix, we find that the critical value of χ^2 for 8 degrees of freedom and $\alpha = .05$ is 15.507, so that we cannot reject the null hypothesis at the .05, or for that matter any reasonable level of significance ($p > .10$). We conclude, therefore, that emergency admissions at this hospital may follow a Poisson distribution with $\lambda = 3$. At least the observed data do not cast any doubt on that hypothesis.

Exercises

10.3.1. The following table shows the distribution of uric acid determinations taken on 250 patients. Test the goodness-of-fit of these data to a normal distribution with $\mu = 5.74$ and $\sigma = 2.01$. Let $\alpha = .01$.

Uric Acid Determination	Observed Frequency
<1	1
1 to 1.99	5
2 to 2.99	15
3 to 3.99	24
4 to 4.99	43
5 to 5.99	50
6 to 6.99	45
7 to 7.99	30
8 to 8.99	22
9 to 9.99	10
10 or higher	5
Total	250

10.3.2. The following data were collected on 300 eight-year-old girls. Test, at the .05 level of significance, the null hypothesis that the data are drawn from a normally distributed population. Use the methods of Chapter 1 to compute the sample mean and standard deviation from grouped data.

Height in Centimeters	Observed Frequency
114 to 115.9	5
116 to 117.9	10
118 to 119.9	14
120 to 121.9	21
122 to 123.9	30
124 to 125.9	40
126 to 127.9	45
128 to 129.9	43
130 to 131.9	42
132 to 133.9	30
134 to 135.9	11
136 to 137.9	5
138 to 139.9	4
	300

10.3.3. The face sheet of patients' records maintained in a local health department contains 10 entries. A sample of 100 records revealed the following distribution of erroneous entries.

Number of Erroneous Entries Out of 10	Number of Records
0	8
1	25
2	32
3	24
4	10
5 or more	1
	100

Test the goodness-of-fit of these data to the binomial distribution with $p = .20$. Find the p-value for this test.

10.3.4. Over the past 10 years the following distribution of accidents was observed by the physician in charge of the employee health clinic of a large industrial firm.

Number of Accidents in a Month	Number of Months This Number Occurred
0	2
1	10
2	15
3	30
4	28
5	15
6	10
7	6
8	2
9	1
10 or more	1
	120

Are these data compatible with the hypothesis that accidents in this firm are Poisson distributed with $\lambda = 4$? What is the p-value for this test?

10.3.5. The following are the numbers of a particular organism found in 100 samples of water from a pond.

Number of Organisms per Sample	Frequency
0	15
1	30
2	25
3	20
4	5
5	4
6	1
7	0
	100

Test the null hypothesis that these data were drawn from a Poisson distribution. Determine the p-value for this test.

10.4 TEST OF INDEPENDENCE

Another, and perhaps the most frequent, use of the chi-square distribution is to test the null hypothesis that two criteria of classification, when applied to the same set of entities, are independent. We say that two criteria of classification are independent if the distribution of one criterion is the same no

Table 10.4.1

Two-Way Classification of a Finite Population of Entities

Second Criterion of Classification Level	**First Criterion of Classification Level** 1	2	3	...	c	**Total**
1	N_{11}	N_{12}	N_{13}	...	N_{1c}	$N_{1.}$
2	N_{21}	N_{22}	N_{23}	...	N_{2c}	$N_{2.}$
3	N_{31}	N_{32}	N_{33}	...	N_{3c}	$N_{3.}$
$\vdots$	$\vdots$	$\vdots$	$\vdots$	$\vdots$	$\vdots$	$\vdots$
r	N_{r1}	N_{r2}	N_{r3}	...	N_{rc}	$N_{r.}$
Total	$N_{.1}$	$N_{.2}$	$N_{.3}$	...	$N_{.c}$	N

matter what the distribution of the other criterion. For example, if average family income and area of residence of the inhabitants of a certain city are independent, we would expect to find the same proportion of families with low, medium, and high average incomes in all areas of the city.

The classification, according to two criteria, of a set of entities, say people, can be shown by a table in which the r rows represent the various levels of one criterion of classification and the c columns represent the various levels of the second criterion. Such a table is generally called a *contingency table.* The classification according to two criteria of a finite population of entities is shown in Table 10.4.1.

We will be interested in testing the null hypothesis that in the population the two criteria of classification are independent. If the hypothesis is rejected, we will conclude that the two criteria of classification are not independent. A sample of size n will be drawn from the population of entities, and the frequency of occurrence of entities in the sample corresponding to the cells formed by the intersections of the rows and columns of Table 10.4.1 along with the marginal totals will be displayed in a table such as Table 10.4.2.

The expected frequencies, under the null hypothesis that the two criteria of classification are independent, are calculated for each cell. The expected frequencies and observed frequencies are compared. If the discrepancy is "small," the null hypothesis is tenable. If the discrepancy is "large," the null hypothesis is rejected, and we conclude that the two criteria of classification are not independent. The decision as to whether the discrepancy between observed and expected frequencies is "large" or "small" will be made on the basis of the size of the quantity computed when we use Equation 10.3.1, where O_i and E_i, refer, respectively, to the observed and expected frequencies in the cells of Table 10.4.2. It would be more logical to designate the observed and expected frequencies in these cells by O_{ij} and E_{ij}, but to keep the notation simple and to avoid the introduction of another formula, we have elected to

Table 10.4.2

Two-Way Classification of a Sample of Entities

Second Criterion of Classification Level	**First Criterion of Classification Level**					
	1	2	3	$\cdots$	c	**Total**
1	n_{11}	n_{12}	n_{13}	$\cdots$	n_{1c}	$n_{1.}$
2	n_{21}	n_{22}	n_{23}	$\cdots$	n_{2c}	$n_{2.}$
3	n_{31}	n_{32}	n_{33}	$\cdots$	n_{3c}	$n_{3.}$
$\vdots$	$\vdots$	$\vdots$	$\vdots$		$\vdots$	$\vdots$
r	n_{r1}	n_{r2}	n_{r3}	$\cdots$	n_{rc}	$n_{r.}$
Total	$n_{.1}$	$n_{.2}$	$n_{.3}$	$\cdots$	$n_{.c}$	n

use the simpler notation. It will be helpful to think of the cells as being numbered from 1 to k where 1 refers to cell 11 and k refers to cell rc. It can be shown that X^2 as defined in this manner is distributed approximately as χ^2 with $(r - 1)(c - 1)$ degrees of freedom when the null hypothesis is true. If the computed value of X^2 is larger than the tabulated value of χ^2 for some α, the null hypothesis is rejected at the α level of significance. The procedure is illustrated with the following example.

Example 10.4.1

A research team studying the relationship between blood type and severity of a certain condition in a population collected data on 1500 subjects as displayed in the contingency table shown as Table 10.4.3.

Table 10.4.3

Fifteen-Hundred Subjects Classified by Severity of Condition and Blood Type

Severity of Condition	**Blood Type**				
	A	B	AB	O	**Total**
Absent	543	211	90	476	1320
Mild	44	22	8	31	105
Severe	28	9	7	31	75
Total	615	242	105	538	1500

The researchers wished to know if these data were compatible with the hypothesis that severity of condition and blood type are independent. The first step in the analysis is to obtain the frequency for each cell that one would expect if, in fact, the two criteria of classification are independent. We may begin by computing estimates of the various marginal probabilities from the marginal totals shown in Table 10.4.3. Our estimate of the probability that a subject picked at random from the population from which the sample was drawn does not have the condition is $1320/1500 = .88$; the probability that a subject picked at random has a mild form of the condition is estimated to be $105/1500 = .07$; and the probability that a subject picked at random has a severe form of the condition is estimated to be $75/1500 = .05$. Similarly, we estimate the probabilities that a subject picked at random from the population under study will have type A, B, AB, and O blood to be $615/1500 = .41$, $242/1500 = .16$, $105/1500 = .07$, and $538/1500 = .36$, respectively.

We learned in Chapter 2 (see Equation 2.6.4) that if two events are independent, the probability of their joint occurrence is equal to the product of their individual probabilities. Under the null hypothesis that blood type and severity of condition are independent, then, we would compute the estimated probability that a subject picked at random is, say, both free of the condition and has blood type A as follows:

$$\begin{aligned} P(\text{free of condition} \cap \text{type A blood}) &= P(\text{free of condition})P(\text{type A blood}) \\ &= \tfrac{1320}{1500} \cdot \tfrac{615}{1500} \\ &= .3608 \end{aligned}$$

The probability just computed is our estimate of the probability that a subject picked at random would fall in the first cell of Table 10.4.3 when the null hypothesis is true. Our estimate of the probability that a subject picked at random would be both free of the condition and have blood type B is

$$\tfrac{1320}{1500} \cdot \tfrac{242}{1500} = .141973$$

The estimated probabilities associated with each of the remaining cells are computed in a similar manner.

After computing the estimated probabilities associated with each cell, we may obtain the corresponding expected frequencies by multiplying each cell probability by 1500, the total sample size. For example, the expected frequency for the first cell is $(.3608)(1500) = 541.2$, and the expected number of subjects out of 1500 who are both free of the condition and have blood type B is $(.141973)(1500) = 212.96$.

A shortcut that saves considerable time may be employed in computing the expected frequencies. Note that the expected frequency for the first cell may be expressed as

$$P(\text{free of condition} \cap \text{type A blood})(1500) = \tfrac{1320}{1500} \cdot \tfrac{615}{1500} \cdot 1500$$

Table 10.4.4

Observed and Expected Frequencies, Example 10.4.1

Severity of Condition	Blood Type				
	A	B	AB	O	Total
Absent	543(541.2)	211(212.96)	90(92.40)	476(473.44)	1320
Mild	44(43.05)	22(16.94)	8(7.35)	31(37.66)	105
Severe	28(30.75)	9(12.10)	7(5.25)	31(26.90)	75
Total	615	242	105	538	1500

One of the denominators of 1500 cancels into the 1500 in the numerator, leaving

$$\frac{(1320)(615)}{1500} = 541.20$$

This leads to the shortcut procedure of obtaining expected cell frequencies by dividing the product of corresponding marginal totals by the total sample size. As another example, note that the expected number of subjects out of 1500 who are both free of the condition and have type B blood is $(242)(1320)/1500 = 212.96$. The observed and expected frequencies for our illustrative example are displayed together in Table 10.4.4 where the expected frequencies are enclosed in parentheses.

From the observed and expected frequencies we may compute

$$\begin{aligned} X^2 &= \sum \frac{(O_i - E_i)^2}{E_i} \\ &= \frac{(543 - 541.2)^2}{541.2} + \frac{(211 - 212.96)^2}{212.96} + \cdots + \frac{(31 - 26.90)^2}{26.90} \\ &= .005987 + .018039 + \cdots + .624907 \\ &= 5.12 \end{aligned}$$

The computed value of $X^2 = 5.12$ is compared with tabulated values of χ^2 with 6 degrees of freedom. It is seen that the computed X^2 is not significant at any reasonable level. For example, the critical value of χ^2 for $\alpha = .10$ and 6 degrees of freedom is 10.645. We conclude, then, that these data are compatible with the hypothesis that severity of the condition and blood type are independent. At least these data, because of the close agreement between observed and expected frequencies, do not provide sufficient evidence to indicate a lack of independence between the two criteria of classification.

The degrees of freedom are determined by multiplying the number of rows, r, minus 1 times the number of columns, c, minus 1. That is, $(r - 1) \times (c - 1) =$

$(3 - 1)(4 - 1) = 6$. The student will note that the number of degrees of freedom is equal to the number of cell frequencies in Table 10.4.1 which could be filled in arbitrarily while maintaining the observed marginal totals. For example, given that 1320 subjects are free of the condition and that 543 of these have blood type A, 211 have blood type B, and 90 have blood type AB, we must enter 476 as the number with blood type O. This accounts for 3 degrees of freedom. On applying the same logic to the second row, we find that we can arbitrarily fill in only three cells, which accounts for 3 more degrees of freedom. When we attempt to fill in the cells of the third row, we find that these frequencies are already determined by the frequencies of the first two rows and, thus, the total degrees of freedom are 6.

The problem of small expected frequencies discussed in the previous section may be encountered when analyzing the data of contingency tables. Although there is a lack of concensus on how to handle this problem, many authors currently follow the rule given by Cochran (5). He suggests that for contingency tables with more than 1 degree of freedom a minimum expectation of 1 is allowable if no more than 20 percent of the cells have expected frequencies of less than 5. To meet this rule, adjacent rows and/or adjacent columns may be combined when to do so is logical in light of other considerations. If X^2 is based on less than 30 degrees of freedom, expected frequencies as small as 2 can be tolerated. We did not experience the problem of small expected frequencies in Example 10.4.1, since they were all greater than 5.

The* 2 × 2 *Contingency Table. Sometimes each of two criteria of classification may be broken down into only two categories, or levels. When data are cross classified in this manner, the result is a contingency table consisting of two rows and two columns. Such a table is commonly referred to as a 2×2 table. When we apply the $(r - 1)(c - 1)$ rule for finding degrees of freedom to a 2×2 table the result is 1 degree of freedom. Let us illustrate this with an example.

Example 10.4.2

A sample of 500 elementary school children in a certain school system were cross classified by nutritional status and academic performance. The results are shown in Table 10.4.5.

The researchers wished to know if they could conclude that there is a relationship between nutritional status and academic performance. A chi-square test is appropriate for reaching a decision. The value of X^2 may be computed by first calculating the expected cell frequencies in the manner discussed above. In the case of a 2×2 contingency table, however, X^2 may

Table 10.4.5

Nutritional Status and Academic Performance of 500 Elementary School Children

Academic Performance	Nutritional Status		
	Poor	**Good**	**Total**
Poor	105	15	120
Satisfactory	80	300	380
Total	185	315	500

Table 10.4.6

A 2 × 2 Contingency Table

Second Criterion of Classification	First Criterion of Classification		
	1	2	**Total**
1	a	b	$a+b$
2	c	d	$c+d$
Total	$a+c$	$b+d$	n

be calculated by the following shortcut formula:

$$X^2 = \frac{n(ad - bc)^2}{(a+c)(b+d)(a+b)(c+d)} \tag{10.4.1}$$

where a, b, c, and d are the observed cell frequencies as shown in Table 10.4.6. For our illustrative example we have

$$X^2 = \frac{500[(105)(300) - (15)(80)]^2}{(185)(315)(120)(308)}$$

$$= 172.746$$

When we compare the calculated value of X^2 with tabulated values of χ^2 with 1 degree of freedom, we find that the probability of getting an X^2 value as large or larger than 172.746, when H_0 is true, is less than .005. The researcher may conclude that there is a relationship between the two characteristics under study.

The problems of how to handle small expected frequencies and small total sample sizes may arise in the analysis of 2 × 2 contingency tables. Cochran (5) suggests that the χ^2 test should not be used if $n < 20$ or if $20 < n < 40$ and any expected frequency is less than 5.

Yates' Correction. The observed frequencies in a contingency table are discrete and thereby give rise to a discrete statistic, X^2, which is approximated by the χ^2 distribution which is continuous. Yates (12) in 1934 proposed a procedure for correcting for this in the case of 2 × 2 tables. The correction consists of subtracting half the total number of observations from the absolute value of the quantity $ad - bc$ before squaring. That is

$$X^2_{\text{corrected}} = \frac{n(|ad - bc| - .5n)^2}{(a + c)(b + d)(a + b)(c + d)} \tag{10.4.2}$$

It is generally agreed that no correction is necessary for larger contingency tables. Although Yates' correction for 2 × 2 tables has been used extensively in the past, recent investigators, see, for example, Grizzle (13), Lancaster (14), Pearson (15), and Plackett (16), have questioned its use. The work of Grizzle, in particular, has strengthened the case against the use of the correction on the basis that it too often results in an overly conservative test, that is, the use of the correction too often leads to nonrejection of the null hypothesis. As a result some practitioners, for example Remington and Schork (17), are recommending against its use. This seems to be a reasonable recommendation to follow.

We may, as a matter of interest, apply the correction to our current example. Using Equation 10.4.2 and the data from Table 10.4.5, we may compute

$$X^2_{\text{corrected}} = \frac{500[|(105)(300) - (15)(80)| - (.5)(500)]^2}{(185)(315)(120)(380)}$$

$$= 169.907$$

As might be expected, with a sample this large, the difference in the two results is not dramatic.

Exercises

In the exercises that follow perform the test at the indicated level of significance and determine the p-value.

10.4.1. A sample of 250 physicians were cross classified according to the size of the community in which they were reared and the size of the community in which they were practicing. The results were as follows.

Size of Community Where Reared	Size of Community Where Practicing <5,000	5,000 to 9,999	10,000 to 49,999	50,000 or more	Total
<5,000	20	18	12	17	67
5,000 to 9,999	6	22	15	13	56
10,000 to 49,999	4	6	14	11	35
50,000 or more	10	19	23	40	92
Total	40	65	64	81	250

Do these data provide sufficient evidence to indicate a lack of independence between the two criteria of classification? Let $\alpha = .01$.

10.4.2. Five-hundred employees of a firm that manufactures a product suspected of being associated with respiratory disorders were cross classified by level of exposure to the product and whether or not they exhibited symptoms of respiratory disorders. The results are shown in this table.

	Level of Exposure			
Symptoms Present	High	Limited	No Known Exposure	Total
Yes	185	33	17	235
No	120	73	72	265
Total	305	106	89	500

Do these data provide sufficient evidence, at the .01 level of significance, to indicate a relationship between level of exposure and the presence of respiratory disorder symptoms?

10.4.3. Five hundred elementary school children were cross classified by socioeconomic group and the presence or absence of a certain speech defect. The results were as follows.

	Socioeconomic Group				
Speech Defect	Upper	Upper Middle	Lower Middle	Lower	Total
Present	8	24	32	27	91
Absent	42	121	138	108	409
Total	50	145	170	135	500

Are these data compatible with the hypothesis that the speech defect is unrelated to socioeconomic status?

10.4.4. A group of 350 adults who participated in a health survey were asked whether or not they were on a diet. The responses by sex are as follows.

	Sex		
	Male	Female	Total
On diet	14	25	39
Not on diet	159	152	311
Total	173	177	350

Do these data suggest that being on a diet is dependent on sex? Let $\alpha = .05$.

10.4.5. A sample of 500 college students participated in a study designed to evaluate the level of college students' knowledge of a certain group of common diseases. The following table shows the students classified by major field of study and level of knowledge of the group of diseases.

	Knowledge of Diseases		
Major	Good	Poor	Total
Premedical	31	91	122
Other	19	359	378
Total	50	450	500

Do these data suggest that there is a relationship between knowledge of the group of diseases and major field of study of the college students from which the present sample was drawn?

10.5 TEST OF HOMOGENEITY

A characteristic of the examples and exercises presented in the last section is that, in each case, the total sample was assumed to have been drawn before the entities were classified according to the two criteria of classification. That is, the observed number of entities falling into each cell was determined after the sample was drawn. As a result, the row and column totals are chance quantities not under the control of the investigator. We think of the sample drawn under these conditions as a single sample drawn from a single population. On occasion, however, either row or column totals may be under the control of the investigator, that is, the investigator may specify that independent samples be drawn from each of several populations. In this case one set of marginal totals is said to be *fixed*, while the other set, corresponding to the criterion of classification applied to the samples, is *random*. The former procedure, as we have seen, leads to a chi-square test of independence. The latter situation leads to a chi-square *test of homogeneity*. The two situations not only involve different sampling procedures; they lead to different questions and null hypotheses. The test of independence is concerned with the question: Are the two criteria of classification independent? The homogeneity test is concerned with the question: Are the samples drawn from populations that are homogeneous with respect to some criterion of classification? In the latter case the null hypothesis states that the samples are drawn from the same population. Despite these differences in concept and sampling procedure, the two tests are mathematically identical as we see when we consider the following example.

Example 10.5.1

A researcher, studying the extent of drug usage among college students who were professed users of drugs, selected from this group a sample of

Table 10.5.1

Extent of Drug Usage Among 510 College Students Classified by Class Standing

	Extent of Drug Usage			
Class Standing	**Experimental**	**Casual**	**Moderate to Heavy**	**Total**
Freshman	57	50	43	150
Sophomore	57	58	20	135
Junior	56	45	24	125
Senior	45	22	33	100
Total	215	175	120	510

150 freshmen, 135 sophomores, 125 juniors, and 100 seniors. Each student completed a questionnaire in which he or she indicated the extent of his or her use of drugs as either experimental, casual, or moderate to heavy. The results are shown in Table 10.5.1. The manner of selecting the samples, that is, selecting a specified number from each population, has the effect of fixing the row totals of the table.

Are these data compatible with the hypothesis that the four populations are homogeneous with respect to the extent of drug usage? The test statistic is the now familiar $X^2 = \sum[(O_i - E_i)^2/E_i]$. To proceed, then, we need expected frequencies for each of the cells in Table 10.5.1.

If the populations are indeed homogeneous, or, equivalently, if the samples are all drawn from the same population, with respect to drug usage, our best estimate of the proportion in the combined population who have used drugs only experimentally is $215/510 = .4216$. By the same token, if the four populations are homogeneous, we interpret this probability as applying to each of the populations individually. For example, under the null hypothesis, 215/510 is our best estimate of the probability that a student picked at random from the drug users will be an experimental user only. We would expect, then, to find $(215/510) \cdot 150 = 63.24$ out of 150 freshmen to be experimental users. Similarly, we would expect $(215/510) \cdot 135 = 56.91$ sophomores, $(215/510) \cdot 125 = 52.70$ juniors, and $(215/510) \cdot 100 = 42.16$ seniors to be experimental users.

We see again that the shortcut procedure of multiplying appropriate marginal totals and dividing by the grand total yields the expected frequencies for the cells. The expected frequencies computed in this manner, along with the observed frequencies, are shown in Table 10.5.2. The expected frequencies are enclosed in parentheses.

Table 10.5.2

Observed and Expected Frequencies, Example 10.5.1

	Extent of Drug Usage			
Class Standing	**Experimental**	**Casual**	**Moderate to Heavy**	**Total**
Freshman	57(63.24)	50(51.47)	43(35.29)	150
Sophomore	57(56.91)	58(46.32)	20(31.76)	135
Junior	56(52.70)	45(42.89)	24(29.41)	125
Senior	45(42.16)	22(34.31)	33(23.53)	100
Total	215	175	120	510

From the data in Table 10.5.2 we compute the following test statistic:

$$X^2 = \frac{(57 - 63.24)^2}{63.24} + \frac{(50 - 51.47)^2}{51.47} + \cdots + \frac{(33 - 23.53)^2}{23.53} = 19.4$$

The degrees of freedom associated with this value are found to be 6 when we apply the $(r - 1)(c - 1)$ rule. We find by consulting Table I that the probability of obtaining a value of X^2 as large or larger than 19.4 when the null hypothesis is true is less than .005. The decision then is to reject the null hypothesis. Consequently, we conclude that the populations are not homogeneous with respect to extent of drug usage.

The rules for small expected frequencies given in the previous section are applicable when carrying out a test of homogeneity.

When the chi-square test of homogeneity is used to test the null hypothesis that two populations are homogeneous, and when there are only two levels of the criterion of classification, the data may be displayed in a 2×2 contingency table. The analysis is identical to the analysis of 2×2 tables given in Section 10.4.

Exercises

In the exercises that follow perform the test at the indicated level of significance and determine the p-value.

10.5.1. In a study of the dental-caries status of children in six communities with varying levels of fluoride in the water supply, a sample of 125 children was selected from each of the communities and given a dental examination. The following table shows the number of caries-free children in each sample.

Community	Number of Children in Sample	Number of Caries-Free Children
A	125	38
B	125	8
C	125	30
D	125	44
E	125	64
F	125	32
Total	750	216

Are these data compatible with the hypothesis that the six populations are homogeneous with respect to the proportion of children who are free of dental caries?

10.5.2. In a study designed to investigate the relationship between nutritional status and ability to perform certain tasks, 400 experimental animals who had been trained to perform these tasks, were divided into four groups. The four groups were fed different diets representing different levels of nutritional deprivation ranging from a well-balanced diet (treatment condition 1) to one highly deficient in essential nutrients (treatment condition 4). After the animals had been on the diets for a period of time, their ability to perform tasks of varying difficulty was tested. Some of the animals were able to perform only the simple tasks, some could perform tasks of moderate difficulty, while others could perform the more difficult tasks. The following table shows the 400 animals classified according to treatment condition and level of difficulty of task performed.

Difficulty of Task Performed	Treatment Condition 1	2	3	4	Total
Simple	3	12	27	49	91
Moderately difficult	13	62	36	48	159
Difficult	84	26	37	3	150
Total	100	100	100	100	400

Should the researchers conclude that there is a lack of homogeneity among the four groups with respect to ability to perform tasks of varying difficulty?

10.5.3. A sample of hospital records was selected from the records of patients with each of five diagnoses. The records were evaluated as to appropriateness of length of stay. The results are shown in the following table.

	Length of Stay Evaluation			
Diagnosis	Appropriate Length of Stay	Understay	Overstay	Total
I	31	6	13	50
II	49	2	4	55
III	55	2	3	60
IV	42	9	24	75
V	33	3	9	45
Total	210	22	53	285

Do these data suggest a lack of homogeneity among the diagnostic groups with respect to length of stay evaluation? Let $\alpha = .05$.

10.5.4. In an air pollution study, a random sample of 200 households was selected from each of two communities. A respondent in each household was asked whether or not anyone in the household was bothered by air pollution. The responses were as follows.

Community	Any Member of Household Bothered by Air Pollution? Yes	No	Total
I	43	157	200
II	81	119	200
Total	124	276	400

Can the researchers conclude that the two communities differ with respect to the variable of interest?

10.6 SUMMARY

In this chapter some uses of the versatile chi-square distribution are discussed. Chi-square goodness-of-fit tests applied to the normal, binomial, and Poisson distributions are presented. We see that the procedure consists of computing a statistic

$$X^2 = \sum \frac{(O_i - E_i)^2}{E_i}$$

which measures the discrepancy between the observed (O_i) and expected (E_i) frequencies of occurrence of values in certain discrete categories. When the appropriate null hypothesis is true, this quantity is distributed approximately as χ^2. When X^2 is greater than the tabulated value of χ^2 for some α, the null hypothesis is rejected at the α level of significance.

Tests of independence and tests of homogeneity are also discussed in this chapter. The tests are mathematically equivalent but conceptually different. Again, these tests essentially test the goodness-of-fit of observed data to expectation under hypotheses, respectively, of independence of two criteria of classifying the data, and homogeneity of proportions among two or more groups.

Review Questions and Exercises

1. Explain how the chi-square distribution may be derived.
2. What are the mean and variance of the chi-square distribution?

3. Explain how the degrees of freedom are computed for the chi-square goodness-of-fit tests.
4. State Cochran's rule for small expected frequencies in goodness-of-fit tests.
5. How does one adjust for small expected frequencies?
6. What is a contingency table?
7. How are the degrees of freedom computed when an X^2 value is computed from a contingency table?
8. Explain the rationale behind the method of computing the expected frequencies in a test of independence.
9. Explain the difference between a test of independence and a test of homogeneity.
10. Explain the rationale behind the method of computing the expected frequencies in a test of homogeneity.
11. A study of 190 pregnancies yielded the following data on the relationship between hypertension of mother and a certain complication of pregnancy.

A Certain Complication of Pregnancy	Mother Hypertensive		
	Yes	No	Total
Present	23	55	78
Absent	12	100	112
Total	35	155	190

Do these data provide sufficient evidence to indicate that the two conditions are not independent? Let $\alpha = .01$. What is the p-value?

12. A sample of 150 chronic carriers of a certain antigen and a sample of 500 noncarriers revealed the following blood group distributions.

Blood Group	Carriers	Noncarriers	Total
O	72	230	302
A	54	192	246
B	16	63	79
AB	8	15	23
Total	150	500	650

Can one conclude from these data that the two populations from which the samples were drawn differ with respect to blood group distribution? Let $\alpha = .05$. What is the p-value for this test?

13. The following table shows 200 males classified according to social class and headache status:

Headache Group	Social Class A	B	C	Total
No Headache (in previous year)	6	30	22	58
Headache	11	35	17	63
Unilateral Headache	4	19	14	37
Migraine	5	25	12	42
Total	26	109	65	200

Do these data provide sufficient evidence to indicate that headache status and social class are related? Let $\alpha = .05$. What is the p-value for this test?

14. The following is the frequency distribution of scores made on an aptitude test by 175 applicants to a physical therapy training facility:

Score	Number of Applicants
10–14	3
15–19	8
20–24	13
25–29	17
30–34	19
35–39	25
40–44	28
45–49	20
50–54	18
55–59	12
60–64	8
65–69	4
Total	175

Do these data provide sufficient evidence to indicate that the population of scores is not normally distributed? Let $\alpha = .05$. What is the p-value for this test?

15. Several studies have contributed evidence to support the hypothesis that handling or "gentling" rats during the early part of their lives has beneficial results. Suppose a study in which a sample of handled rats

and a sample of unhandled rats compared with respect to overall health status were to yield the following results:

Health Status	Group		
	Handled	Unhandled	Total
High	37	23	60
Low	13	27	40
Total	50	50	100

Would these data support the hypothesis? Let $\alpha = .05$.

16. A local health department sponsored a VD information program that was open to high school juniors and seniors who ranged in age from 16 through 19 years. Since each year of age was about equally represented in the area served, the program director hypothesized that each age would be equally represented by those who attended. The age breakdown of those attending was as follows.

Age	Number Attending
16	26
17	50
18	44
19	40

Should the hypothesis be rejected? Let $\alpha = .05$. What is the p-value for this test?

17. A survey of children under 15 years of age residing in the inner city area of a large city were classified according to ethnic group and hemoglobin level. The results were as follows:

Ethnic Group	Hemoglobin Level (gms/100 ml)			
	10.0 or Greater	9.0–9.9	<9.0	Total
A	80	100	20	200
B	99	190	96	385
C	70	30	10	110
Total	249	320	126	695

Do these data provide sufficient evidence to indicate, at the .05 level of significance that the two variables are related? What is the p-value for this test?

18. A sample of reported cases of mumps in preschool children showed the following distribution by age:

Age (years)	Number of Cases
Under 1	6
1	20
2	35
3	41
4	48
Total	150

Test the hypothesis that cases occur with equal frequency in the five age categories. Let $\alpha = .05$. What is the p-value for this test?

19. Each of a sample of 250 men drawn from a population of suspected joint disease victims was asked which of three symptoms bother him most. The same question was asked of a sample of 300 suspected women joint disease victims. The results were as follows:

Symptom by which Bothered Most	Men	Women
Morning Stiffness	111	102
Nocturnal Pain	59	73
Joint Swelling	80	125
	250	300

Do these data provide sufficient evidence to indicate that the two populations are not homogeneous with respect to major symptoms? Let $\alpha = .05$. What is the p-value for this test?

For each of the following situations, indicate whether a chi-square test of homogeneity or a chi-square test of independence is appropriate.

20. A researcher wished to compare the status of three communities with respect to immunity against polio in preschool children. A sample of preschool children was drawn from each of the three communities.

21. In a study of the relationship between smoking and respiratory illness, a random sample of adults were classified according to consumption of tobacco and extent of respiratory symptoms.

22. A physician, who wished to know more about the relationship between smoking and birth defects studies the health records of a sample of mothers and their children, including still births and spontaneously aborted fetuses where possible.

23. A health research team believes that the incidence of depression is higher among people with hypoglycemia than among people who do not suffer from this condition.

References

References cited

1. Karl Pearson, "On the Criterion that a Given System of Deviations from the Probable in the Case of a Correlated System of Variables is such that it can be Reasonably Supposed to Have Arisen from Random Sampling," *The London, Edinburgh and Dublin Philosophical Magazine and Journal of Science*, Fifth Series, *50* (1900), 157–175. Reprinted in *Karl Pearson's Early Statistical Papers*, Cambridge University Press, 1948.
2. H. O. Lancaster, *The Chi-Squared Distribution*, Wiley, New York, 1969.
3. Harald Cramer, *Mathematical Methods of Statistics*, Princeton University Press, Princeton, N.J., 1958.
4. William G. Cochran, "The χ^2 Test of Goodness of Fit," *Annals of Mathematical Statistics*, *23* (1952), 315–345.
5. William G. Cochran, "Some Methods for Strengthening the Common χ^2 Tests," *Biometrics*, *10* (1954), 417–451.
6. John T. Roscoe and Jackson A. Byars, "An Investigation of the Restraints with Respect to Sample Size Commonly Imposed on the Use of the Chi-Square Statistic," *Journal of the American Statistical Association*, *66* (1971), 755–759.
7. James K. Yarnold, "The Minimum Expectation in X^2 Goodness-of-Fit Tests and the Accuracy of Approximations for the Null Distribution," *Journal of the American Statistical Association*, *65* (1970), 864–886.
8. Merle W. Tate and Leon A. Hyer, "Significance Values for an Exact Multinomial Test and Accuracy of the Chi-Square Approximation," U.S. Department of Health Education, and Welfare, Office of Education Bureau of Research, August 1969.
9. Malcolm J. Slakter, "Comparative Validity of the Chi-Square and Two Modified Chi-Square Goodness-of-Fit Tests for Small but Equal Expected Frequencies," *Biometrika*, *53* (1966), 619–23.
10. Malcolm J. Slakter, "A Comparison of the Pearson Chi-Square and Kolmogorov Goodness-of-Fit Tests with Respect to Validity," *Journal of the American Statistical Association*, *60* (1965), 854–858.
11. R. C. Lewontin and J. Felsenstein, "The Robustness of Homogeneity Tests in 2 × *N* Tables," *Biometrics*, *21* (1965), 19–33.

12. F. Yates, "Contingency Tables Involving Small Numbers and the χ^2 Tests," *Journal of the Royal Statistical Society Supplement*, *1* 1934 (Series B), 217–235.

13. J. E. Grizzle, "Continuity Correction in the χ^2 Test for 2×2 Tables," *The American Statistician*, *21* (October 1967), 28–32.

14. H. O. Lancaster, "The Combination of Probabilities Arising from Data in Discrete Distributions," *Biometrika*, *36* (1949), 370–382.

15. E. S. Pearson, "The Choice of Statistical Test Illustrated on the Interpretation of Data in a 2×2 Table," *Biometrika*, *34* (1947), 139–167.

16. R. L. Plackett, "The Continuity Correction in 2×2 Tables," *Biometrika*, *51* (1964), 427–338.

17. Richard D. Remington and M. Anthony Schork, *Statistics With Applications to the Biological and Health Sciences*, Prentice-Hall, Englewood Cliffs, N.J., 1970.

11

NONPARAMETRIC AND DISTRIBUTION-FREE STATISTICS

11.1 INTRODUCTION

The statistical inference procedures we have discussed up to this point, with one exception, are classified as *parametric statistics.* The one exception is our uses of chi-square: as a test of goodness-of-fit, as a test of homogeneity, and as a test of independence. These uses of chi-square come under the heading of *nonparametric statistics.*

The obvious question now is: What is the difference? In answer, let us recall the nature of the inferential procedures that we have categorized as *parametric.* In each case, our interest was focused on estimating or testing a hypothesis about one or more population parameters. Furthermore, central to these procedures was a knowledge of the functional form of the population from which were drawn the samples providing the basis for the inference.

An example of a parametric statistical test is the widely used t test. The most common uses of this test are for testing a hypothesis about a single population mean or the difference between two population means. One of the assumptions underlying the valid use of this test is that the sampled population or populations be, at least, approximately normally distributed.

As we shall learn, the procedures that we discuss in this chapter either are not concerned with population parameters or do not depend on knowledge of the sampled population. Strictly speaking, only those procedures that test hypotheses that are not statements about population parameters are classified as *nonparametric,* while those that make no assumption about the sampled population are called *distribution-free* procedures. Despite this distinction, it is customary to use the terms *nonparametric* and *distribution-free* interchangeably and to discuss the various procedures of both types under the heading of *nonparametric statistics.* We will follow this convention. This point is discussed by Kendall and Sundrum (1) and Gibbons (2).

The above discussion implies the following two advantages of nonparametric statistics.

1. They allow for the testing of hypotheses that are not statements about population parameter values. The chi-square tests of goodness-of-fit, homogeneity, and independence are examples of tests possessing this advantage.
2. Nonparametric tests may be used when the form of the sampled population is unknown.

Other advantages have been listed by several writers, for example, Gibbons (2), Blum and Fattu (3), Moses (4), and Siegel (5). In addition to the two already mentioned, the following are most frequently given.

3. Nonparametric procedures are computationally easier and consequently more quickly applied than parametric procedures. This can be a desirable feature in certain cases, but when time is not at a premium, it merits a low priority as a criterion for choosing a nonparametric test.
4. Nonparametric procedures may be applied when the data being analyzed consist merely of rankings or classifications. That is, the data may not be based on a measurement scale strong enough to allow the arithmetic operations necessary for carrying out parameteric procedures. The subject of measurement scales is discussed in more detail in the next section.

Although nonparametric statistics enjoy a number of advantages, their disadvantages must also be recognized. Moses (4) has noted the following.

1. The use of nonparametric procedures with data that can be handled with a parametric procedure results in a waste of data.
2. The application of some of the nonparametric tests may be laborious for large samples.

In a general introductory textbook, space limitations prevent the presentation of more than a sampling of nonparametric procedures. Additional procedures discussed at an introductory or intermediate level may be found in the books by Conover (6), Siegel (5), Bradley (7), Kraft and Van Eeden (8), Tate and Clelland (9), Gibbons (10), Mosteller and Rourke (11), Pierce (12), Noether (13), Hollander and Wolfe (14), and Lehmann (15). More mathematically rigorous books have been written by Gibbons (2), Hajek (16), and Walsh (17, 18). Savage (19) has prepared a bibliography of nonparametric statistics.

11.2 MEASUREMENT SCALES

As was pointed out in the previous section, one of the advantages of nonparameteric statistical procedures is that they can be used with data that are based on a weak measurement scale. To understand fully the meaning of this statement, it is necessary to know and understand the meaning of measurement and the various measurement scales most frequently used. This subject is discussed in considerable detail in the literature. Refer, in particular, to the writings of Stevens (20, 21).

Measurement. This may be defined as the assignment of numbers to objects or events according to a set of rules. The various measurement scales result from the fact that measurement may be carried out under different sets of rules.

The Nominal Scale. The lowest measurement scale is the *nominal scale*. As the name implies it consists of "naming" observations or classifying them into various mutually exclusive and collectively exhaustive categories. The practice of using numbers to distinguish among the various medical diagnoses constitutes measurement on a nominal scale. Other examples include such dichotomies as male–female, well–sick, under 65 years of age–65 and over child–adult, and married–not married. As we have seen, under certain conditions the chi-square test may be used for testing hypotheses regarding the frequency of occurrence of observations in various nominal categories.

The Ordinal Scale. Whenever observations are not only different from category to category, but when they can be ranked according to some criterion, they are said to be measured on an ordinal scale. Convalescing patients may be characterized as unimproved, improved, and much improved. Individuals may be classified according to socioeconomic status as low, medium, or high. The intelligence of children may be above average, average or below average. In each of these examples the members of any one category are all considered equal, but the members of one category are considered lower, worse, or smaller than those in another category, which in turn bears a similar relationship to another category. For example, a much improved patient is in better health than one classified as improved, while a patient who has improved is in better condition than one who has not improved. It is usually impossible to infer that the difference between members of one category, and the next adjacent category is equal to the difference between members of that category and the members of the category adjacent to it. The degree of improvement between unimproved and improved is probably not the same as that between improved and much improved. The implication is that if a finer breakdown were made resulting in more categories, these, too, could be ordered in a similar manner. The function of numbers assigned to ordinal data is to order (or rank) the observations from lowest to highest and, hence, the term ordinal. Numerous nonparametric statistical tests have been developed for use with ordinal data.

The Interval Scale. The *interval scale* is a more sophisticated scale than the nominal or ordinal in that with this scale it is not only possible to order measurements, but the distance between any two measurements is also known. We know, say, that the difference between a measurement of 20 and a measurement of 30 is equal to the difference between measurements of 30 and 40. The ability to do this implies the use of a unit distance and a zero point, both of which are arbitrary. The selected zero point is not a true zero in that it does not indicate a total absence of the quantity being measured. Perhaps the best example of an interval scale is provided by the way in which temperature is usually measured. The unit of measurement is the degree and the point of comparison is the arbitrarily chosen "zero degrees." The interval scale unlike the nominal and ordinal scales is a truly quantitative scale. When the interval scale of measurement has been achieved, and when the assumptions of the model are met, the usual parametric statistical procedures such as the t test and the F test may be used.

The Ratio Scale. The highest level of measurement is the *ratio scale.* This scale is characterized by the fact that equality of ratios as well as equality of intervals may be determined. Fundamental to the ratio scale is a true zero point. The measurement of such familiar traits as height, weight, and length, make use of the ratio scale. When the ratio scale of measurement has been achieved, any statistical procedure may be used provided that the assumptions of the particular model employed are met.

11.3 THE SIGN TEST

The familiar t test is not strictly valid for testing (a) the null hypothesis that a population mean is equal to some particular value, or (b) the null hypothesis that the mean difference between two populations is equal to zero unless it is known (or the researcher is willing to assume) that the relevant populations are normally distributed. Case b will be recognized as a situation that was analyzed by the paired comparisons test in Chapter 6. When the normality assumptions cannot be made or when the data at hand are ranks rather than measurements on an interval or ratio scale, an alternative test must be sought. Although the t test is known to be rather insensitive to violations of the normality assumption, there are times when an alternative test is desirable.

A frequently used nonparametric test that does not depend on the assumptions of the t test, or measurement beyond the ordinal scale, is the *sign test.* This test focuses on the median rather than the mean as a measure of central tendency or location. The median and mean will be equal in symmetric distributions. The only assumption underlying the test is that the distribution of the variable of interest is continuous.

The sign test gets its name from the fact that plusses and minuses, rather than numerical values, provide the raw data used in the calculations. We illustrate the use of the sign test, first in the case of a single sample, and then by an example involving paired samples.

Example 11.3.1

In a school for the mentally retarded, 10 girls selected at random received special instruction in personal care and grooming. Two weeks after completion of the course of instruction the girls were interviewed by a nurse and a social worker who assigned each girl a score based on her general appearance. The investigators believed that at best the scores achieved the level of an ordinal scale. They felt that although a score of, say, 8 represented a better appearance than a score of 6, they were unwilling to say that the difference between scores of 6 and 8 was equal to the difference between, say, scores of 8 and 10; or that the difference between scores of 6 and 8 represented twice as much improvement as the difference between scores of 5 and 6. The scores are shown in Table 11.3.1.

Let us use these data to test, at the .05 level of significance, the null hypothesis that the median score of the hypothetical population from which we assume this sample to have been drawn is 5 against the alternative that the

Table 11.3.1

General Appearance Scores of 10 Mentally Retarded Girls

Girl	**Score**	**Girl**	**Score**
1	4	6	6
2	5	7	10
3	8	8	7
4	8	9	6
5	9	10	6

Table 11.3.2

Scores Above (+) and Below (−) the Hypothesized Median Based on Data of Example 11.3.1

Girl	1	2	3	4	5	6	7	8	9	10
Score relative to hypothesized median	−	0	+	+	+	+	+	+	+	+

median is not 5. This statement of the alternative hypothesis implies a two-sided test.

As a first step in testing the hypothesis, we examine the data in Table 11.3.1 to determine which scores lie above and which ones lie below the hypothesized median of 5. If we assign a plus sign to those scores that lie above the hypothesized median and a minus to those that fall below, we have the results shown in Table 11.3.2.

If the null hypothesis were true, that is, if the median were, in fact, 5, we would expect the number of scores falling above and below 5 to be approximately equal. This line of reasoning suggests an alternative way in which we could have stated the null hypothesis, namely, that the probability of a plus is equal to the probability of a minus, and these probabilities are each equal to .5. Stated symbolically, the hypothesis would be

$$H_0: P(+) = P(-) = .5$$

In other words, we would expect about the same number of plus signs as minus signs in Table 11.3.2 when H_0 is true. A look at Table 11.3.2 reveals a preponderance of plusses; specifically, we observe eight plusses, one minus, and one zero, which was assigned to the score that fell exactly on the median. The usual procedure for handling zeros is to eliminate them from the analysis and reduce n, the sample size, accordingly. If we follow this procedure our problem reduces to one consisting of nine observations of which eight are plus and one is minus.

Since the number of plusses and minuses is not the same, we wonder if the distribution of signs is sufficiently disproportionate to cast doubt on our hypothesis. Stated another way, we wonder if this small a number of minuses could have come about by chance alone when the null hypothesis is true; or if the number is so small that something other than chance (that is, a false null hypothesis) is responsible for the results.

Based on what we learned in Chapter 3, it seems reasonable to conclude that the observations in Table 11.3.2 constitute a set of n independent random variables from the Bernoulli population with parameter, p. If we let $k =$ the number of minus signs, the sampling distribution of k is the binomial probability distribution with parameter $p = .5$ if the null hypothesis is true.

We may determine the probability of observing x or fewer minus signs when given a sample of size n and parameter p by evaluating the following expression:

$$P(k \leq x | n, p) = \sum_{k=0}^{x} \binom{n}{k} p^k q^{n-k} \tag{11.3.1}$$

For our example we would compute

$$\binom{9}{0}(.5)^0(.5)^{9-0} + \binom{9}{1}(.5)^1(.5)^{9-1} = .00195 + .01758 = .0195$$

We can use Table C and find

$$P(k \leq 1 | 9, .5) = 1 - \sum_{k=2}^{9} \binom{9}{k}(.5)^k(.5)^{9-k} = 1 - .9805 = .0195$$

With a two-sided test either a very small number of minuses or a very small number of plusses would cause rejection of the null hypothesis. Since, in our example, there are fewer minuses, we focus our attention on minuses rather than plusses. By setting α equal to .05, we are saying that if the number of minuses is so small that the probability of observing this few or fewer is less than .025 (half of α), we will reject the null hypothesis. The probability we have computed, .0195, is less than .025. We, therefore, reject the null hypothesis and conclude that the median score is not 5. The p-value for this test is 2(.0195) = .0390.

When the data to be analyzed consist of observations in matched pairs, and the assumptions underlying the t test are not met, or the measurement scale is weak, the sign test may be employed to test the null hypothesis that the median difference is 0. An alternative way of stating the null hypothesis is

$$P(X_i > Y_i) = P(X_i < Y_i) = .5$$

One of the matched scores, say Y_i, is subtracted from the other score, X_i. If Y_i is less than X_i, the sign of the difference is +, and if Y_i is greater than X_i, the sign of the difference is −. If the median difference is 0, we would expect a pair picked at random to be just as likely to yield a + as a − when the subtraction is performed. We may state the null hypothesis, then, as

$$P(+) = P(-) = .5$$

In a random sample of matched pairs we would expect the number of +'s and −'s to be about equal. If there are too many +'s or too many −'s than can be accounted for by chance alone when the null hypothesis is true, we will entertain some doubt about the truth of our null hypothesis. By means of the sign test, we can decide how many of one sign constitutes more than can be accounted for by chance alone.

Table 11.3.3

Oral Hygiene Scores of 12 Subjects Receiving Oral Hygiene Instruction (X_i) and 12 Subjects Not Receiving Instruction (Y_i)

	Score	
Pair Number	**Instructed** (X_i)	**Not Instructed** (Y_i)
1	1.5	2.0
2	2.0	2.0
3	3.5	4.0
4	3.0	2.5
5	3.5	4.0
6	2.5	3.0
7	2.0	3.5
8	1.5	3.0
9	1.5	2.5
10	2.0	2.5
11	3.0	2.5
12	2.0	2.5

Example 11.3.2

Twelve pairs of patients seen in a dental clinic were obtained by carefully matching on such factors as age, sex, intelligence, and initial oral hygiene scores. One member of each pair received instruction on how to brush the teeth and on other oral hygiene matters. Six months later all 24 subjects were examined and assigned an oral hygiene score by a dental hygienist unaware of which subjects had received the instruction. A low score indicates a high level of oral hygiene. The results are shown in Table 11.3.3.

The researcher wished to know if the instruction had produced a beneficial effect. If so, this fact would be reflected in the scores assigned to the members of each pair. If we take the differences $X_i - Y_i$ we would expect to observe more $-$'s than $+$'s if instruction had been beneficial, since a low score indicates a higher level of oral hygiene. If, in fact, instruction is beneficial, the median of the hypothetical population of all such differences would be less than 0, that is, negative. If, on the other hand, instruction has no effect, the median of this population would be zero. The null and alternate hypotheses, then, are

H_0: the median of the differences is zero

H_A: the median of the differences is negative

Table 11.3.4

Signs of Differences ($X_i - Y_i$) in Oral Hygiene Scores of 12 Subjects Instructed (X_i) and 12 Matched Subjects Not Instructed (Y_i)

Pair	1	2	3	4	5	6	7	8	9	10	11	12
Sign of score differences	−	0	−	+	−	−	−	−	−	−	+	−

Let us use a .05 level of significance and proceed to test the null hypothesis. As will be seen, the procedure is identical to the single sample procedure once the score differences have been obtained for each pair. Performing the subtractions and observing signs yields the results shown in Table 11.3.4.

The nature of the hypothesis indicates a one-sided test so that all of $\alpha = .05$ is associated with the rejection region which consists of all values of k (where k is equal to the number of + signs) for which the probability of obtaining that many or fewer plusses due to chance alone when H_0 is true is equal to or less than .05. We see in Table 11.3.4 that the experiment yielded one zero, two plusses, and nine minuses. When we eliminate the zero, the effective sample size is $n = 11$ with two plusses and nine minuses. In other words, since only a few plus signs will cause rejection of the null hypothesis, we want to know the probability of obtaining no more than two plusses out of eleven tries when the null hypothesis is true. As we have seen, the answer is obtained by evaluating the appropriate binomial expression. In this example we find

$$P(k \leq 2 | 11, .5) = \sum_{k=0}^{2} \binom{11}{k} (.5)^k (.5)^{11-k}$$

$$= 1 - \sum_{k=3}^{11} \binom{11}{k} (.5)^k (.5)^{11-k}$$

By consulting Table C, we find this probability to be

$$1 - .9673 = .0327$$

Since .0327 is less than .05, we must reject H_0 and conclude that the median difference is negative. That is, we conclude that the instruction was beneficial. For this test, $p = .0327$.

As has been demonstrated, the sign test may be used with a single sample or with two samples in which each member of one sample is matched with a member of the other sample to form a sample of matched pairs. We have also seen that the alternative hypothesis may lead to either a one-sided or a two-sided test. In either case we concentrate on the less frequently occurring sign and calculate the probability of obtaining that few or fewer of that sign.

Sample Size. We saw in Chapter 4 that when the sample size is large and when p is close to .5, the binomial distribution may be approximated by the normal distribution. The rule of thumb used was that the normal approximation is appropriate when both np and nq are greater than 5. When $p = .5$, as was hypothesized in our two examples, a sample of size 12 would satisfy the rule of thumb. Following this guideline, one could use the normal approximation when the sign test is used to test the null hypothesis that the median or median difference is 0 and n is equal to or greater than 12. Gibbons (2) concurs in this recommendation, although Siegel (5) recommends that n be, at least, 25. Since the procedure involves approximating a continuous distribution by a discrete distribution, the continuity correction of .5 is generally used. The test statistic then is

$$z = \frac{(k \pm .5) - .5n}{.5\sqrt{n}} \tag{11.3.2}$$

which is compared with the value of z from the unit normal distribution corresponding to the chosen level of significance. In Equation 11.3.2, $k + .5$ is used when $k < n/2$ and $k - .5$ is used when $k > n/2$.

In addition to the references already cited, the sign test is discussed in considerable detail by Dixon and Mood (22).

Exercises

11.3.1. A random sample of 15 student nurses were given a test to measure their level of authoritarianism with the following results.

Student number	1	2	3	4	5	6	7	8	9	10	11	12
Authoritarianism score	75	90	85	110	115	95	132	74	82	104	88	124
Student number	13	14	15									
Authoritarianism score	110	76	98									

Test at the .05 level of significance, the null hypothesis that the median score for the population sampled is 100. Determine the p-value.

11.3.2. A group of 20 patients seen in a physical therapy clinic were given a test, designed to measure their level of motivation, prior to participation in an experimental remotivation program. At the end of the program the patients were retested. The before and after scores were as follows.

Patient	Score Before	Score After	Patient	Score Before	Score After
1	10	15	11	16	24
2	8	10	12	10	23
3	5	10	13	15	25
4	14	14	14	5	15
5	15	25	15	24	20
6	22	20	16	20	25
7	17	20	17	14	24
8	10	22	18	10	23
9	8	16	19	15	25
10	20	18	20	14	25

Would you conclude that the remotivation program is effective? Let $\alpha = .05$. A high score indicates a high level of motivation. Determine the p-value.

11.4 THE MEDIAN TEST

The sign test for two samples given in the preceding section required that the samples be related. It is frequently of interest to make inferences based on two samples that are not related, that is, samples that are independent. To test the null hypothesis that two samples are drawn from populations with equal means, one employs the t or z statistic (depending on the sample sizes and/or whether the population variances are known or unknown) when the conditions for these parametric tests are met. A nonparametric counterpart is provided by the median test that may be used to test the null hypothesis that two independent samples have been drawn from populations with equal medians. The test, attributed mainly to Mood (23) and Westenberg (24), is also discussed by Brown and Mood (25) and Moses (4) as well as in several other references already cited.

The assumptions underlying the test are (a) the samples are selected at random from their respective populations, (b) the populations are of the same form, differing only in location, and (c) the variable of interest is continuous. The level of measurement must be, at least, ordinal. The two samples do not have to be of equal size. The test procedure can be demonstrated best by means of an example.

Example 11.4.1

Each of a random sample of 12 male students from a rural junior high school and 16 male students from an urban junior high school was given a

Table 11.4.1

Level of Mental Health Scores of Junior High Boys			
School			
Urban	**Rural**	**Urban**	**Rural**
35	29	25	50
26	50	27	37
27	43	45	34
21	22	46	31
27	42	33	
38	47	26	
23	42	46	
25	32	41	

test to measure their level of mental health. The results are shown in Table 11.4.1.

We wish to determine if we can conclude that there is a difference in median mental health scores between rural and urban junior high school boys. Suppose we choose a .05 level of significance.

The first step in the procedure is to compute the common median of the two samples combined. This is done by arranging the observations in ascending order and, since the total number of observations is even, obtaining the mean of the two middle numbers. For our example the median is $(33 + 34)/2 = 33.5$.

We now determine for each group the number of observations falling above and below the common median. The resulting frequencies are arranged in a 2×2 table. For the present example we obtain Table 11.4.2.

If the two samples are, in fact, from populations with the same median, we would expect about one half the scores in each sample to be above the combined median and about one half to be below. If the conditions relative

Table 11.4.2

Level of Mental Health Scores of Junior High School Boys			
	Urban	**Rural**	**Total**
Number of scores above median	6	8	14
Number of scores below median	10	4	14
Total	16	12	28

to sample size and expected frequencies for a 2×2 contingency table as discussed in Chapter 10 are met, the chi-square test with 1 degree of freedom may be used to test the null hypothesis of equal population medians. For example we have, by Formula 10.4.1,

$$X^2 = \frac{28[(6)(4) - (8)(10)]^2}{(16)(12)(14)(14)} = 2.33$$

Since $2.33 < 3.841$, the critical value of χ^2 with $\alpha = .05$ and 1 degree of freedom, we are unable to reject the null hypothesis on the basis of these data. We conclude, then, that the two samples may have been drawn from populations with equal medians. Since $2.33 < 2.706$, we have $p > .10$.

Sometimes one or more observed values will be exactly equal to the computed median and, hence, will fall neither above nor below the median. We note that if $n_1 + n_2$ is odd, at least one value will always be exactly equal to the median. This raises the question of what to do with observations of this kind. Siegel (5) recommends dropping them from the analysis if $n_1 + n_2$ is large and there are only a few values that fall at the combined median, or dichotomizing the scores into those that exceed the median and those that do not, in which case the observations that equal the median will be counted in the second category. Alternative procedures are suggested by Senders (26) and Hays and Winkler (27). The problem is discussed in considerable detail by Bradley (7).

Before we use the chi-square test, it should be determined that the necessary conditions for a 2×2 contingency table discussed in Chapter 10 are met. If they are not, a procedure known as Fisher's exact test (28) may be used. This test is discussed and illustrated by Siegel (5).

The median test extends logically to the case where it is desired to test the null hypothesis that $k \geq 3$ samples are from populations with equal medians. For this test a $2 \times k$ contingency table may be constructed by using the frequencies that fall above and below the median computed from combined samples. If conditions as to sample size and expected frequencies are met, X^2 may be computed and compared with the critical χ^2 with $k - 1$ degrees of freedom. Senders (26) and Conover (6) give numerical examples for the case where more than two samples are involved.

Exercises

11.4.1. Fifteen patient records from each of two hospitals were reviewed and assigned a score designed to measure level of care. The scores were as follows:

Hospital A: 99, 85, 73, 98, 83, 88, 99, 80, 74, 91, 80, 94, 94, 98, 80

Hospital B: 78, 74, 69, 79, 57, 78, 79, 68, 59, 91, 89, 55, 60, 55, 79

Would you conclude, at the .05 level of significance, that the two population medians are different? Determine the *p*-value.

11.4.2. The following serum albumin values were obtained from 17 normal and 13 hospitalized subjects.

Serum Albumin (g/100 ml)			
Normal Subjects		Hospitalized Subjects	
2.4	3.0	1.5	3.1
3.5	3.2	2.0	1.3
3.1	3.5	3.4	1.5
4.0	3.8	1.7	1.8
4.2	3.9	2.0	2.0
3.4	4.0	3.8	1.5
4.5	3.5	3.5	
5.0	3.6		
2.9			

Would you conclude at the .05 level of significance that the medians of the two populations sampled are different? Determine the *p*-value.

11.5 THE KOLMOGOROV–SMIRNOV GOODNESS-OF-FIT TEST

When one wishes to examine how well the distribution of sample data conforms to some theoretical distribution, a test known as the Kolmogorov-Smirnov goodness-of-fit test provides an alternative to the chi-square goodness-of-fit test discussed in Chapter 10. The test gets its name from A. Kolmogorov and N. V. Smirnov, two Russian mathematicians who introduced two closely related tests in the 1930s.

Kolmogorov's work (29) is concerned with the one-sample case as discussed here. Smirnov's work (30) deals with the case involving two samples in which interest centers on testing the hypothesis that the distributions of the two parent populations are identical. The test for the first situation is frequently referred to as the Kolmogorov-Smirnov one-sample test. The test for the two-sample case, commonly referred to as the Kolmogorov-Smirnov two-sample test, will not be discussed here. Those interested in this topic should refer to Conover (6), Gibbons (2, 10), and Siegel (5).

In using the Kolmogorov-Smirnov goodness-of-fit test a comparison is made between some theoretical cumulative distribution function, $F_T(x)$, and a sample cumulative distribution function, $F_S(x)$. The sample is a random sample from a population with unknown cumulative distribution function $F(x)$. It will be recalled (Section 3.2) that a cumulative distribution function gives the probability that X is equal to or less than a particular value, x. That is, by means of the sample cumulative distribution function, $F_S(x)$, we may determine $P(X \leq x)$. If there is close agreement between the theoretical and sample cumulative distributions, the hypothesis that the sample was drawn from the population with the specified cumulative distribution function, $F_T(x)$, is supported. If, however, there is a discrepancy between the theoretical and observed cumulative distribution functions too great to be attributed to chance alone, when H_0 is true, the hypothesis is rejected.

The difference between the theoretical cumulative distribution function $F_T(x)$, and the sample cumulative distribution function, $F_S(x)$ is measured by the statistic D, which is the greatest vertical distance between $F_S(x)$ and $F_T(x)$. When a two-sided test is appropriate, that is, when the hypotheses are

$$H_0: F(x) = F_T(x) \qquad \text{for all } x \text{ from } -\infty \text{ to } +\infty$$

$$H_A: F(x) \neq F_T(x), \qquad \text{for at least one } x \text{ the statistic is}$$

$$D = \sup_x |F_S(x) - F_T(x)| \tag{11.5.1}$$

which is read, "D equals the supremum, (greatest) over all x, of the absolute value of the differcnce $F_S(x)$ minus $F_T(x)$."

The null hypothesis is rejected at the α level of significance if the computed value of D exceeds the value shown in Table M for $1 - \alpha$ (two sided) and the sample size n. Tests in which the alternative is one sided are possible. Numerical examples are given by Conover (6) and Goodman (31).

The assumptions underlying the Kolmogorov-Smirnov test include the following.

1. The sample is a random sample.

2. The hypothesized distribution $F_T(x)$ is continuous.

Noether (32) has shown that when values of D are based on a discrete theoretical distribution, the test is conservative. When the test is used with discrete data, then, the investigator should bear in mind that the true probability of committing a Type I error is, at most, equal to α, the stated level of significance. The test is also conservative if one or more parameters have to be estimated from sample data.

Example 11.5.1

Fasting blood glucose determinations made on 36 nonobese, apparently healthy, adult males are shown in Table 11.5.1. We wish to test the null hypothesis that these data are from a normally distributed population with a mean of 80 and a standard deviation of 6. The appropriate hypotheses are

$$H_0: F(x) = F_T(x) \qquad \text{for all } x \text{ from } -\infty \text{ to } +\infty$$

$$H_A: F(x) \neq F_T(x) \qquad \text{for at least one } x$$

Our first step is to compute values of $F_S(x)$ as shown in Table 11.5.2.

Table 11.5.1

Fasting Blood Glucose Values (mg/100 ml) for 36 Nonobese, Apparently Healthy, Adult Males

75	92	80	80	84	72
84	77	81	77	75	81
80	92	72	77	78	76
77	86	77	92	80	78
68	78	92	68	80	81
87	76	80	87	77	86

Table 11.5.2

Values of $F_S(x)$ for Example 11.5.1

x	**Frequency**	**Cumulative Frequency**	$F_S(x)$
68	2	2	.0556
72	2	4	.1111
75	2	6	.1667
76	2	8	.2222
77	6	14	.3889
78	3	17	.4722
80	6	23	.6389
81	3	26	.7222
84	2	28	.7778
86	2	30	.8333
87	2	32	.8889
92	4	36	1.0000
	36		

We obtain values of $F_T(x)$ by first converting each observed value of x to a value of the unit normal variable, z. From Appendix Table F we then find the area between 0 and z. From these areas we are able to compute values of $F_T(x)$. The procedure, which is similar to that used to obtain expected relative frequencies in the chi-square goodness-of-fit test is summarized in Table 11.5.3.

The test statistic D may be computed algebraically, or it may be determined graphically by actually measuring the largest vertical distance between the curves of $F_S(x)$ and $F_T(x)$ on a graph. The graphs of the two distributions are shown in Figure 11.5.1.

Examination of the graphs of $F_S(x)$ and $F_T(x)$ reveals that $D \approx .16 = (.72 - .56)$. Reference to Table M reveals that a computed D of .16 is not

Table 11.5.3

Steps in Calculation of $F_T(x)$ for Example 11.5.1

x	$z = (x - 80)/6$	**Area Between** 0 **and** z	$F_T(x)$
68	-2.00	.4772	$.0228 = .5 - .4772$
72	-1.33	.4082	$.0918 = .5 - .4082$
75	$-.83$	.2967	$.2033 = .5 - .2967$
76	$-.67$	.2486	$.2514 = .5 - .2486$
77	$-.50$	.1915	$.3085 = .5 - .1915$
78	$-.33$	.1293	$.3707 = .5 - .1293$
80	.00	.0000	$.5000 = .5 - .0000$
81	.17	.0675	$.5675 = .5 + .0675$
84	.67	.2486	$.7486 = .5 + .2486$
86	1.00	.3413	$.8413 = .5 + .3413$
87	1.17	.3790	$.8790 = .5 + .3790$
92	2.00	.4772	$.9772 = .5 + .4772$

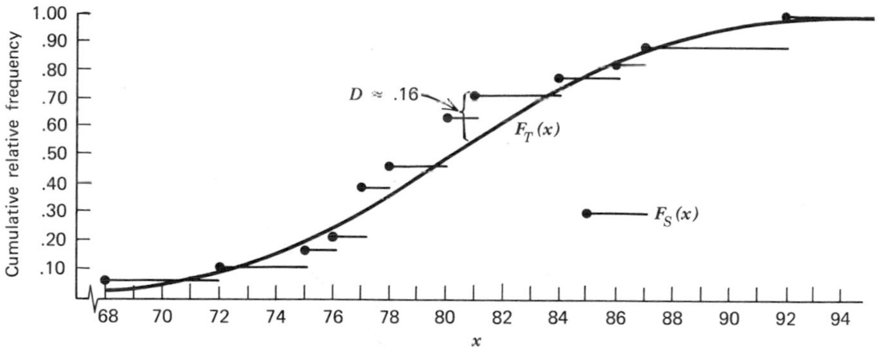

Figure 11.5.1 $F_S(x)$ *and* $F_T(x)$ *for Example 11.5.1.*

significant at any reasonable level. Therefore, we are not willing to reject H_0. The sample may have come from the specified distribution. Since we have a two-sided test, and since $.16 < .174$, we have $p > .20$.

Now let us compute the value of D algebraically. The possible values of $|F_S(x) - F_T(x)|$ are shown in Table 11.5.4. This table shows that the exact value of D is .1547.

The reader should be aware that in determining the value of D *it is not always sufficient to compute and choose from the possible values of* $|F_S(x) - F_T(x)|$. *The largest vertical distance between* $F_S(x)$ *and* $F_T(x)$ *may not occur at an observed value,* x. *but at some other value of* X. Such a situation is illustrated in Figure 11.5.2. We see that if only values of $|F_S(x) - F_T(x)|$

Table 11.5.4

Calculation of $|F_S(x) - F_T(x)|$ for Example 11.5.1

x	$F_S(x)$	$F_T(x)$	$\|F_S(x) - F_T(x)\|$
68	.0556	.0228	.0328
72	.1111	.0918	.0193
75	.1667	.2033	.0366
76	.2222	.2514	.0292
77	.3889	.3085	.0804
78	.4722	.3707	.1015
80	.6389	.5000	.1389
81	.7222	.5675	.1547
84	.7778	.7486	.0292
86	.8333	.8413	.0080
87	.8889	.8790	.0099
92	1.0000	.9772	.0228

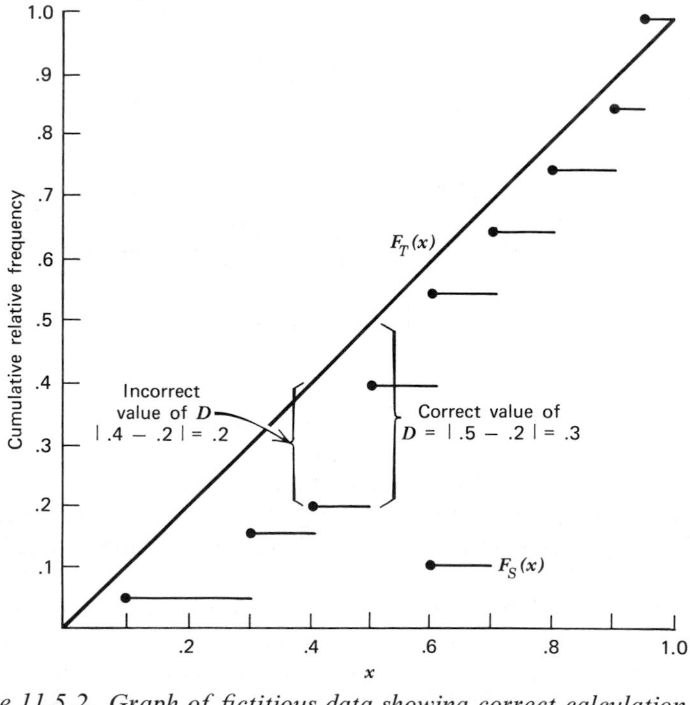

Figure 11.5.2. Graph of fictitious data showing correct calculation of D.

at the left endpoints of the horizontal bars are considered we would incorrectly compute D as $|.2 - .4| = .2$. One can see by examining the graph, however, that the largest vertical distance between $F_S(x)$ and $F_T(x)$ occurs at the right endpoint of the horizontal bar originating at the point corresponding to $x = .4$, and the correct value of D is $|.5 - .2| = .3$.

One can determine the correct value of D algebraically by computing, in addition to the differences $|F_S(x) - F_T(x)|$, the differences $|F_S(x_{i-1}) - F_T(x_i)|$ for all values of $i = 1, 2, \ldots, r + 1$, where $r =$ the number of different values of x and $F_S(x_0) = 0$. The correct value of the test statistic will then be

$$D = \underset{1 \le i \le r}{\text{maximum}} \{\text{maximum}\,[|F_S(x_i) - F_T(x_i)|, |F_S(x_{i-1}) - F_T(x_i)|]\} \quad (11.5.2)$$

The advantages and disadvantages of the Kolmogorov-Smirnov goodness-of-fit test in comparison with the chi-square test have been discussed by Goodman (31), Massey (33), Birnbaum (34), and Slakter (35). The following are some important points of comparison.

1. The Kolmogorov-Smirnov test does not require that the observations be grouped as is the case with the chi-square test. The consequence of this difference is that the Kolmogorov-Smirnov test makes use of all the information present in a set of data.
2. The Kolmogorov-Smirnov test can be used with any size sample. It will be recalled that certain minimum sample sizes are required for the use of the chi-square test.
3. As has been noted the Kolmogorov-Smirnov test is not applicable when parameters have to be estimated from the sample. The chi-square test may be used in these situations by reducing the degrees of freedom by 1 for each parameter estimated.
4. The problem of the assumption of a continuous theoretical distribution has already been mentioned.

Exercises

11.5.1. The weights at autopsy of the brains of 25 adults suffering from a certain disease were as follows:

Weight of Brain (grams)

859	1073	1041	1166	1117
962	1051	1064	1141	1202
973	1001	1016	1168	1255
904	1012	1002	1146	1233
920	1039	1086	1140	1348

Can one conclude from these data that the sampled population is not normally distributed with a mean of 1050 and a standard deviation of 50? Determine the p-value for this test.

11.5.2. IQs of a sample of 30 adolescents arrested for drug abuse in a certain metropolitan jurisdiction were as follows:

IQ

95	100	91	106	109	110
98	104	97	100	107	119
92	106	103	106	105	112
101	91	105	102	101	110
101	95	102	104	107	118

Do these data provide sufficient evidence that the sampled population of IQ scores is not normally distributed with a mean of 105 and a standard deviation of 10? Determine the p-value.

11.5.3. For a sample of apparently normal subjects who served as controls in an experiment, the following systolic blood pressure readings were recorded at the beginning of the experiment:

162	177	151	167
130	154	179	146
147	157	141	157
153	157	134	143
141	137	151	161

Can one conclude on the basis of these data that the population of blood pressures from which the sample was drawn is not normally distributed? Determine the p-value.

11.6 THE KRUSKAL–WALLIS ONE-WAY ANALYSIS OF VARIANCE BY RANKS

In Chapter 7 we discuss how one-way analysis of variance may be used to test the null hypothesis that several group means are equal. When the assumptions underlying this technique are not met, that is, when the populations from which the samples are drawn are not normally distributed with equal variances, or when the data for analysis consist only of ranks, a nonparametric alternative to the one-way analysis of variance may be used to test the hypothesis of equal location parameters. As was pointed out in Section 11.4, the median test may be extended to accommodate the situation involving more than two groups. A deficiency of this test, however, is the fact that it uses only a small amount of the information available, that is, whether or not the observations are above or below a single number, the median of the combined samples. Several nonparametric analogs to analysis of variance are available that use more information by taking into account the magnitude of each observation relative to the magnitude of every other observation. Perhaps the best known of these procedures is the Kruskal-Wallis one-way analysis of variance by ranks (36).

The application of the test involves the following steps.

1. The $n_1, n_2, \ldots, n_k$ observations from the k groups are combined into a single series of size n and arranged in order of magnitude from smallest to largest. The observations are then replaced by ranks from 1, which is assigned to the smallest observation, to n, which is assigned to the largest observation. When two or more observations have the same value, each observation is given the mean of the ranks for which it is tied.
2. The ranks assigned to observations in each of the k groups are added separately to give k rank sums.
3. The test statistic

$$H = \frac{12}{n(n+1)} \sum_{j=1}^{k} \frac{R_j^2}{n_j} - 3(n+1) \qquad (11.6.1)$$

is computed.

In Equation 11.6.1

k = the number of groups

n_j = the number of observations in the jth group

n = the number of observations in all groups combined

R_j = the sum of the ranks in the jth group

4. When there are three groups and five or fewer observations in each group, the significance of the computed H is determined by consulting Appendix Table N. When there are more than five observations in one or more of the groups, H is compared with tabulated values of χ^2 with $k - 1$ degrees of freedom. The adequacy of the chi-square approximation for small samples is discussed by Gabriel and Lachenbruch (37).

Example 11.6.1

The effects of two drugs on reaction time to a certain stimulus were studied in three groups of experimental animals. Group III served as a control while the animals in Group I were treated with drug A and those in Group II were treated with drug B prior to the application of the stimulus. Table 11.6.1 shows the reaction times in seconds of the 13 animals.

Table 11.6.1

Reaction Time in Seconds of 13 Experimental Animals

Group I	Group II	Group III
17	8	2
20	7	5
40	9	4
31	8	3
35		

Table 11.6.2

The Data of Table 11.6.1 Replaced by Ranks

Group I	Group II	Group III
9	6.5	1
10	5	4
13	8	3
11	6.5	2
12		
$R_1 = 55$	$R_2 = 26$	$R_3 = 10$

Can we conclude that the three groups differ with respect to reaction time? We can so conclude if we can reject the null hypothesis that the three groups do not differ in their reaction times.

When the three groups are combined into a single series and ranked, the table of ranks shown in Table 11.6.2 may be constructed.

The null hypothesis implies that the observations in the three groups constitute a sample of size 13 from a single population. If this be true, we would expect the ranks to be well distributed among the three groups. Consequently, we would expect the total sum of ranks to be divided among the three groups in proportion to group size. Departures from these conditions are reflected in the magnitude of the test statistic H. The null hypothesis will be rejected if the computed value of H is so large that the probability of obtaining a value that large or larger when H_0 is true is equal to or less than the chosen significance level, α.

From the data in Table 11.6.2 and Equation 11.6.1 we obtain

$$H = \frac{12}{13(13+1)}\left[\frac{(55)^2}{5} + \frac{(26)^2}{4} + \frac{(10)^2}{4}\right] - 3(13+1)$$

$$= 10.68$$

Table N shows that when the n_j's are 5, 4, and 4, the probability of obtaining a value of $H \geq 10.68$ is less than .009. The null hypothesis can be rejected at the .01 level of significance, and we conclude that there is a difference in the average reaction time among the three groups. For this test, $p < .009$.

It will be noted that the two values in group II were each assigned the rank of 6.5. We may adjust the value of H for this tie by dividing it by

$$1 - \frac{\sum T}{n^3 - n} \tag{11.6.2}$$

where $T = t^3 - t$. The letter t is used to designate the number of tied observations in a group of tied values. In our present example there is only one group of tied values but, in general, there may be several groups of tied values resulting in several values of T. Since there were only two tied observations in our one group of ties, we have $T = 2^3 - 2 = 6$ and $\sum T = 6$, so that Expression 11.6.2 is

$$1 - \frac{6}{13^3 - 13} = .9973$$

and

$$\frac{H}{1 - \dfrac{\sum T}{n^3 - n}} = \frac{10.68}{.9973} = 10.71$$

which, of course, is also significant at the .01 level.

As is the case here, the effect of the adjustment for ties is usually negligible. Note also that the effect of the adjustment is to increase H, so that if the unadjusted H is significant at the chosen level, there is no need to apply the adjustment.

Now let us illustrate the procedure when there are more than three groups and, at least, one of the n_j's is greater than 5.

Example 11.6.2

Table 11.6.3 shows the net book value of equipment capital per bed for a sample of hospitals from each of five types of hospitals. We wish to determine, by means of the Kruskal-Wallis test, if we can conclude that the average net

Table 11.6.3

Net Book Value of Equipment per Bed by Hospital Type

Type Hospital				
A	B	C	D	E
\$1735(11)	\$5260(35)	\$2790(20)	\$3475(26)	\$6090(40)
1520(2)	4455(28)	2400(12)	3115(22)	6000(38)
1476(1)	4480(29)	2655(16)	3050(21)	5894(37)
1688(7)	4325(27)	2500(13)	3125(23)	5705(36)
1702(10)	5075(32)	2755(19)	3275(24)	6050(39)
2667(17)	5225(34)	2592(14)	3300(25)	6150(41)
1575(4)	4613(30)	2601(15)	2730(18)	5110(33)
1602(5)	4887(31)	1648(6)		
1530(3)		1700(9)		
1698(8)				
$R_1 = 68$	$R_2 = 246$	$R_3 = 124$	$R_4 = 159$	$R_5 = 264$

book value of equipment capital per bed differs among the five types of hospital. The ranks of the 41 values, along with the sum of ranks for each group, are shown in the table.

From the sums of the ranks we compute

$$H = \frac{12}{41(41+1)}\left[\frac{(68)^2}{10} + \frac{(246)^2}{8} + \frac{(124)^2}{9} + \frac{(159)^2}{7} + \frac{(264)^2}{7}\right] - 3(41+1)$$

$$= 36.39$$

Reference to Table I with $k - 1 = 4$ degrees of freedom indicates that the probability of obtaining a value of H as large or larger than 36.39, due to chance alone, when there is no difference among the groups is less than .005. We conclude, then, that there is a difference among the groups with respect to the average value of the variable of interest.

Exercises

For the following exercises, perform the test at the indicated level of significance and determine the p-value.

11.6.1. The following table shows the pesticide residue levels (ppb) in blood samples from four groups of human subjects. Use the Kruskal-Wallis test to test at the .05 level of significance the null hypothesis that there is no difference among the groups with respect to average level of pesticide residue.

Group			
A	B	C	D
10	4	15	7
37	35	5	11
12	32	10	10
31	19	12	8
11	33	6	2
9	18	6	5
44	11	9	4
12	7	11	5
15	32	9	2
42	17	14	6
23	8	15	3

11.6.2. The following are average daily charges made to patients hospitalized for a certain surgical procedure by samples of hospitals located in three different parts of the country.

	Group	
I	II	III
\$80.75	\$58.63	\$84.21
78.15	72.70	101.76
85.40	64.20	107.74
71.94	62.50	115.30
82.05	63.24	126.15

Can we conclude at the .05 level of significance that the groups differ with respect to the average daily charges?

11.6.3. Refer to the data in Table 7.2.1 (Example 7.2.1) and apply the Kruskal-Wallis test. Compare the results with those obtained when the F test was used.

11.6.4. Refer to Exercise 7.2.1 and apply the Kruskal-Wallis Test.

11.6.5. Refer to Exercise 7.2.2 and apply the Kruskal-Wallis Test.

11.6.6. Refer to Exercise 7.2.3 and apply the Kruskal-Wallis Test.

11.6.7. Refer to Exercise 7.2.4 and apply the Kruskal-Wallis Test.

11.7 THE FRIEDMAN TWO-WAY ANALYSIS OF VARIANCE BY RANKS

Just as we may on occasion have need of a nonparametric analog to the parametric one-way analysis of variance, we may also find it necessary to analyze the data in a two-way classification by nonparametric methods analogous to the two-way analysis of variance. Such a need may arise because the assumptions necessary for parametric analysis of variance are not met, because the measurement scale employed is weak, or because results are needed in a hurry. A test frequently employed under these circumstances is the Friedman two-way analysis of variance by ranks (38, 39). This test is appropriate whenever the data are measured on, at least, an ordinal scale and can be meaningfully arranged in a two-way classification as is given for the randomized block experiment discussed in Chapter 7. The following example illustrates this procedure.

Example 11.7.1

Nine physical therapists were asked to rank three models of low-volt electrical stimulator in order of preference. A rank of 1 indicates first preference. The results are shown in Table 11.7.1.

The null hypothesis to be tested is that there is no difference in preferences for the models. The alternative hypothesis is that the models are not preferred equally. By means of the Friedman test we will be able to determine if it is reasonable to assume that the columns of ranks have been drawn from the same population. If the null hypothesis is true we would expect the observed distribution of ranks within any column to be the product of chance factors

Table 11.7.1

Physical Therapists' Rankings of Three Models of Low-Volt Electrical Stimulator

	Model		
Therapist	**A**	**B**	**C**
1	2	3	1
2	2	3	1
3	2	3	1
4	1	3	2
5	3	2	1
6	1	2	3
7	2	3	1
8	1	3	2
9	1	3	2
R_j	15	25	14

and, hence, we would expect the numbers 1, 2, and 3 to occur with approximately the same frequency in each column. If, on the other hand, the null hypothesis is false (that is, the models are not equally preferred), we would expect a preponderance of relatively high (or low) ranks in at least one column. This condition would be reflected in the sums of the ranks. The Friedman test will tell us whether or not the observed sums of ranks are so discrepant that it is not likely they are a result of chance when H_0 is true.

Since the data already consist of rankings within blocks (rows), our first step is to sum the ranks within each column (treatment). These sums are the R_j's shown in Table 11.7.1. A test statistic, denoted by Friedman as χ_r^2 is computed as follows:

$$\chi_r^2 = \frac{12}{nk(k+1)} \sum_{j=1}^{k} (R_j)^2 - 3n(k+1) \qquad (11.7.1)$$

where $n =$ the number of rows (blocks) and $k =$ the number of columns (treatments). Critical values for various values of n and k are given in Table O.

For our illustrative example we compute

$$\chi_r^2 = \frac{12}{9(3)(3+1)}[(15)^2 + (25)^2 + (14)^2] - 3(9)(3+1)$$
$$= 8.222$$

When we consult Appendix Table O*a*, we find that the probability of obtaining a value of χ_r^2 as large as 8.222 due to chance alone, when the null hypothesis is true, is .016. We are able, therefore, to reject the null hypothesis and conclude that the three models of low-volt electrical stimulator are not equally preferred. For this test, $p = .016$.

When the original data consist of measurements on an interval or a ratio scale instead of ranks, the measurements are assigned ranks based on their relative magnitudes within blocks. If ties occur each value is assigned the mean of the ranks for which it is tied.

When the values of k and or n exceed those given in Table O of the Appendix, the critical value of χ_r^2 is obtained by consulting the χ^2 table (Table I) with the chosen α and $k - 1$ degrees of freedom.

Example 11.7.2

Table 11.7.2 shows the responses, in percent decrease in salivary flow, of 16 experimental animals following different dose levels of atropine. The ranks (in parentheses) and the sum of the ranks are also given in the table. We wish to see if we may conclude that the different dose levels produce different responses. That is, we test the null hypothesis of no difference in response among the four dose levels.

Table 11.7.2

Percent Decrease in Salivary Flow of Experimental Animals Following Different Dose Levels of Atropine

	Dose Level			
Animal Number	**A**	**B**	**C**	**D**
1	29(1)	48(2)	75(3)	100(4)
2	72(2)	30(1)	100(3.5)	100(3.5)
3	70(1)	100(4)	86(2)	96(3)
4	54(2)	35(1)	90(3)	99(4)
5	5(1)	43(3)	32(2)	81(4)
6	17(1)	40(2)	76(3)	81(4)
7	74(1)	100(3)	100(3)	100(3)
8	6(1)	34(2)	60(3)	81(4)
9	16(1)	39(2)	73(3)	79(4)
10	52(2)	34(1)	88(3)	96(4)
11	8(1)	42(3)	31(2)	79(4)
12	29(1)	47(2)	72(3)	99(4)
13	71(1)	100(3.5)	97(2)	100(3.5)
14	7(1)	33(2)	58(3)	79(4)
15	68(1)	99(4)	84(2)	93(3)
16	70(2)	30(1)	99(3.5)	99(3.5)
R_j	20	36.5	44	59.5

From the data we compute

$$\chi_r^2 = \frac{12}{16(4)(4+1)}[(20)^2 + (36.5)^2 + (44)^2 + (59.5)^2] - 3(16)(4+1)$$

$$= 30.32$$

Reference to Table I indicates that with $k - 1 = 3$ degrees of freedom the probability of getting a value of χ_r^2 as large as 30.32 due to chance alone is, when H_0 is true, less than .005. We reject the null hypothesis and conclude that the different dose levels do produce different responses.

Exercises

For the following exercises perform the test at the indicated level of significance and determine the p-value.

11.7.1. The following table shows the scores made by nine randomly selected student nurses on final examinations in three subject areas.

Student Number	Fundamentals	Subject Area Physiology	Anatomy
1	98	95	77
2	95	71	79
3	76	80	91
4	95	81	84
5	83	77	80
6	99	70	93
7	82	80	87
8	75	72	81
9	88	81	83

Test the null hypothesis that student nurses constituting the population from which the above sample was drawn perform equally well in all three subject areas against the alternative hypothesis that they perform better in, at least, one area. Let $\alpha = .05$.

11.7.2. Fifteen randomly selected physical therapy students were given the following instructions: "Assume that you will marry a person with one of the following handicaps (the handicaps were listed and designated by the letters A to J). Rank these handicaps from 1 to 10 according to your first, second, third (and so on) choice of a handicap for your marriage partner." The results are shown in the following table.

Student Number	Handicap A	B	C	D	E	F	G	H	I	J
1	1	3	5	9	8	2	4	6	7	10
2	1	4	5	7	8	2	3	6	9	10
3	2	3	7	8	9	1	4	6	5	10
4	1	4	7	8	9	2	3	6	5	10
5	1	4	7	8	10	2	3	6	5	9
6	2	3	7	9	8	1	4	5	6	10
7	2	4	6	9	8	1	3	7	5	10
8	1	5	7	9	10	2	3	4	6	8
9	1	4	5	7	8	2	3	6	9	10
10	2	3	6	8	9	1	4	7	5	10
11	2	4	5	8	9	1	3	7	6	10
12	2	3	6	8	10	1	4	5	7	9
13	3	2	6	9	8	1	4	7	5	10
14	2	5	7	8	9	1	3	4	6	10
15	2	3	6	7	8	1	5	4	9	10

Test the null hypothesis of no preference for handicaps against the alternative that some handicaps are preferred over others. Let $\alpha = .05$.

11.7.3. Refer to Example 7.3.1. Work the example using the Friedman test and compare the results with those obtained using the parametric two-way analysis of variance.

11.7.4. Refer to Exercise 7.3.1. Work this exercise by using the Friedman test.

11.7.5. Use the Friedman test to work Exercise 7.3.2.

11.7.6. Use the Friedman test to work Exercise 7.3.3.

11.7.7. Use the Friedman test to work Exercise 7.3.4.

11.8 THE SPEARMAN RANK CORRELATION COEFFICIENT

Several nonparametric measures of correlation are available to the researcher. Refer to Kendall (40), Kruskal (41), and Hotelling and Pabst (42) for detailed discussions of the various methods.

A frequently used procedure that is attractive because of the simplicity of the calculations involved is due to Spearman (43). The measure of correlation computed by this method is called the Spearman rank correlation coefficient and is designated by r_s. This procedure makes use of the two sets of ranks which may be assigned to the sample values of X and Y, the independent and continuous variables of a bivariate distribution. The usually tested hypotheses and their alternatives are as follows.

(1) H_0: X and Y are mutually independent.
H_A: X and Y are not mutually independent.

(2) H_0: X and Y are mutually independent.
H_A: There is a tendency for large values of X and large values of Y to be paired together.

(3) H_0: X and Y are mutually independent.
H_A: There is a tendency for large values of X to be paired with small values of Y.

The hypotheses specified in no. 1 lead to a two-sided test and are used when it is desired to detect any departure from independence. The one-sided tests indicated by nos. 2 and 3 are used, respectively, when investigators wish to know if they can conclude that the variables are directly or inversely correlated.

The hypothesis-testing procedure involves the following steps.

1. Rank the values of X from 1 to n (the number of pairs of values of X and Y in the sample). Rank the values of Y from 1 to n.
2. Compute d_i for each pair of observations by subtracting the rank of Y_i from the rank of X_i.
3. Square each d_i and compute $\sum d_i^2$, the sum of the squared values.

4. Compute

$$r_s = 1 - \frac{6\sum d_i^2}{n(n^2 - 1)} \qquad (11.8.1)$$

5. If n is between 4 and 30 compare the computed value of r_s with the critical values, r_s^*, of Table P. For the two-sided test, H_0 is rejected at the α significance level if r_s is greater than r_s^* or less than $-r_s^*$ where r_s^* is at the intersection of the column headed $\alpha/2$ and the row corresponding to n. For the one-sided test with H_A specifying direct correlation, H_0 is rejected at the α significance level if r_s is greater than r_s^* for α and n. The null hypothesis is rejected at the significance level in the other one-sided test if r_s is less than $-r_s^*$ for α and n.
6. If n is greater than 30, one may compute

$$z = r_s\sqrt{n - 1} \qquad (11.8.2)$$

and use Table F to obtain critical values.
7. Tied observations present rather a problem. Glasser and Winter (44) point out that the use of Table P is strictly valid only when the data do not contain any ties (unless some random procedure for breaking ties is employed). In practice, however, the table is frequently used after some other method for handling ties has been employed. If the number of ties is large, a correction for ties found in Siegel (5) may be employed. The correction factor for ties is

$$T = \frac{t^3 - t}{12} \qquad (11.8.3)$$

where t = the number of observations that are tied for some particular rank. When this correction factor is used r_s is computed from

$$r_s = \frac{\sum x^2 + \sum y^2 - \sum d_i^2}{2\sqrt{\sum x^2 \sum y^2}} \qquad (11.8.4)$$

instead of from Equation 11.8.1.

In Equation 11.8.4

$$\sum x^2 = \frac{n^3 - n}{12} - \sum T_x$$

$$\sum y^2 = \frac{n^3 - n}{12} - \sum T_y$$

T_x = the sum of the values of T for the various tied ranks in X, and

T_y = the sum of the values of T for the various tied ranks in Y

Gibbons (2), as well as Siegel (5), points out that unless the number of ties is excessive the correction makes very little difference in the value of r_s. When the number of ties is small, we can follow the usual procedure of assigning the tied observations the mean of the ranks for which they are tied and proceed with steps 2 to 6 above. Edgington (45) discusses the problem of ties in some detail.

Example 11.8.1

In a study of the relationship between age and the EEG, data were collected on 20 subjects between the ages of 20 and 60 years. Table 11.8.1 shows the age and a particular EEG output value for each of the 20 subjects.

The investigator wishes to know if it can be concluded that this particular EEG output is inversely correlated with age. The hypotheses for the one-sided test, then, are

H_0: This EEG output and age are mutually independent.

H_A: There is a tendency for this EEG output to decrease with age.

Suppose we let $\alpha = .05$.

When the X and Y values are ranked we have the results shown in Table 11.8.2.

Table 11.8.1

Age and EEG Output Value for 20 Subjects

Subject Number	**Age** (X)	**EEG Output Value** (Y)
1	20	98
2	21	75
3	22	95
4	24	100
5	27	99
6	30	65
7	31	64
8	33	70
9	35	85
10	38	74
11	40	68
12	42	66
13	44	71
14	46	62
15	48	69
16	51	54
17	53	63
18	55	52
19	58	67
20	60	55

Table 11.8.2

Ranks for Data of Example 11.8.1

Subject Number	**Rank** (X)	**Rank** (Y)	d_i	d_i^2
1	1	18	−17	289
2	2	15	−13	169
3	3	17	−14	196
4	4	20	−16	256
5	5	19	−14	196
6	6	7	−1	1
7	7	6	1	1
8	8	12	−4	16
9	9	16	−7	49
10	10	14	−4	16
11	11	10	1	1
12	12	8	4	16
13	13	13	0	0
14	14	4	10	100
15	15	11	4	16
16	16	2	14	196
17	17	5	12	144
18	18	1	17	289
19	19	9	10	100
20	20	3	17	289
				$\sum d_i^2 = 2340$

The d_i, d_i^2 and $\sum d_i^2$ are shown in the same table.

Substitution of the data from Table 11.8.2 into Equation 11.8.1 gives

$$r_s = 1 - \frac{6(2340)}{20[(20)^2 - 1]} = -.76$$

Reference to Table P shows that for a one-sided test, $\alpha = .05$ and $n = 20$, the critical value of r_s^* is $-.3789$. Since our computed $r_s = -.76$ is less than the critical r_s^* we reject the null hypothesis and conclude that the two variables are inversely related. Since $-.76 < -.6586$, we have for this test $p < .001$.

Let us now illustrate the procedure for a sample with $n > 30$ and some tied observations.

Example 11.8.2

In Table 11.8.3 are shown the ages and concentrations (ppm) of a certain mineral in the tissue of 35 subjects on whom autopsies were performed as part of a large research project.

Table 11.8.3

Age and Mineral Concentration (ppm) in Tissue of 35 Subjects

Subject Number	**Age** (X)	**Mineral Concentration** (Y)	**Subject Number**	**Age** (X)	**Mineral Concentration** (Y)
1	82	169.63	19	50	4.48
2	85	48.94	20	71	46.93
3	83	41.16	21	54	30.91
4	64	63.95	22	62	34.27
5	82	21.09	23	47	41.44
6	53	5.40	24	66	109.88
7	26	6.33	25	34	2.78
8	47	4.26	26	46	4.17
9	37	3.62	27	27	6.57
10	49	4.82	28	54	61.73
11	65	108.22	29	72	47.59
12	40	10.20	30	41	10.46
13	32	2.69	31	35	3.06
14	50	6.16	32	75	49.57
15	62	23.87	33	50	5.55
16	33	2.70	34	76	50.23
17	36	3.15	35	28	6.81
18	53	60.59			

The ranks, d_i, d_i^2, and $\sum d_i^2$ are shown in Table 11.8.4. Let us test, at the .05 level of significance, the null hypothesis that X and Y are mutually independent against the two-sided alternative that they are not mutually independent.

From the data in Table 11.8.4 we compute

$$r_s = 1 - \frac{6(1788.5)}{35[(35^2 - 1]} = .75$$

To test the significance of r_s we compute

$$z = .75\sqrt{35 - 1} = 4.37$$

Since 4.37 is greater than $z = 3.09$, $p < 2(.001) = .002$, and we reject H_0 and conclude that the two variables under study are not mutually independent.

For comparative purposes let us correct for ties using Equation 11.8.3 and then compute r_s by Equation 11.8.4.

Table 11.8.4

Ranks for Data of Example 11.8.2

Subject Number	Rank (X)	Rank (Y)	d_i	d_i^2	Subject Number	Rank (X)	Rank (Y)	d_i	d_i^2
1	32.5	35	−2.5	6.25	19	17	9	8	64.00
2	35	27	8	64.00	20	28	25	3	9.00
3	34	23	11	121.00	21	21.5	21	.5	.25
4	25	32	−7	49.00	22	23.5	22	1.5	2.25
5	32.5	19	13.5	182.25	23	13.5	24	−10.5	110.25
6	19.5	11	8.5	72.25	24	27	34	−7	49.00
7	1	14	−13	169.00	25	6	3	3	9.00
8	13.5	8	5.5	30.25	26	12	7	5	25.00
9	9	6	3	9.00	27	2	15	−13	169.00
10	15	10	5	25.00	28	21.5	31	−9.5	90.25
11	26	33	−7	49.00	29	29	26	3	9.00
12	10	17	−7	49.00	30	11	18	−7	49.00
13	4	1	3	9.00	31	7	4	3	9.00
14	17	13	4	16.00	32	30	28	2	4.00
15	23.5	20	3.5	12.25	33	17	12	5	25.00
16	5	2	3	9.00	34	31	29	2	4.00
17	8	5	3	9.00	35	3	16	−13	169.00
18	19.5	30	−10.5	110.25					
									$\sum d_i^2 = 1788.5$

In the rankings of X we had six groups of ties that were broken by assigning the values 13.5, 17, 19.5, 21.5, 23.5, and 32.5. In five of the groups two observations tied, and in one group three observations tied. We, therefore, compute five values of

$$T_x = \frac{2^3 - 2}{12} = \frac{6}{12} = .5$$

and one value of

$$T_x = \frac{3^3 - 3}{12} = \frac{24}{12} = 2$$

From these computations, we have $\sum T_x = 5(.5) + 2 = 4.5$, so that

$$\sum x^2 = \frac{35^3 - 35}{12} - 4.5 = 3565.5$$

Since no ties occurred in the Y rankings, we have $\sum T_y = 0$ and

$$\sum y^2 = \frac{35^3 - 35}{12} - 0 = 3570.0$$

From Table 11.8.4 we have $\sum d_i^2 = 1788.5$. From these data we may now compute by Equation 11.8.4

$$r_s = \frac{3565.5 + 3570.0 - 1788.5}{2\sqrt{(3565.5)(3570)}} = .75$$

We see that in this case the correction for ties does not make any difference in the value of r_s.

Exercises

For the following exercises perform the test at the indicated level of significance and determine the p-value.

11.8.1. The following table shows 15 randomly selected geographic areas ranked by population density and age-adjusted death rate. Can we conclude at the .05 level of significance that population density and age-adjusted death rate are not mutually independent?

	Rank by	
Area	Population Density (X)	Age-Adjusted Death Rate (Y)
1	8	10
2	2	14
3	12	4
4	4	15
5	9	11
6	3	1
7	10	12
8	5	7
9	6	8
10	14	5
11	7	6
12	1	2
13	13	9
14	15	3
15	11	13

11.8.2. The following table shows 10 communities ranked by DMF teeth per 100 children and fluoride concentration in ppm in the public water supply.

	Rank by	
Community	DMF Teeth per 100 Children (X)	Fluoride Concentration (Y)
1	8	1
2	9	3
3	7	4
4	3	9
5	2	8
6	4	7
7	1	10
8	5	6
9	6	5
10	10	2

Do these data present sufficient evidence to indicate that the number of DMF Teeth per 100 children tends to decrease as fluoride concentration increases? Let $\alpha = .05$.

11.8.3. Refer to Example 8.7.1. Compute r_s and test the null hypothesis that the two methods are mutually independent. Compare the results with those obtained by using the methods of Chapter 8.

11.8.4. Compute r_s for the data of Exercise 8.7.3 and test the null hypothesis that the two variables are mutually independent. Compare the results with those obtained using the methods of Chapter 8.

11.8.5. Compute r_s for the data of Exercise 8.7.4. Do the data provide sufficient evidence to indicate that CO concentration increases as traffic volume increases?

11.8.6. Compute r_s for the data of Exercise 8.7.5 and test the null hypothesis that the two variables are mutually independent.

11.9 SUMMARY

This chapter is concerned with nonparametric statistical tests. These tests may be used either when the assumptions underlying the parametric tests are not realized or when the data to be analyzed are measured on a scale too weak for the arithmetic procedures necessary for the parametric tests.

The four measurement scales—nominal, ordinal, interval, and ratio—are defined and illustrated.

Finally, six nonparametric tests are described and illustrated. Except for the Kolmogorov-Smirnov goodness-of-fit test, each test provides a nonparametric alternative to a well-known parametric test. There are a number of other nonparametric tests available, many of which are described and illustrated in the references cited at the end of this chapter.

Review Questions and Exercises

1. Define nonparametric statistics.
2. What is meant by the term distribution-free statistical tests?
3. What are the advantages of using nonparametric statistical tests?
4. What are some of the disadvantages of the nonparametric tests?
5. Define the word measurement.
6. List in order of sophistication and describe the four measurement scales.
7. Describe a situation in your particular area of interest where each of the following tests could be used. Use real or realistic data and test an appropriate hypothesis using each test.
   (a) The sign test
   (b) The median test
   (c) The Kolmogorov-Smirnov goodness-of-fit test
   (d) The Kruskal-Wallis one-way analysis of variance by ranks
   (e) The Friedman two-way analysis of variance by ranks
   (f) The Spearman rank correlation coefficient
8. The following are the ranks of the ages (X) of 20 surgical patients and the dose (Y) of an analgesic agent required to block one spinal segment.

Rank of Age in Years (X)	Rank of Dose Requirement (Y)	Rank of Age in Years (X)	Rank of Dose Requirement (Y)
1	1	11	13
2	7	12	5
3	2	13	11
4	4	14	16
5	6	15	20
6	8	16	18
7	3	17	19
8	15	18	17
9	9	19	10
10	12	20	14

Compute r_S and test (two-sided) for significance. Let $\alpha = .05$. Determine the p-value for this test.

9. The following pulmonary function data were collected on children with muscular dystrophy before and after a period of respiratory therapy. Scores are expressed as percent of predicted normal values for height, weight, and body surface measurement.

Forced Vital Capacity (Liters)

Before:	74	65	84	89	84	65	78	86	83	82
After:	79	78	100	92	104	70	81	84	85	90

Use the sign test to determine whether one should conclude that the therapy is effective. Let $\alpha = .05$. What is the p-value?

10. Three methods of reducing skin bacterial load by bathing were compared. Bacteria counts were made on the right foot of subjects before and after treatment. The variable of interest was percent reduction of bacteria. Twenty-seven nursing student volunteers participated in the experiment. The three methods of bathing the foot were whirlpool agitation, spraying, and soaking. The results were as follows:

Whirlpool		Spraying		Soaking	
91	80	18	16	6	10
87	92	22	15	6	12
88	81	20	26	8	5
84	93	29	19	9	9
86		25		13	

Can one conclude on the basis of these data that the three methods are not equally effective? Let $\alpha = .05$. What is the p-value for this test?

11. Ten subjects with bronchial asthma participated in an experiment to evaluate the relative effectiveness of three drugs. The following table shows the change in FEV_1 (forced expired volume in 1 second) values (expressed as liters) two hours after drug administration.

		Drug	
Subject	A	B	C
1	.00	.13	.26
2	.04	.17	.23
3	.02	.20	.21
4	.02	.27	.19
5	.04	.11	.36
6	.03	.18	.25
7	.05	.21	.32
8	.02	.23	.38
9	.00	.24	.30
10	.12	.08	.30

Are these data sufficient to indicate a difference in drug effectiveness? Let $\alpha = .05$. What is the p-value for this test?

12. Sera from two groups of subjects following streptococcal infection were assayed for neutralizing antibodies to streptolysin O (ASO). The results were as follows:

ASO (Measured in Todd Units)

Group A	Group B
324	558
275	108
349	291
604	863
566	303
810	640
340	358
295	503
357	646
580	689
344	250
655	540
380	630
503	190
314	

Do these data provide sufficient evidence to indicate a difference in population medians? Let $\alpha = .05$. What is the p-value for this test?

13. The following are the $PaCO_2$ (mm Hg) values in 16 patients with bronchopulmonary disease:

39, 40, 45, 48, 49, 56, 60, 75, 42, 48, 32, 37, 32, 33, 33, 36

Use the Kolmogorov-Smirnov test to test the null hypothesis that $PaCO_2$ values in the sampled population are normally distributed.

14. The following table shows, the caloric intake (cal/day/kg) and oxygen consumption, VO_2 (ml/min/kg) in 10 infants.

Caloric Intake (X)	VO_2 (Y)
50	7.0
70	8.0
90	10.5
120	11.0
40	9.0
100	10.8
150	12.0
110	10.0
75	9.5
160	11.9

Test the null hypothesis that the two variables are mutually independent against the alternative that they are directly related. Let $\alpha = .05$. What is the p-value for this test?

References

References cited

1. M. G. Kendall and R. M. Sundrum, "Distribution-Free Methods and Order Properties," *Review of the International Statistical Institute, 21:3* (1953), 124–134.
2. Jean Dickinson Gibbons, *Nonparametric Statistical Inference*, McGraw-Hill, New York, 1971.
3. J. R. Blum and N. A. Fattu, "Nonparametric Methods," *Review of Educational Research, 24* (1954), 467–487.
4. L. E. Moses, "Nonparametric Statistics for Psychological Research," *Psychological Bulletin, 49* (1952), 122–143.
5. Sidney Siegel, *Nonparametric Statistics for the Behaviorial Sciences*, McGraw-Hill, New York, 1956.
6. W. J. Conover, *Practical Nonparametric Statistics*, Wiley, New York, 1971.
7. James V. Bradley, *Distribution Free Statistics*, Prentice-Hall, Englewood Cliffs, N.J., 1968.
8. Charles H. Kraft and Constance Van Eeden, *A Nonparametric Introduction to Statistics*, Macmillan, New York, 1968.
9. Merle W. Tate and Richard C. Clelland, *Nonparametric and Shortcut Statistics in the Social, Biological, and Medical Sciences*, Interstate Printers and Publishers, Danville, Ill., 1957.
10. Jean Dickinson Gibbons, *Nonparametric Methods for Quantitative Analysis*, Holt, Rinehart and Winston, New York, 1976.
11. Frederick Mosteller and Robert E. K. Rourke, *Sturdy Statistics: Nonparametric and Order Statistics*, Reading, Mass., Addison-Wesley, 1973.
12. Albert Pierce, *Fundamentals of Nonparametric Statistics*, Belmont, Cal., Dickensen, 1970.
13. G. E. Noether, *Introduction to Statistics: A Fresh Approach*, Boston, Houghton Mifflin, 1971.
14. Myles Hollander and Douglas A. Wolfe, *Nonparametric Statistical Methods*, Wiley, New York, 1973.
15. E. L. Lehmann, *Nonparametrics, Statistical Methods Based on Ranks*, Holden-Day, San Francisco, 1975.

16. Jaroslav Hajek, *A Course in Nonparametric Statistics*, Holden-Day, San Francisco, 1969.

17. John Edward Walsh, *Handbook of Nonparametric Statistics*, Van Nostrand, Princeton, N.J., 1962.

18. John E. Walsh, *Handbook of Nonparametric Statistics*, II, Van Nostrand, Princeton, N.J., 1965.

19. I. R. Savage, *Bibliography of Nonparametric Statistics*, Harvard University Press, Cambridge, Mass. (1962).

20. S. S. Stevens, "On the Theory of Scales of Measurement," *Science*, *103* (1946), 677–680.

21. S. S. Stevens, "Mathematics, Measurement and Psychophysics," in S. S. Stevens (editor), *Handbook of Experimental Psychology*, Wiley, New York, 1951.

22. W. J. Dixon and A. M. Mood, "The Statistical Sign Test," *Journal of the American Statistical Association*, *41* (1946), 557–566.

23. A. M. Mood, *Introduction to the Theory of Statistics*, McGraw-Hill, New York, 1950.

24. J. Westenberg, "Significance Test for Median and Interquartile Range in Samples from Continuous Populations of Any Form," *Proceedings Koninklijke Nederlandse Akademie Van Wetenschappen*, *51* (1948), 252–261.

25. G. W. Brown and A. M. Mood, "On Median Tests for Linear Hypotheses," *Proceedings of the Second Berkeley Symposium on Mathematical Statistics and Probability*, University of California Press, Berkeley, 1951, pp. 159–166.

26. V. L. Senders, *Measurement and Statistics*, Oxford University Press, New York, 1958.

27. William L. Hays and Robert L. Winkler, *Statistics: Probability, Inference, and Decision*, Holt, Rinehart and Winston, New York, 1971.

28. Ronald A. Fisher, *Statistical Methods for Research Workers*, Thirteenth Edition, Hafner, New York, 1958.

29. A. N. Kolmogorov, "Sulla Determinazione Empirica di una Legge di Distribuizione," *Giornale dell' Istitute Italiano degli Altuari*, *4* (1933), 83–91.

30. N. V. Smirnov, "Estimate of Deviation Between Empirical Distribution Functions in Two Independent Samples," (in Russian) *Bulletin Moscow University*, *2* (1939), 3–16.

31. L. A. Goodman, "Kolmogorov-Smirnov Tests for Psychological Research," *Psychological Bulletin*, *51* (1954), 160–168.

32. Gottfried E. Noether, *Elements of Nonparametric Statistics*, Wiley, New York, 1967.

33. F. J. Massey, "The Kolmogorov-Smirnov Test for Goodness of Fit," *Journal of the American Statistical Association*, *46* (1951), 68–78.

34. Z. W. Birnbaum, "Numerical Tabulation of the Distribution of Kolmogorov's Statistic for Finite Sample Size," *Journal of the American Statistical Association*, *47* (1952), 425–441.

35. M. J. Slakter, A "Comparison of the Pearson Chi-Square and Kolmogorov Goodness-of-Fit Tests with Respect to Validity," *Journal of the American Statistical Association*, *60* (1965), 854–58.

36. W. H. Kruskal and W. A. Wallis, "Use of Ranks in One-Criterion Analysis of Variance," *Journal of the American Statistical Association* *47* (1952), 583–621; errata, ibid., *48* (1953), 907–911.

37. K. R. Gabriel and P. A. Lachenbruch, "Nonparametric ANOVA in Small Samples: A Monte Carlo Study of the Adequacy of the Asymptotic Approximation," *Biometrics*, *25* (1969), 593–596.

38. M. Friedman, "The Use of Ranks to Avoid the Assumption of Normality Implicit in the Analysis of Variance," *Journal of the American Statistical Association*, *32* (1937), 675–701.

39. M. Friedman, "A Comparison of Alternative Tests of Significance for the Problem of *m* Rankings," *Annals of Mathematical Statistics*, *11* (1940) 86–92.

40. M. G. Kendall, *Rank Correlation Methods*, Second Edition, Hafner, New York, 1955.

41. W. H. Kruskal, "Ordinal Measures of Association," *Journal of the American Statistical Association*, *53* (1958), 814–861.

42. Harold Hotelling and Margaret R. Pabst, "Rank Correlation and Tests of Significance Involving No Assumption of Normality," *Annals of Mathematical Statistics*, *7* (1936), 29–43.

43. C. Spearman, "The Proof and Measurement of Association Between Two Things," *American Journal of Psychology*, *15* (1904), 72–101.

44. G. J. Glasser and R. F. Winter, "Critical Values of the Coefficient of Rank Correlation for Testing the Hypothesis of Independence," *Biometrika*, *48* (1961), 444–448.

45. Eugene S. Edgington, *Statistical Inference: The Distribution-Free Approach*, McGraw-Hill, New York, 1969.

Additional references: journal articles

1. Olive Jean Dunn, "Multiple Comparisons Using Rank Sums," *Technometrics*, *6* (1964), 241–252.

2. J. Gaito, "Nonparametric Methods in Psychological Research," *Psychological Reports*, *5* (1959), 115–125.

3. F. M. Lord, "On the Statistical Treatment of Football Numbers," *American Psychologist*, *8* (1953), 750–751.

4. B. J. McDonald and W. A. Thompson, "Rank Sum Multiple Comparisons in One- and Two-Way Classifications," *Biometrika*, *54* (1967), 487–498.

5. Wayne W. Daniel and Carol E. Coogler, "Some Quick and Easy Statistical Procedures for the Physical Therapist," *Physical Therapy*, *54* (1974), 135–140.

6. Wayne W. Daniel and Beaufort B. Longest, "Some Practical Statistical Procedures," *Journal of Nursing Administration*, *5* (1975), 23–27.

12

VITAL STATISTICS

12.1 INTRODUCTION

The private physician arrives at a diagnosis and treatment plan for an individual patient by means of a case history, a physical examination, and various laboratory tests. The community may be thought of as a living complex organism for which the public health team is the physician. To carry out this role satisfactorily the public health team must also make use of appropriate tools and techniques for evaluating the health status of the community. Traditionally these tools and techniques have consisted of the community's vital statistics, which include the counts of births, deaths, illnesses, and the various rates and ratios that may be computed from them.

In succeeding sections we give some of the more useful and widely used rates and ratios. Before proceeding, however, let us distinguish between the terms *rate* and *ratio* by defining each as follows.

1. *Rate*. Although there are some exceptions, the term rate usually is reserved to refer to those calculations that imply the probability of the occurrence of some event. A rate is expressed in the form

$$\left(\frac{a}{a+b}\right)k \qquad (12.1.1)$$

where

$a =$ the frequency with which an event has occurred during some specified period of time.

$a + b =$ the number of persons exposed to the risk of the event during the same period of time

$k =$ some number such as 10, 100, 1000, 10,000, or 100,000.

As indicated by Expression 12.1.1 the numerator of a rate is a component part of the denominator. The purpose of the multiplier, k, called the base, is to avoid results involving the very small numbers that may arise in the calculation of rates, and to facilitate comprehension of the rate. The value chosen for k will depend on the magnitudes of the numerator and denominator.

2. *Ratio.* A ratio is a fraction of the form

$$\left(\frac{c}{d}\right)k \tag{12.1.2}$$

where k is some base as already defined and both c and d refer to the frequency of occurrence of some event or item. In the case of a ratio, as opposed to a rate, the numerator is not a component part of the denominator. We can speak, for example, of the person-doctor ratio or the person-hospital-bed ratio of a certain geographical area. The values of k most frequently used in ratios are 1 and 100.

12.2 DEATH RATES AND RATIOS

The rates and ratios discussed in this section are concerned with the occurrence of death. Death rates express the relative frequency of the occurrence of death within some specified interval of time in a specific population. The denominator of a death rate is referred to as the population at risk. The numerator represents only those deaths that occurred in the population specified by the denominator.

1. *Annual Crude Death Rate.* The annual crude death rate is defined as

$$\frac{\text{total number of deaths during year (January 1 to December 31)}}{\text{total population as of July 1}} \cdot k$$

where the value of k is usually chosen as 1000. This is the most widely used rate for measuring the overall health of a community. To compare the crude death rates of two communities is hazardous, unless it is known that the communities are comparable with respect to the many characteristics, other than health conditions, that influence the death rate. Variables that enter into the picture include age, race, sex, and socioeconomic status. When two populations must be compared on the basis of death rates, adjustments may be made to reconcile the population differences with respect to these variables. The same precautions should be exercised when comparing the annual death rates for the same community for two different years.

2. *Annual Specific Death Rates.* It is usually more meaningful and enlightening to observe the death rates of small, well-defined subgroups of the total population. Rates of this type are called *specific death rates* and are defined as

$$\frac{\text{total number of deaths in a specific subgroup during a year}}{\text{total population in the specific subgroup as of July 1}} \cdot k$$

where k is usually equal to 1000. Subgroups for which specific death rates may be computed include those groups that may be distinguished on the basis of sex, race, and age. Specific rates may be computed for two or more characteristics simultaneously. For example, we may compute the death rate for white males, thus obtaining a race-sex specific rate. Cause-specific death rates may also be computed by including in the numerator only those deaths due to a particular cause of death, say cancer, heart disease, or accidents. Because of the small fraction that results, the base, k, for a cause specific rate, is usually 100,000 or 1,000,000.

3. *Adjusted or Standardized Death Rates.* As we have already pointed out, the usefulness of the crude death rate is restricted by the fact that it does not reflect the composition of the population with respect to certain characteristics by which it is influenced. We have seen that by means of specific death rates various segments of the population may be investigated individually. If, however, we attempt to obtain an overall impression of the health of a population by looking at individual specific death rates, we are soon overwhelmed by their great number.

What is wanted is a single figure that measures the forces of mortality in a population while holding constant one or more of the compositional factors such as age, race, or sex. Such a figure, called an *adjusted death rate*, is available. It is most commonly obtained by what is known as the *direct method* of adjustment. The method consists essentially of applying to a *standard population* specific rates observed in the population of interest. From the resulting expected numbers we may compute an overall rate that tells us what the rate for the population of interest would be if that population had the same composition as the standard population. This method is not restricted to the computation of adjusted death rates only, but it may be used to obtain other adjusted rates, for example, an adjusted birth rate. If two or more populations are adjusted in this manner, they are then directly comparable on the basis of the adjustment factors. Opinions differ as to what population should be used as the standard. The population of the United States as of the last decennial census is frequently used. For adjustment calculations a population of 1,000,000, reflecting the composition of the standard population and called the *standard million*, is usually used. In the following example we illustrate the direct method of adjustment to obtain an age-adjusted death rate.

Table 12.2.1

Calculation of Age-Adjusted Death Rate for Georgia, 1970, by Direct Method

1 Age (Years)	2 Population[a]	3 Deaths[a]	4 Age-Specific Death Rates (per *100,000*)	5 Standard Population Based on U.S. Population *1970*[b]	6 Number of Expected Deaths in Standard Population
0 to 4	424,600	2,483	584.8	84,416	494
5 to 14	955,000	449	47.0	200,508	94
15 to 24	863,000	1,369	158.6	174,406	277
25 to 34	608,100	1,360	223.6	122,569	274
35 to 44	518,400	2,296	442.9	113,614	503
45 to 54	486,400	4,632	952.3	114,265	1,088
55 to 64	384,400	7,792	2,027.1	91,480	1,854
65 to 74	235,900	9,363	3,969.1	61,195	2,429
75 and over	132,900	12,042	9,060.9	37,547	3,402
Total	4,608,700	41,786[c]		1,000,000	10,415

[a] *Georgia Vital and Morbidity Statistics* **1970**, Georgia Department of Public Health, Atlanta, Georgia.

[b] *1970 Census of Population*, PC(1)-B1, Table 49.

[c] Excludes 44 deaths at unknown age.

Example 12.2.1

The 1970 crude death rate for Georgia was 9.1 deaths per 1000 population. Let us obtain an age-adjusted death rate for Georgia by using the 1970 United States census as the standard population. In other words, we want a death rate that could have been expected in Georgia if the age composition of the Georgia population had been the same as that of the United States in 1970. The data necessary for the calculations are shown in Table 12.2.1.

The procedure for calculating an age-adjusted death rate by the direct method consists of the following steps.

1. The population of interest is listed (column 2) according to age group (column 1).
2. The deaths in the population of interest are listed (column 3) by age group.

3. The age-specific death rates (column 4) for each age group are calculated by dividing column 3 by column 2 and multiplying by 100,000.
4. The standard population (column 5) is listed by age group.
5. The expected number of deaths in the standard population for each group (column 6) is computed by multiplying column 4 by column 5 and dividing by 100,000. The entries in column 6 are the deaths that would be expected in the standard population if the persons in this population had been exposed to the same risk of death experienced by the population being adjusted.
6. The entries in column 6 are summed to obtain the total number of expected deaths in the standard population.
7. The age-adjusted death rate is computed in the same manner as a crude death rate. That is, the age-adjusted death rate is equal to

$$\frac{\text{total number of expected deaths}}{\text{total standard population}} \cdot 1000$$

In the present example we have an age-adjusted death rate of

$$\frac{10{,}415}{1{,}000{,}000} \cdot 1000 = 10.4$$

We see, then, that the crude death rate has been increased from 9.1 per 1000 to 10.4 per 1000 by adjusting the 1970 population of Georgia to the age distribution of the standard population. This increase in the death rate following adjustment reflects the fact that in 1970 the population of Georgia was slightly younger than the population of the United States as a whole. For example, only 8 percent of the Georgia population was 65 years of age or older whereas 10 percent of the United States population was in that age group.

4. *Maternal Mortality Rate.* This rate is defined as

$$\frac{\text{deaths from all puerperal causes during a year}}{\text{total live births during the year}} \cdot k$$

where k is taken as 1000 or 100,000. The preferred denominator for this rate is the number of women who were pregnant during the year. This denominator, however, is impossible to determine.

A death from a puerperal cause is a death that can be ascribed to some phase of childbearing. Because of the decline in the maternal mortality rate in the United States, it is more convenient to use $k = 100{,}000$. In some countries, however, $k = 1000$ results in a more convenient rate. The decline in the maternal mortality rate in this country also has had the effect of reducing its usefulness as a discriminator among communities with varying qualities of medical care and health facilities.

Some limitations of the maternal mortality rate include the following.

(a) Fetal deaths are not included in the denominator. This results in an inflated rate, since a mother can die from a puerperal cause without producing a live birth.
(b) A maternal death can be counted only once, although twins or larger multiple births may have occurred. Such cases cause the denominator to be too large and, hence, there is a too small rate.
(c) Under-registration of live births, which result in a too small denominator, causes the rate to be too large.
(d) A maternal death may occur in a year later than the year in which the birth occurred. Although there are exceptions, in most cases the transfer of maternal deaths will balance out in a given year.

5. *Infant Mortality Rate.* This rate is defined as

$$\frac{\text{number of deaths under 1 year of age during a year}}{\text{total number of live births during the year}} \cdot k$$

where k is generally taken as 1000. Use and interpretation of this rate must be made in light of its limitations which are similar to those that characterize the maternal mortality rate. Many of the infants who die in a given calendar year were born during the previous year; and, similarly, many children born in a given calendar year will die during the following year. In populations with a stable birthrate this does not pose a serious problem. In periods of rapid change, however, some adjustment should be made. One way to make an adjustment is to allocate the infant deaths to the calendar year in which the infants were born before computing the rate.

6. *Neonatal Mortality Rate.* In an effort to better understand the nature of infant deaths, rates for ages less than a year are frequently computed. Of these, the one most frequently computed is the *neonatal mortality rate*, which is defined as

$$\frac{\text{number of deaths under 28 days of age during a year}}{\text{total number of live births during the year}} \cdot k$$

where $k = 1000$.

7. *Fetal Death Rate.* This rate is defined as

$$\frac{\text{total number of fetal deaths during a year}}{\text{total deliveries during the year}} \cdot k$$

where k is usually taken to be 1000. A fetal death is defined as a product of conception that shows no sign of life after complete birth. There are several problems associated with the use and interpretation of this rate. There is variation among reporting areas with respect to the duration of gestation. Some areas report all fetal deaths regardless of length of gestation while others have a minimum gestation period that must be reached before reporting is required. Another objection to the fetal death rate is that it does not take into account the extent to which a community is trying to reproduce. The ratio to be considered next has been proposed to overcome this objection.

8. *Fetal Death Ratio.* This ratio is defined as

$$\frac{\text{total number of fetal deaths during a year}}{\text{total number of live births during the year}} \cdot k$$

where k is taken as 100 or 1000.

Some authorities have suggested that the number of fetal deaths as well as live births be included in the denominator in an attempt to include all pregnancies in the computation of the ratio. The objection to this suggestion rests on the incompleteness of fetal death reporting.

9. *Perinatal Mortality Rate.* Since fetal deaths occurring late in pregnancy and neonatal deaths frequently have the same underlying causes, it has been suggested that the two be combined to obtain what is known as the *perinatal mortality rate.* This rate is computed as

$$\frac{\begin{gathered}\text{(number of fetal deaths of 28 weeks or more)}\\ + \text{(infant deaths under 7 days)}\end{gathered}}{\begin{gathered}\text{(number of fetal deaths of 28 weeks or more)}\\ + \text{(number of live births)}\end{gathered}} \cdot k$$

where $k = 1000$.

10. *Cause-of-Death Ratio.* This ratio is defined as

$$\frac{\text{number of deaths due to a specific disease during a year}}{\text{total number of deaths due to all causes during the year}} \cdot k$$

where $k = 100$. This index is used to measure the relative importance of a given cause of death. It should be used with caution in comparing one community with another. A higher cause-of-death ratio in one community than that in another may be because the first community has a low mortality from other causes.

11. *Proportional Mortality Ratio.* This index has been suggested as a single measure for comparing the overall health conditions of different communities. It is defined as

$$\frac{\text{number of deaths of persons 50 years of age and older}}{\text{total number of deaths}} \cdot k$$

where $k = 100$. The specified class is usually an age group such as 50 years and over, or a cause of death category, such as accidents. The proportional mortality ratio exhibits certain defects as noted by Linder and Grove (1).

Exercises

12.2.1. The following annual data were reported for a certain geographic area

	Number		
	Total	White	Nonwhite
Estimated population as of July 1	597,500	361,700	235,800
Total live births	12,437	6,400	6,037
Immature births	1,243	440	803
Fetal deaths:			
Total	592	365	227
Under 20 weeks gestation	355	269	86
20 to 27 weeks gestation	103	42	61
28 weeks and more	123	49	74
Unknown length of gestation	11	5	6
Deaths			
Total all ages	6,219	3,636	2,583
Under 1 year	267	97	170
Under 28 days	210	79	131
Deaths from immaturity	16	12	4
Maternal Deaths	2	—	2
Cause of death			
Malignant neoplasms	948	626	322
Ischaemic heart disease	1,697	1,138	559

Source: *Georgia Vital and Morbidity Statistics 1970*, Georgia Department of Public Health, Atlanta, p. 47.

From these data compute the following rates and ratios: (a) crude death rate, (b) race-specific death rates for white and nonwhite, (c) maternal mortality rate, (d) infant mortality rate, (e) neonatal mortality rate, (f) fetal death ratio, (g) cause of death ratios for malignant neoplasms and ischaemic heart disease.

12.2.2. The following table shows the deaths and estimated population by age for the state of Georgia for 1971. Use these data to compute the age-adjusted death rate for Georgia, 1971. Use the same standard population that was used in Example 12.2.1.

Age (Years)	Estimated Population	Deaths
0 to 4	423,700	2,311
5 to 14	947,900	480
15 to 24	891,300	1,390
25 to 34	623,700	1,307
35 to 44	520,000	2,137
45 to 54	494,200	4,640
55 to 64	388,600	7,429
65 to 74	243,000	9,389
75 and over	136,000	12,411
Total	4,668,400	41,494[a]

Source: Statistics Section, Office of Evaluation and Research, Georgia Department of Human Resources, Atlanta.
[a] Excludes 42 deaths at unknown age.

12.3 MEASURES OF FERTILITY

The term *fertility* as used by American demographers refers to the actual bearing of children as opposed to the capacity to bear children for which phenomenon the term *fecundity* is used. A knowledge of the "rate" of child-bearing in a community is important to the health worker in planning services and facilities for mothers, infants, and children. The following are the six basic measures of fertility.

1. *Crude Birth Rate.* This rate is the most widely used of the fertility measures. It is obtained from

$$\frac{\text{total number of live births during a year}}{\text{total population as of July 1}} \cdot k$$

   where $k = 1000$. For an illustration of the computation of this and the other five rates, see Table 12.3.1.

2. *General Fertility Rate.* This rate is defined as

$$\frac{\text{number of live births during a year}}{\text{total number of women of childbearing age}} \cdot k$$

   where $k = 1000$, and the childbearing age is usually defined as ages 15 through 44 or ages 15 through 49. The attractive feature of this rate, when compared to the crude birth rate, is the fact that the denominator approximates the number of persons actually exposed to the risk of bearing a child.

3. *Age-Specific Fertility Rate.* Since the rate of childbearing is not uniform throughout the childbearing ages, a rate that permits the analysis of fertility rates for shorter maternal age intervals is desirable. The rate used

Table 12.3.1

Illustration of Procedures for Computing Six Basic Measures of Fertility, for Georgia, 1970

(1) Age of Woman (Years)	(2) Number of Women in Population[a]	(3) Number of Births to Women of Specified Age[b]	(4) Age Specific Birthrate per 1000 Women	(5) Standard Population Based on U.S. Population 1970[c]	(6) Expected Births	(7) Cumulative Fertility Rate
15 to 19	220,100	21,790	99.0	193,762	19,182	495.0
20 to 24	209,500	37,051	176.9	173,583	30,707	1,379.5
25 to 29	170,100	22,135	130.1	140,764	18,313	2,030.0
30 to 34	139,100	9,246	66.5	119,804	7,967	2,362.5
35 to 39	135,400	3,739	27.6	116,925	3,227	2,500.5
40 to 49	261,700	1,044	4.0	255,162	1,021	2,540.5
Total	1,135,900	95,005		1,000,000	80,417	

Computation of six basic rates:

(1) Crude birth rate = total births divided by total population
= (95,584/4,608,700)(1000) = 21.

(2) General fertility rate = (95,584/1,135,900)(1000) = 84.1.

(3) Age-specific fertility rates = entries in column 3 divided by entries in column 2 multiplied by 1000 for each age group. Results appear in column 4.

(4) Total fertility rate = the sum of each age-specific rate multiplied by the age interval width = (99.0)(5) + (176.9)(5) + (130.1)(5) + (66.5)(5) + (27.6)(5) + (4.0)(10) = 2,540.5.

(5) Cumulative fertility rate = age-specific birth rate multiplied by age interval width cumulated by age. See column 7.

(6) Standardized general fertility rate = (80,417/1,000,000)(1000) = 80.4.

[a] Statistics Section, Office of Evaluation and Research, Georgia Department of Human Resources, Atlanta.

[b] *Georgia Vital and Morbidity Statistics 1970*, Georgia Department of Public Health, Atlanta.

[c] 1970 Census of Population, PC(1)-B1.

is the age-specific fertility rate which is defined as

$$\frac{\text{number of births to women of a certain age in a year}}{\text{total number of women of the specified age}} \cdot k$$

where $k = 1000$. Age-specific rates may be computed for single years of age, or any age interval. Rates for five-year age groups are the ones most frequently computed. Specific fertility rates may be computed also for other population subgroups such as those defined by race, socioeconomic status, and various demographic characteristics.

4. *Total Fertility Rate.* If the age-specific fertility rates for all ages are added and multiplied by the interval into which the ages were grouped, the result is called the *total fertility rate.* The resulting figure is an estimate of the number of children a cohort of 1000 women would have if, during their reproductive years, they reproduced at the rates represented by the age-specific fertility rates from which the total fertility rate is computed.
5. *Cumulative-Fertility Rate.* The cumulative fertility rate is computed in the same manner as the total fertility rate except that the adding process can terminate at the end of any desired age group. The numbers in column 7 of Table 12.3.1 are the cumulative fertility rates through the ages indicated in column 1. The final entry in the cumulative fertility rate column is the total fertility rate.
6. *Standardized Fertility Rate.* Just as the crude death rate may be standardized or adjusted, so may we standardize the general fertility rate. The procedure is identical to that discussed in Section 12.2 for adjusting the crude death rate. The necessary computations for computing the age-standardized fertility rate are shown in Table 12.3.1.

Exercises

12.3.1. The data in the following table are for the state of Georgia for the year 1971.

Age of Woman (Years)	Number of Women in Population	Number of Births to Women of Specified Age
15 to 19	225,200	21,834
20 to 24	217,600	35,997
25 to 29	173,400	21,670
30 to 34	143,300	8,935
35 to 39	134,100	3,464
40 to 49	267,800	925[a]

Source: Statistics Section, Office of Evaluation and Research, Georgia Department of Human Resources, Atlanta.
[a] May include some births to women over 49 years of age.

From the above data compute the following rates:
(a) Age-specific fertility rates for each age group.
(b) Total fertility rate.
(c) Cumulative fertility rate through each age group.
(d) General fertility rate standardized by age.
Use the standard population shown in Table 12.3.1.

12.3.2. There were a total of 95,546 live births in Georgia in 1971. The estimated total population as of July 1, 1971 was 4,668,400, and the number of women between the ages of 15 and 49 was 1,161,400. Use these data to compute:

(a) The crude birth rate.

(b) The general fertility rate.

12.4 MEASURES OF MORBIDITY

Another area that concerns the health worker who is analyzing the health of a community is *morbidity*. Data for the study of the morbidity of a community are not, as a rule, as readily available and complete as are the data on births and deaths because of incompleteness of reporting and differences among states with regard to laws requiring the reporting of diseases. The two rates most frequently used in the study of diseases in a community are the *incidence rate* and the *prevalence rate*.

1. *Incidence Rate*. This rate is defined as

$$\frac{\text{total number of new cases of a specific disease during a year}}{\text{total population as of July 1}} \cdot k$$

   where the value of k depends on the magnitude of the numerator. A base of 1000 is used when convenient, but 100 can be used for the more common diseases, and 10,000 or 100,000 can be used for those less common or rare. This rate, which measures the degree to which new cases are occurring in the community, is useful in helping determine the need for initiation of preventive measures. It is a meaningful measure for both chronic and acute diseases.

2. *Prevalence Rate*. Although it is referred to as a rate, the *prevalence rate* is really a ratio, since it is computed from

$$\frac{\text{total number of cases, new or old, existing at a point in time}}{\text{total population at that point in time}} \cdot k$$

   where the value of k is selected by the same criteria as for the incidence rate. This rate is especially useful in the study of chronic diseases, but it may also be computed for acute diseases.

3. *Case-Fatality Ratio*. This ratio is useful in determining how well the treatment program for a certain disease is succeeding. It is defined as

$$\frac{\text{total number of deaths due to a disease}}{\text{total number of cases due to the disease}} \cdot k$$

   where $k = 100$. The period of time covered is arbitrary, depending on the nature of the disease, and it may cover several years for an endemic disease.

Note that this ratio can be interpreted as the probability of dying following contraction of the disease in question and, as such, reveals the seriousness of the disease.

4. *Immaturity Ratio.* This ratio is defined as

$$\frac{\text{number of live births under 2500 grams during a year}}{\text{total number of live births during the year}} \cdot k$$

where $k = 100$.

5. *Secondary Attack Rate.* This rate measures the occurrence of a contagious disease among susceptible persons who have been exposed to a primary case and is defined as

$$\frac{\begin{array}{c}\text{number of additional cases among contacts of a}\\ \text{primary case within the maximum incubation period}\end{array}}{\text{total number of susceptible contacts}} \cdot k$$

where $k = 100$. This rate is used to measure the spread of infection and is usually applied to closed groups such as a household or classroom where it can be reasonably assumed that all members were, indeed, contacts.

12.5 SUMMARY

This chapter is concerned with the computation and interpretation of various rates and ratios that are useful in studying the health of a community. More specifically, we discuss the more important rates and ratios relating to births, deaths, and morbidity. Individuals who wish to continue their reading in this area should consult the references.

References

References cited

1. Forest E. Linder and Robert D. Grove, *Vital Statistics Rates in the United States, 1900–1940*, United States Government Printing Office, Washington, D.C., 1947.

Other references

1. Donald J. Bogue, *Principles of Demography*, Wiley, New York, 1969.
2. John P. Fox, Carrie E. Hall, and Lila R. Elveback, *Epidemiology*, Macmillian, New York, 1970, Chapter 7.

3. Bernard G. Greenberg, "Biostatistics," in Hugh Rodman Leavell and E. Gurney Clark, *Preventive Medicine*, Third Edition, McGraw-Hill, New York, 1965.
4. Mortimer Spiegelman, *Introduction to Demography*, Revised Edition, Harvard University Press, Cambridge, Massachusetts, 1968.

APPENDIX

List of Tables

Table A

Squares and Square Roots

n	n^2	$\sqrt{n}$	$\sqrt{10n}$	$(10n)^2$
1.0	1.00	1.00000	3.16228	100
1.1	1.21	1.04881	3.31662	121
1.2	1.44	1.09545	3.46410	144
1.3	1.69	1.14018	3.60555	169
1.4	1.96	1.18322	3.74166	196
1.5	2.25	1.22474	3.87298	225
1.6	2.56	1.26491	4.00000	256
1.7	2.89	1.30384	4.12311	289
1.8	3.24	1.34164	4.24264	324
1.9	3.61	1.37840	4.35890	361
2.0	4.00	1.41421	4.47214	400
2.1	4.41	1.44914	4.58258	441
2.2	4.84	1.48324	4.69042	484
2.3	5.29	1.51658	4.79583	529
2.4	5.76	1.54919	4.89898	576
2.5	6.25	1.58114	5.00000	625
2.6	6.76	1.61245	5.09902	676
2.7	7.29	1.64317	5.19615	729
2.8	7.84	1.67332	5.29150	784
2.9	8.41	1.70294	5.38516	841
3.0	9.00	1.73205	5.47723	900
3.1	9.61	1.76068	5.56776	961
3.2	10.24	1.78885	5.65685	1024
3.3	10.89	1.81659	5.74456	1089
3.4	11.56	1.84391	5.83095	1156
3.5	12.25	1.87083	5.91608	1225
3.6	12.96	1.89737	6.00000	1296
3.7	13.69	1.92354	6.08276	1369
3.8	14.44	1.94936	6.16441	1444
3.9	15.21	1.97484	6.24500	1521
4.0	16.00	2.00000	6.32456	1600
4.1	16.81	2.02485	6.40312	1681
4.2	17.64	2.04939	6.48074	1764
4.3	18.49	2.07364	6.55744	1849
4.4	19.36	2.09762	6.63325	1936
4.5	20.25	2.12132	6.70820	2025
4.6	21.16	2.14476	6.78233	2116
4.7	22.09	2.16795	6.85565	2209
4.8	23.04	2.19089	6.92820	2304
4.9	24.01	2.21359	7.00000	2401
5.0	25.00	2.23607	7.07107	2500
5.1	26.01	2.25832	7.14143	2601
5.2	27.04	2.28035	7.21110	2704
5.3	28.09	2.30217	7.28011	2809

(*Table A continued*)

n	n^2	$\sqrt{n}$	$\sqrt{10n}$	$(10n)^2$
5.4	29.16	2.32379	7.34847	2916
5.5	30.25	2.34521	7.41620	3025
5.6	31.36	2.36643	7.48331	3136
5.7	32.49	2.38747	7.54983	3249
5.8	33.64	2.40832	7.61577	3364
5.9	34.81	2.42899	7.68115	3481
6.0	36.00	2.44949	7.74597	3600
6.1	37.21	2.46982	7.81025	3721
6.2	38.44	2.48998	7.87401	3844
6.3	39.69	2.50998	7.93725	3969
6.4	40.96	2.52982	8.00000	4096
6.5	42.25	2.54951	8.06226	4225
6.6	43.56	2.56905	8.12404	4356
6.7	44.89	2.58844	8.18535	4489
6.8	46.24	2.60768	8.24621	4624
6.9	47.61	2.62679	8.30662	4761
7.0	49.00	2.64575	8.36660	4900
7.1	50.41	2.66458	8.42615	5041
7.2	51.84	2.68328	8.48528	5184
7.3	53.29	2.70185	8.54400	5329
7.4	54.76	2.72029	8.60233	5476
7.5	56.25	2.73861	8.66025	5625
7.6	57.76	2.75681	8.71780	5776
7.7	59.29	2.77489	8.77496	5929
7.8	60.84	2.79285	8.83176	6084
7.9	62.41	2.81069	8.88819	6241
8.0	64.00	2.82843	8.94427	6400
8.1	65.61	2.84605	9.00000	6561
8.2	67.24	2.86356	9.05539	6724
8.3	68.89	2.88097	9.11043	6889
8.4	70.56	2.89828	9.16515	7056
8.5	72.25	2.91548	9.21954	7225
8.6	73.96	2.93258	9.27362	7396
8.7	75.69	2.94958	9.32738	7569
8.8	77.44	2.96648	9.38083	7744
8.9	79.21	2.98329	9.43398	7921
9.0	81.00	3.00000	9.48683	8100
9.1	82.81	3.01662	9.53939	8281
9.2	84.64	3.03315	9.59166	8464
9.3	86.49	3.04959	9.64365	8649
9.4	88.36	3.06594	9.69536	8836
9.5	90.25	3.08221	9.74679	9025
9.6	92.16	3.09839	9.79796	9216
9.7	94.09	3.11448	9.84886	9409
9.8	96.04	3.13050	9.89949	9604
9.9	98.01	3.14643	9.94987	9801

Table B

Logarithms

N	0	1	2	3	4	5	6	7	8	9
10	0000	0043	0086	0128	0170	0212	0253	0294	0334	0374
11	0414	0453	0492	0531	0569	0607	0645	0682	0719	0755
12	0792	0828	0864	0899	0934	0969	1004	1038	1072	1106
13	1139	1173	1206	1239	1271	1303	1335	1367	1399	1430
14	1461	1492	1523	1553	1584	1614	1644	1673	1703	1732
15	1761	1790	1818	1847	1875	1903	1931	1959	1987	2014
16	2041	2068	2095	2122	2148	2175	2201	2227	2253	2279
17	2304	2330	2355	2380	2405	2430	2455	2480	2504	2529
18	2553	2577	2601	2625	2648	2672	2695	2718	2742	2765
19	2788	2810	2833	2856	2878	2900	2923	2945	2967	2989
20	3010	3032	3054	3075	3096	3118	3139	3160	3181	3201
21	3222	3243	3263	3284	3304	3324	3345	3365	3385	3404
22	3424	3444	3464	3483	3502	3522	3541	3560	3579	3598
23	3617	3636	3655	3674	3692	3711	3729	3747	3766	3784
24	3802	3820	3838	3856	3874	3892	3909	3927	3945	3962
25	3979	3997	4014	4031	4048	4065	4082	4099	4116	4133
26	4150	4166	4183	4200	4216	4232	4249	4265	4281	4298
27	4314	4330	4346	4362	4378	4393	4409	4425	4440	4456
28	4472	4487	4502	4518	4533	4548	4564	4579	4594	4609
29	4624	4639	4654	4669	4683	4698	4713	4728	4742	4757
30	4771	4786	4800	4814	4829	4843	4857	4871	4886	4900
31	4914	4928	4942	4955	4969	4983	4997	5011	5024	5038
32	5051	5065	5079	5092	5105	5119	5132	5145	5159	5172
33	5185	5198	5211	5224	5237	5250	5263	5276	5289	5302
34	5315	5328	5340	5353	5366	5378	5391	5403	5416	5428
35	5441	5453	5465	5478	5490	5502	5514	5527	5539	5551
36	5563	5575	5587	5599	5611	5623	5635	5647	5658	5670
37	5682	5694	5705	5717	5729	5740	5752	5763	5775	5786
38	5798	5809	5821	5832	5843	5855	5866	5877	5888	5899
39	5911	5922	5933	5944	5955	5966	5977	5988	5999	6010
40	6021	6031	6042	6053	6064	6075	6085	6096	6107	6117
41	6128	6138	6149	6160	6170	6180	6191	6201	6212	6222
42	6232	6243	6253	6263	6274	6284	6294	6304	6314	6325
43	6335	6345	6355	6365	6375	6385	6395	6405	6415	6425
44	6435	6444	6454	6464	6474	6484	6493	6503	6513	6522
45	6532	6542	6551	6561	6571	6580	6590	6599	6609	6618
46	6628	6637	6646	6656	6665	6675	6684	6693	6702	6712
47	6721	6730	6739	6749	6758	6767	6776	6785	6794	6803
48	6812	6821	6830	6839	6848	6857	6866	6875	6884	6893
49	6902	6911	6920	6928	6937	6946	6955	6964	6972	6981
50	6990	6998	7007	7016	7024	7033	7042	7050	7059	7067
51	7076	7084	7093	7101	7110	7118	7126	7135	7143	7152
52	7160	7168	7177	7185	7193	7202	7210	7218	7226	7235
53	7243	7251	7259	7267	7275	7284	7292	7300	7308	7316

(*Table B continued*)

N	0	1	2	3	4	5	6	7	8	9
54	7324	7332	7340	7348	7356	7364	7372	7380	7388	7396
55	7404	7412	7419	7427	7435	7443	7451	7459	7466	7474
56	7482	7490	7497	7505	7513	7520	7528	7536	7543	7551
57	7559	7566	7574	7582	7589	7597	7604	7612	7619	7627
58	7634	7642	7649	7657	7664	7672	7679	7686	7694	7701
59	7709	7716	7723	7731	7738	7745	7752	7760	7767	7774
60	7782	7789	7796	7803	7810	7818	7825	7832	7839	7846
61	7853	7860	7868	7875	7882	7889	7896	7903	7910	7917
62	7924	7931	7938	7945	7952	7959	7966	7973	7980	7987
63	7993	8000	8007	8014	8021	8028	8035	8041	8048	8055
64	8062	8069	8075	8082	8089	8096	8102	8109	8116	8122
65	8129	8136	8142	8149	8156	8162	8169	8176	8182	8189
66	8195	8202	8209	8215	8222	8228	8235	8241	8248	8254
67	8261	8267	8274	8280	8287	8293	8299	8306	8312	8319
68	8325	8331	8338	8344	8351	8357	8363	8370	8376	8382
69	8388	8395	8401	8407	8414	8420	8426	8432	8439	8445
70	8451	8457	8463	8470	8476	8482	8488	8494	8500	8506
71	8513	8519	8525	8531	8537	8543	8549	8555	8561	8567
72	8573	8579	8585	8591	8597	8603	8609	8615	8621	8627
73	8633	8639	8645	8651	8657	8663	8669	8675	8681	8686
74	8692	8698	8704	8710	8716	8722	8727	8733	8739	8745
75	8751	8756	8762	8768	8774	8779	8785	8791	8797	8802
76	8808	8814	8820	8825	8831	8837	8842	8848	8854	8859
77	8865	8871	8876	8882	8887	8893	8899	8904	8910	8915
78	8921	8927	8932	8938	8943	8949	8954	8960	8965	8971
79	8976	8982	8987	8993	8998	9004	9009	9015	9020	9025
80	9031	9036	9042	9047	9053	9058	9063	9069	9074	9079
81	9085	9090	9096	9101	9106	9112	9117	9122	9128	9133
82	9138	9143	9149	9154	9159	9165	9170	9175	9180	9186
83	9191	9196	9201	9206	9212	9217	9222	9227	9232	9238
84	9243	9248	9253	9258	9263	9269	9274	9279	9284	9289
85	9294	9299	9304	9309	9315	9320	9325	9330	9335	9340
86	9345	9350	9355	9360	9365	9370	9375	9380	9385	9390
87	9395	9400	9405	9410	9415	9420	9425	9430	9435	9440
88	9445	9450	9455	9460	9465	9469	9474	9479	9484	9489
89	9494	9499	9504	9509	9513	9518	9523	9528	9533	9538
90	9542	9547	9552	9557	9562	9566	9571	9576	9581	9586
91	9590	9595	9600	9605	9609	9614	9619	9624	9628	9633
92	9638	9643	9647	9652	9657	9661	9666	9671	9675	9680
93	9685	9689	9694	9699	9703	9708	9713	9717	9722	9727
94	9731	9736	9741	9745	9750	9754	9759	9763	9768	9773
95	9777	9782	9786	9791	9795	9800	9805	9809	9814	9818
96	9823	9827	9832	9836	9841	9845	9850	9854	9859	9863
97	9868	9872	9877	9881	9886	9890	9894	9899	9903	9908
98	9912	9917	9921	9926	9930	9934	9939	9943	9948	9952
99	9956	9961	9965	9969	9974	9978	9983	9987	9991	9996

combination of n things taken x at a time $\binom{n}{x} = \dfrac{n!}{x!\,(n-x)!}$

Table C

Cumulative Binomial Probability Distribution

$$P(X \geq x|n, p) = \sum_{X=x}^{n} \binom{n}{x} p^x q^{n-x}$$

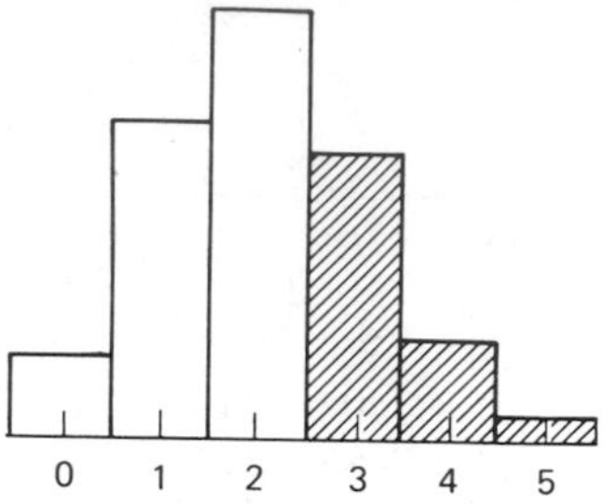

$P(X \geqslant 3 \mid 5, .40) = .3174$

$n = 5$

x \ p	.01	.02	.03	.04	.05	.06	.07	.08	.09	.10
1	.0490	.0961	.1413	.1846	.2262	.2661	.3043	.3409	.3760	.4095
2	.0010	.0038	.0085	.0148	.0226	.0319	.0425	.0544	.0674	.0815
3	.0000	.0001	.0003	.0006	.0012	.0020	.0031	.0045	.0063	.0086
4	.0000	.0000	.0000	.0000	.0000	.0001	.0001	.0002	.0003	.0005
	.11	.12	.13	.14	.15	.16	.17	.18	.19	.20
1	.4416	.4723	.5016	.5296	.5563	.5818	.6061	.6293	.6513	.6723
2	.0965	.1125	.1292	.1467	.1648	.1835	.2027	.2224	.2424	.2627
3	.0112	.0143	.0179	.0220	.0266	.0318	.0375	.0437	.0505	.0579
4	.0007	.0009	.0013	.0017	.0022	.0029	.0036	.0045	.0055	.0067
5	.0000	.0000	.0000	.0001	.0001	.0001	.0001	.0002	.0002	.0003
	.21	.22	.23	.24	.25	.26	.27	.28	.29	.30
1	.6923	.7113	.7293	.7464	.7627	.7781	.7927	.8065	.8196	.8319
2	.2833	.3041	.3251	.3461	.3672	.3883	.4093	.4303	.4511	.4718
3	.0659	.0744	.0836	.0933	.1035	.1143	.1257	1376	.1501	.1631
4	.0081	.0097	.0114	.0134	.0156	.0181	.0208	.0238	.0272	.0308
5	.0004	.0005	.0006	.0008	.0010	.0012	.0014	.0017	.0021	.0024
	.31	.32	.33	.34	.35	.36	.37	.38	.49	.40
1	.8436	.8546	.8650	.8748	.8840	.8926	.9008	.9084	.9155	.9222
2	.4923	.5125	.5325	.5522	.5716	.5906	.6093	.6276	.6455	.6630
3	.1766	.1905	.2050	.2199	.2352	.2509	.2670	.2835	.3003	.3174
4	.0347	.0390	.0436	.0486	.0540	.0598	.0660	.0726	.0796	.0870
5	.0029	.0034	.0039	.0045	.0053	.0060	.0069	.0079	.0090	.0102
	.41	.42	.43	.44	.45	.46	.47	.48	.49	.50
1	.9285	.9344	.9398	.9449	.9497	.9541	.9582	.9620	.9655	.9688
2	.6801	.6967	.7129	.7286	.7438	.7585	.7728	.7865	.7998	.8125
3	.3349	.3525	.3705	.3886	.4069	.4253	.4439	.4625	.4813	.5000
4	.0949	.1033	.1121	.1214	.1312	.1415	.1522	.1635	.1752	.1875
5	.0116	.0131	.0147	.0165	.0185	.0206	.0229	.0255	.0282	.0312

(*Table C continued*)

n = 6

x \ p	.01	.02	.03	.04	.05	.06	.07	.08	.09	.10
1	.0585	.1142	.1670	.2172	.2649	.3101	.3530	.3936	.4321	.4686
2	.0015	.0057	.0125	.0216	.0328	.0459	.0608	.0773	.0952	.1143
3	.0000	.0002	.0005	.0012	.0022	.0038	.0058	.0085	.0118	.0158
4	.0000	.0000	.0000	.0000	.0001	.0002	.0003	.0005	.0008	.0013
5	.0000	.0000	.0000	.0000	.0000	.0000	.0000	.0000	.0000	.0001
	.11	.12	.13	.14	.15	.16	.17	.18	.19	.20
1	.5030	.5356	.5664	.5954	.6229	.6487	.6731	.6960	.7176	.7379
2	.1345	.1556	.1776	.2003	.2235	.2472	.2713	.2956	.3201	.3446
3	.0206	.0261	.0324	.0395	.0476	.0560	.0655	.0759	.0870	.0989
4	.0018	.0025	.0034	.0045	.0059	.0075	.0094	.0116	.0141	.0170
5	.0001	.0001	.0002	.0003	.0004	.0005	.0007	.0010	.0013	.0016
6	.0000	.0000	.0000	.0000	.0000	.0000	.0000	.0000	.0000	.0001
	.21	.22	.23	.24	.25	.26	.27	.28	.29	.30
1	.7569	.7748	.7916	.8073	.8220	.8358	.8487	.8607	.8719	.8824
2	.3692	.3937	.4180	.4422	.4661	.4896	.5128	.5356	.5580	.5798
3	.1115	.1250	.1391	.1539	.1694	.1856	.2023	.2196	.2374	.2557
4	.0202	.0239	.0280	.0326	.0376	.0431	.0492	.0557	.0628	.0705
5	.0020	.0025	.0031	.0038	.0046	.0056	.0067	.0079	.0093	.0109
6	.0001	.0001	.0001	.0002	.0002	.0003	.0004	.0005	.0006	.0007
	.31	.32	.33	.34	.35	.36	.37	.38	.39	.40
1	.8921	.9011	.9095	.9173	.9246	.9313	.9375	.9432	.9485	.9533
2	.6012	.6220	.6422	.6619	.6809	.6994	.7172	.7343	.7508	.7667
3	.2744	.2936	.3130	.3328	.3529	.3732	.3937	.4143	.4350	.4557
4	.0787	.0875	.0969	.1069	.1174	.1286	.1404	.1527	.1657	.1792
5	.0127	.0148	.0170	.0195	.0223	.0254	.0228	.0325	.0365	.0410
6	.0009	.0011	.0013	.0015	.0018	.0022	.0026	.0030	.0035	.0041
	.41	.42	.43	.44	.45	.46	.47	.48	.49	.50
1	.9578	.9619	.9657	.9692	.9723	.9752	.9778	.9802	.9824	.9844
2	.7819	.7965	.8105	.8238	.8364	.8485	.8599	.8707	.8810	.8906
3	.4764	.4971	.5177	.5382	.5585	.5786	.5985	.6180	.6373	.6562
4	.1933	.2080	.2232	.2390	.2553	.2721	.2893	.3070	.3252	.3438
5	.0458	.0510	.0566	.0627	.0692	.0762	.0837	.0917	.1003	.1094
6	.0048	.0055	.0063	.0073	.0083	.0095	.0108	.0122	.0138	.0156

(*Table C continued*)

$n = 7$

x \ p	.01	.02	.03	.04	.05	.06	.07	.08	.09	.10
1	.0679	.1319	.1920	.2486	.3017	.3515	.3983	.4422	.4832	.5217
2	.0020	.0079	.0171	.0294	.0444	.0618	.0813	.1026	.1255	.1497
3	.0000	.0003	.0009	.0020	.0038	.0063	.0097	.0140	.0193	.0257
4	.0000	.0000	.0000	.0001	.0002	.0004	.0007	.0012	.0018	.0027
5	.0000	.0000	.0000	.0000	.0000	.0000	.0000	.0001	.0001	.0002

x \ p	.11	.12	.13	.14	.15	.16	.17	.18	.19	.20
1	.5577	.5913	.6227	.6521	.6794	.7049	.7286	.7507	.7712	.7903
2	.1750	.2012	.2281	.2556	.2834	.3115	.3396	.3677	.3956	.4233
3	.0331	.0416	.0513	.0620	.0738	.0866	.1005	.1154	.1313	.1480
4	.0039	.0054	.0072	.0094	.0121	.0153	.0189	.0231	.0279	.0333
5	.0003	.0004	.0006	.0009	.0012	.0017	.0022	.0029	.0037	.0047
6	.0000	.0000	.0000	.0000	.0001	.0001	.0001	.0002	.0003	.0004

x \ p	.21	.22	.23	.24	.25	.26	.27	.28	.29	.30
1	.8080	.8243	.8395	.8535	.8665	.8785	.8895	.8997	.9090	.9176
2	.4506	.4775	.5040	.5298	.5551	.5796	.6035	.6266	.6490	.6706
3	.1657	.1841	.2033	.2231	.2436	.2646	.2861	.3081	.3304	.3529
4	.0394	.0461	.0536	.0617	.0706	.0802	.0905	.1016	.1134	.1260
5	.0058	.0072	.0088	.0107	.0129	.0153	.0181	.0213	.0248	.0288
6	.0005	.0006	.0008	.0011	.0013	.0017	.0021	.0026	.0031	.0038
7	.0000	.0000	.0000	.0000	.0001	.0001	.0001	.0001	.0002	.0002

x \ p	.31	.32	.33	.34	.35	.36	.37	.38	.39	.40
1	.9255	.9328	.9394	.9454	.9510	.9560	.9606	.9648	.9686	.9720
2	.6914	.7113	.7304	.7487	.7662	.7828	.7987	.8137	.8279	.8414
3	.3757	.3987	.4217	.4447	.4677	.4906	.5134	.5359	.5581	.5801
4	.1394	.1534	.1682	.1837	.1998	.2167	.2341	.2521	.2707	.2898
5	.0332	.0380	.0434	.0492	.0556	.0625	.0701	.0782	.0869	.0963
6	.0046	.0055	.0065	.0077	.0090	.0105	.0123	.0142	.0164	.0188
7	.0003	.0003	.0004	.0005	.0006	.0008	.0009	.0011	.0014	.0016

x \ p	.41	.42	.43	.44	.45	.46	.47	.48	.49	.50
1	.9751	.9779	.9805	.9827	.9848	.9866	.9883	.9897	.9910	.9922
2	.8541	.8660	.8772	.8877	.8976	.9068	.9153	.9233	.9307	.9375
3	.6017	.6229	.6436	.6638	.6836	.7027	.7213	.7393	.7567	.7734
4	.3094	.3294	.3498	.3706	.3917	.4131	.4346	.4563	.4781	.5000
5	.1063	.1169	.1282	.1402	.1529	.1663	.1803	.1951	.2105	.2266
6	.0216	.0246	.0279	.0316	.0357	.0402	.0451	.0504	.0562	.0625
7	.0019	.0023	.0027	.0032	.0037	.0044	.0051	.0059	.0068	.0078

(*Table C continued*)

$n = 8$

x \ p	.01	.02	.03	.04	.05	.06	.07	.08	.09	.10
1	.0773	.1492	.2163	.2786	.3366	.3904	.4404	.4868	.5297	.5695
2	.0027	.0103	.0223	.0381	.0572	.0792	.1035	.1298	.1577	.1869
3	.0001	.0004	.0013	.0031	.0058	.0096	.0147	.0211	.0289	.0381
4	.0000	.0000	.0001	.0002	.0004	.0007	.0013	.0022	.0034	.0050
5	.0000	.0000	.0000	.0000	.0000	.0000	.0001	.0001	.0003	.0004
	.11	.12	.13	.14	.15	.16	.17	.18	.19	.20
1	.6063	.6404	.6718	.7008	.7275	.7521	.7748	.7956	.8147	.8322
2	.2171	.2480	.2794	.3111	.3428	.3744	.4057	.4366	.4670	.4967
3	.0487	.0608	.0743	.0891	.1052	.1226	.1412	.1608	.1815	.2031
4	.0071	.0097	.0129	.0168	.0214	.0267	.0328	.0397	.0476	.0563
5	.0007	.0010	.0015	.0021	.0029	.0038	.0050	.0065	.0083	.0104
6	.0000	.0001	.0001	.0002	.0002	.0004	.0005	.0007	.0009	.0012
7	.0000	.0000	.0000	.0000	.0000	.0000	.0000	.0000	.0001	.0001
	.21	.22	.23	.24	.25	.26	.27	.28	.29	.30
1	.8483	.8630	.8764	.8887	.8999	.9101	.9194	.9278	.9354	.9424
2	.5257	.5538	.5811	.6075	.6329	.6573	.6807	.7031	.7244	.7447
3	.2255	.2486	.2724	.2967	.3215	.3465	.3718	.3973	.4228	.4482
4	.0659	.0765	.0880	.1004	.1138	.1281	.1433	.1594	.1763	.1941
5	.0129	.0158	.0191	.0230	.0273	.0322	.0377	.0438	.0505	.0580
6	.0016	.0021	.0027	.0034	.0042	.0052	.0064	.0078	.0094	.0113
7	.0001	.0002	.0002	.0003	.0004	.0005	.0006	.0008	.0010	.0013
8	.0000	.0000	.0000	.0000	.0000	.0000	.0000	.0000	.0001	.0001
	.31	.32	.33	.34	.35	.36	.37	.38	.39	.40
1	.9486	.9543	.9594	.9640	.9681	.9719	.9752	.9782	.9808	.9832
2	.7640	.7822	.7994	.8156	.8309	.8452	.8586	.8711	.8828	.8936
3	.4736	.4987	.5236	.5481	.5722	.5958	.6189	.6415	.6634	.6846
4	.2126	.2319	.2519	.2724	.2936	.3153	.3374	.3599	.3828	.4059
5	.0661	.0750	.0846	.0949	.1061	.1180	.1307	.1443	.1586	.1737
6	.0134	.0159	.0187	.0218	.0253	.0293	.0336	.0385	.0439	.0498
7	.0016	.0020	.0024	.0030	.0036	.0043	.0051	.0061	.0072	.0085
8	.0001	.0001	.0001	.0002	.0002	.0003	.0004	.0004	.0005	.0007
	.41	.42	.43	.44	.45	.46	.47	.48	.49	.50
1	.9853	.9872	.9889	.9903	.9916	.9928	.9938	.9947	.9954	.9961
2	.9037	.9130	.9216	.9295	.9368	.9435	.9496	.9552	.9602	.9648
3	.7052	.7250	.7440	.7624	.7799	.7966	.8125	.8276	.8419	.8555
4	.4292	.4527	.4762	.4996	.5230	.5463	.5694	.5922	.6146	.6367
5	.1895	.2062	.2235	.2416	.2604	.2798	.2999	.3205	.3416	.3633
6	.0563	.0634	.0711	.0794	.0885	.0982	.1086	.1198	.1318	.1445
7	.0100	.0117	.0136	.0157	.0181	.0208	.0239	.0272	.0310	.0352
8	.0008	.0010	.0012	.0014	.0017	.0020	.0024	.0028	.0033	.0039

(*Table C continued*)

$n = 9$

x \ p	.01	.02	.03	.04	.05	.06	.07	.08	.09	.10
1	.0865	.1663	.2398	.3075	.3698	.4270	.4796	.5278	.5721	.6126
2	.0034	.0131	.0282	.0478	.0712	.0978	.1271	.1583	.1912	.2252
3	.0001	.0006	.0020	.0045	.0084	.0138	.0209	.0298	.0405	.0530
4	.0000	.0000	.0001	.0003	.0006	.0013	.0023	.0037	.0057	.0083
5	.0000	.0000	.0000	.0000	.0000	.0001	.0002	.0003	.0005	.0009
6	.0000	.0000	.0000	.0000	.0000	.0000	.0000	.0000	.0000	.0001
	.11	.12	.13	.14	.15	.16	.17	.18	.19	.20
1	.6496	.6835	.7145	.7427	.7684	.7918	.8131	.8324	.8499	.8658
2	.2599	.2951	.3304	.3657	.4005	.4348	.4685	.5012	.5330	.5638
3	.0672	.0833	.1009	.1202	.1409	.1629	.1861	.2105	.2357	.2618
4	.0117	.0158	.0209	.0269	.0339	.0420	.0512	.0615	.0730	.0856
5	.0014	.0021	.0030	.0041	.0056	.0075	.0098	.0125	.0158	.0196
6	.0001	.0002	.0003	.0004	.0006	.0009	.0013	.0017	.0023	.0031
7	.0000	.0000	.0000	.0000	.0000	.0001	.0001	.0002	.0002	.0003
	.21	.22	.23	.24	.25	.26	.27	.28	.29	.30
1	.8801	.8931	.9048	.9154	.9249	.9335	.9411	.9480	.9542	.9596
2	.5934	.6218	.6491	.6750	.6997	.7230	.7452	.7660	.7856	.8040
3	.2885	.3158	.3434	.3713	.3993	.4273	.4552	.4829	.5102	.5372
4	.0994	.1143	.1304	.1475	.1657	.1849	.2050	.2260	.2478	.2703
5	.0240	.0291	.0350	.0416	.0489	.0571	.0662	.0762	.0870	.0988
6	.0040	.0051	.0065	.0081	.0100	.0122	.0149	.0179	.0213	.0253
7	.0004	.0006	.0008	.0010	.0013	.0017	.0022	.0028	.0035	.0043
8	.0000	.0000	.0001	.0001	.0001	.0001	.0002	.0003	.0003	.0004
	.31	.32	.33	.34	.35	.36	.37	.38	.39	.40
1	.9645	.9689	.9728	.9762	.9793	.9820	.9844	.9865	.9883	.9899
2	.8212	.8372	.8522	.8661	.8789	.8908	.9017	.9118	.9210	.9295
3	.5636	.5894	.6146	.6390	.6627	.6856	.7076	.7287	.7489	.7682
4	.2935	.3173	.3415	.3662	.3911	.4163	.4416	.4669	.4922	.5174
5	.1115	.1252	.1398	.1553	.1717	.1890	.2072	.2262	.2460	.2666
6	.0298	.0348	.0404	.0467	.0536	.0612	.0696	.0787	.0886	.0994
7	.0053	.0064	.0078	.0094	.0112	.0133	.0157	.0184	.0215	.0250
8	.0006	.0007	.0009	.0011	.0014	.0017	.0021	.0026	.0031	.0038
9	.0000	.0000	.0000	.0001	.0001	.0001	.0001	.0002	.0002	.0003

(*Table C continued*)

$n = 9$ (Continued)

x \ p	.41	.42	.43	.44	.45	.46	.47	.48	.49	.50
1	.9913	.9926	.9936	.9946	.9954	.9961	.9967	.9972	.9977	.9980
2	.9372	.9442	.9505	.9563	.9615	.9662	.9704	.9741	.9775	.9805
3	.7866	.8039	.8204	.8359	.8505	.8642	.8769	.8889	.8999	.9102
4	.5424	.5670	.5913	.6152	.6386	.6614	.6836	.7052	.7260	.7461
5	.2878	.3097	.3322	.3551	.3786	.4024	.4265	.4509	.4754	.5000
6	.1109	.1233	.1366	.1508	.1658	.1817	.1985	.2161	.2346	.2539
7	.0290	.0334	.0383	.0437	.0498	.0564	.0637	.0717	.0804	.0898
8	.0046	.0055	.0065	.0077	.0091	.0107	.0125	.0145	.0169	.0195
9	.0003	.0004	.0005	.0006	.0008	.0009	.0011	.0014	.0016	.0020

$n = 10$

x \ p	.01	.02	.03	.04	.05	.06	.07	.08	.09	.10
1	.0956	.1829	.2626	.3352	.4013	.4614	.5160	.5656	.6106	.6513
2	.0043	.0162	.0345	.0582	.0861	.1176	.1517	.1879	.2254	.2639
3	.0001	.0009	.0028	.0062	.0115	.0188	.0283	.0401	.0540	.0702
4	.0000	.0000	.0001	.0004	.0010	.0020	.0036	.0058	.0088	.0128
5	.0000	.0000	.0000	.0000	.0001	.0002	.0003	.0006	.0010	.0016
6	.0000	.0000	.0000	.0000	.0000	.0000	.0000	.0000	.0001	.0001

x \ p	.11	.12	.13	.14	.15	.16	.17	.18	.19	.20
1	.6882	.7215	.7516	.7787	.8031	.8251	.8448	.8626	.8784	.8926
2	.3028	.3417	.3804	.4184	.4557	.4920	.5270	.5608	.5932	.6242
3	.0884	.1087	.1308	.1545	.1798	.2064	.2341	.2628	.2922	.3222
4	.0178	.0239	.0313	.0400	.0500	.0614	.0741	.0883	.1039	.1209
5	.0025	.0037	.0053	.0073	.0099	.0130	.0168	.0213	.0266	.0328
6	.0003	.0004	.0006	.0010	.0014	.0020	.0027	.0037	.0049	.0064
7	.0000	.0000	.0001	.0001	.0001	.0002	.0003	.0004	.0006	.0009
8	.0000	.0000	.0000	.0000	.0000	.0000	.0000	.0000	.0001	.0001

x \ p	.21	.22	.23	.24	.25	.26	.27	.28	.29	.30
1	.9053	.9166	.9267	.9357	.9437	.9508	.9570	.9626	.9674	.9718
2	.6536	.6815	.7079	.7327	.7560	.7778	.7981	.8170	.8345	.8507
3	.3526	.3831	.4137	.4442	.4744	.5042	.5335	.5622	.5901	.6172
4	.1391	.1587	.1794	.2012	.2241	.2479	.2726	.2979	.3239	.3504
5	.0399	.0479	.0569	.0670	.0781	.0904	.1037	.1181	.1337	.1503
6	.0082	.0104	.0130	.0161	.0197	.0239	.0287	.0342	.0404	.0473
7	.0012	.0016	.0021	.0027	.0035	.0045	.0056	.0070	.0087	.0106
8	.0001	.0002	.0002	.0003	.0004	.0006	.0007	.0010	.0012	.0016
9	.0000	.0000	.0000	.0000	.0000	.0000	.0001	.0001	.0001	.0001

(*Table C continued*)

$n = 10$ (Continued)

x \ p	.31	.32	.33	.34	.35	.36	.37	.38	.39	.40
1	.9755	.9789	.9818	.9843	.9865	.9885	.9902	.9916	.9929	.9940
2	.8656	.8794	.8920	.9035	.9140	.9236	.9323	.9402	.9473	.9536
3	.6434	.6687	.6930	.7162	.7384	.7595	.7794	.7983	.8160	.8327
4	.3772	.4044	.4316	.4589	.4862	.5132	.5400	.5664	.5923	.6177
5	.1679	.1867	.2064	.2270	.2485	.2708	.2939	.3177	.3420	.3669
6	.0551	.0637	.0732	.0836	.0949	.1072	.1205	.1348	.1500	.1662
7	.0129	.0155	.0185	.0220	.0260	.0305	.0356	.0413	.0477	.0548
8	.0020	.0025	.0032	.0039	.0048	.0059	.0071	.0086	.0103	.0123
9	.0002	.0003	.0003	.0004	.0005	.0007	.0009	.0011	.0014	.0017
10	.0000	.0000	.0000	.0000	.0000	.0000	.0000	.0001	0001	.0001

x \ p	.41	.42	.43	.44	.45	.46	.47	.48	.49	.50
1	.9949	.9957	.9964	.9970	.9975	.9979	.9983	.9986	.9988	.9990
2	.9594	.9645	.9691	.9731	.9767	.9799	.9827	.9852	.9874	.9893
3	.8483	.8628	.8764	.8889	.9004	.9111	.9209	.9298	.9379	.9453
4	.6425	.6665	.6898	.7123	.7340	.7547	.7745	.7933	.8112	.8281
5	.3922	.4178	.4436	.4696	.4956	.5216	.5474	.5730	.5982	.6230
6	.1834	.2016	.2207	.2407	.2616	.2832	.3057	.3288	.3526	.3770
7	.0626	.0712	.0806	.0908	.1020	.1141	.1271	.1410	.1560	.1719
8	.0146	.0172	.0202	.0236	.0274	.0317	.0366	.0420	.0480	.0547
9	.0021	.0025	.0031	.0037	.0045	.0054	.0065	.0077	.0091	.0107
10	.0001	.0002	.0002	.0003	.0003	.0004	.0005	.0006	.0008	.0010

$n = 11$

x \ p	.01	.02	.03	.04	.05	.06	.07	.08	.09	.10
1	.1047	.1993	.2847	.3618	.4312	.4937	.5499	.6004	.6456	.6862
2	.0052	.0195	.0413	.0692	.1019	.1382	.1772	.2181	.2601	.3026
3	.0002	.0012	.0037	.0083	.0152	.0248	.0370	.0519	.0695	.0896
4	.0000	.0000	.0002	.0007	.0016	.0030	.0053	.0085	.0129	.0185
5	.0000	.0000	.0000	.0000	.0001	.0003	.0005	.0010	.0017	.0028
6	.0000	.0000	.0000	.0000	.0000	.0000	.0000	.0001	.0002	.0003

x \ p	.11	.12	.13	.14	.15	.16	.17	.18	.19	.20
1	.7225	.7549	.7839	.8097	.8327	.8531	.8712	.8873	.9015	.9141
2	.3452	.3873	.4286	.4689	.5078	.5453	.5811	.6151	.6474	.6779
3	.1120	.1366	.1632	.1915	.2212	.2521	.2839	.3164	.3494	.3826
4	.0256	.0341	.0442	.0560	.0694	.0846	.1013	.1197	.1397	.1611
5	.0042	.0061	.0087	.0119	.0159	.0207	.0266	.0334	.0413	.0504
6	.0005	.0008	.0012	.0018	.0027	.0037	.0051	.0068	.0090	.0117
7	.0000	.0001	.0001	.0002	.0003	.0005	.0007	.0010	.0014	.0020
8	.0000	.0000	.0000	.0000	.0000	.0000	.0001	.0001	.0002	.0002

(*Table C continued*)

$n = 11$ (Continued)

x \ p	.21	.22	.23	.24	.25	.26	.27	.28	.29	.30
1	.9252	.9350	.9436	.9511	.9578	.9636	.9686	.9730	.9769	.9802
2	.7065	.7333	.7582	.7814	.8029	.8227	.8410	.8577	.8730	.8870
3	.4158	.4488	.4814	.5134	.5448	.5753	.6049	.6335	.6610	.6873
4	.1840	.2081	.2333	.2596	.2867	.3146	.3430	.3719	.4011	.4304
5	.0607	.0723	.0851	.0992	.1146	.1313	.1493	.1685	.1888	.2103
6	.0148	.0186	.0231	.0283	.0343	.0412	.0490	.0577	.0674	.0782
7	.0027	.0035	.0046	.0059	.0076	.0095	.0119	.0146	.0179	.0216
8	.0003	.0005	.0007	.0009	.0012	.0016	.0021	.0027	.0034	.0043
9	.0000	.0000	.0001	.0001	.0001	.0002	.0002	.0003	.0004	.0006

x \ p	.31	.32	.33	.34	.35	.36	.37	.38	.39	.40
1	.9831	.9856	.9878	.9896	.9912	.9926	.9938	.9948	.9956	.9964
2	.8997	.9112	.9216	.9310	.9394	.9470	.9537	.9597	.9650	.9698
3	.7123	.7361	.7587	.7799	.7999	.8186	.8360	.8522	.8672	.8811
4	.4598	.4890	.5179	.5464	.5744	.6019	.6286	.6545	.6796	.7037
5	.2328	.2563	.2807	.3059	.3317	.3581	.3850	.4122	.4397	.4672
6	.0901	.1031	.1171	.1324	.1487	.1661	.1847	.2043	.2249	.2465
7	.0260	.0309	.0366	.0430	.0501	.0581	.0670	.0768	.0876	.0994
8	.0054	.0067	.0082	.0101	.0122	.0148	.0177	.0210	.0249	.0293
9	.0008	.0010	.0013	.0016	.0020	.0026	.0032	.0039	.0048	.0059
10	.0001	.0001	.0001	.0002	.0002	.0003	.0004	.0005	.0006	.0007

x \ p	.41	.42	.43	.44	.45	.46	.47	.48	.49	.50
1	.9970	.9975	.9979	.9983	.9986	.9989	.9991	.9992	.9994	.9995
2	.9739	.9776	.9808	.9836	.9861	.9882	.9900	.9916	.9930	.9941
3	.8938	.9055	.9162	.9260	.9348	.9428	.9499	.9564	.9622	.9673
4	.7269	.7490	.7700	.7900	.8089	.8266	.8433	.8588	.8733	.8867
5	.4948	.5223	.5495	.5764	.6029	.6288	.6541	.6787	.7026	.7256
6	.2690	.2924	.3166	.3414	.3669	.3929	.4193	.4460	.4729	.5000
7	.1121	.1260	.1408	.1568	.1738	.1919	.2110	.2312	.2523	.2744
8	.0343	.0399	.0461	.0532	.0610	.0696	.0791	.0895	.1009	.1133
9	.0072	.0087	.0104	.0125	.0148	.0175	.0206	.0241	.0282	.0327
10	.0009	.0012	.0014	.0018	.0022	.0027	.0033	.0040	.0049	.0059
11	.0001	.0001	.0001	.0001	.0002	.0002	.0002	.0003	.0004	.0005

$n = 12$

x \ p	.01	.02	.03	.04	.05	.06	.07	.08	.09	.10
1	.1136	.2153	.3062	.3873	.4596	.5241	.5814	.6323	.6775	.7176
2	.0062	.0231	.0486	.0809	.1184	.1595	.2033	.2487	.2948	.3410
3	.0002	.0015	.0048	.0107	.0196	.0316	.0468	.0652	.0866	.1109
4	.0000	.0001	.0003	.0010	.0022	.0043	.0075	.0120	.0180	.0256
5	.0000	.0000	.0000	.0001	.0002	.0004	.0009	.0016	.0027	.0043
6	.0000	.0000	.0000	.0000	.0000	.0000	.0001	.0002	.0003	.0005
7	.0000	.0000	.0000	.0000	.0000	.0000	.0000	.0000	.0000	.0001

(*Table C continued*)

$n = 12$ (Continued)

x \ p	.11	.12	.13	.14	.15	.16	.17	.18	.19	.20
1	.7530	.7843	.8120	.8363	.8578	.8766	.8931	.9076	.9202	.9313
2	.3867	.4314	.4748	.5166	.5565	.5945	.6304	.6641	.6957	.7251
3	.1377	.1667	.1977	.2303	.2642	.2990	.3344	.3702	.4060	.4417
4	.0351	.0464	.0597	.0750	.0922	.1114	.1324	.1552	.1795	.2054
5	.0065	.0095	.0133	.0181	.0239	.0310	.0393	.0489	.0600	.0726
6	.0009	.0014	.0022	.0033	.0046	.0065	.0088	.0116	.0151	.0194
7	.0001	.0002	.0003	.0004	.0007	.0010	.0015	.0021	.0029	.0039
8	.0000	.0000	.0000	.0000	.0001	.0001	.0002	.0003	.0004	.0006
9	.0000	.0000	.0000	.0000	.0000	.0000	.0000	.0000	.0000	.0001

x	.21	.22	.23	.24	.25	.26	.27	.28	.29	.30
1	.9409	.9493	.9566	.9629	.9683	.9730	.9771	.9806	.9836	.9862
2	.7524	.7776	.8009	.8222	.8416	.8594	.8755	.8900	.9032	.9150
3	.4768	.5114	.5450	.5778	.6093	.6397	.6687	.6963	.7225	.7472
4	.2326	.2610	.2904	.3205	.3512	.3824	.4137	.4452	.4765	.5075
5	.0866	.1021	.1192	.1377	.1576	.1790	.2016	.2254	.2504	.2763
6	.0245	.0304	.0374	.0453	.0544	.0646	.0760	.0887	.1026	.1178
7	.0052	.0068	.0089	.0113	.0143	.0178	.0219	.0267	.0322	.0386
8	.0008	.0011	.0016	.0021	.0028	.0036	.0047	.0060	.0076	.0095
9	.0001	.0001	.0002	.0003	.0004	.0005	.0007	.0010	.0013	.0017
10	.0000	.0000	.0000	.0000	.0000	.0001	.0001	.0001	.0002	.0002

x	.31	.32	.33	.34	.35	.36	.37	.38	.39	.40
1	.9884	.9902	.9918	.9932	.9943	.9953	.9961	.9968	.9973	.9978
2	.9256	.9350	.9435	.9509	.9576	.9634	.9685	.9730	.9770	.9804
3	.7704	.7922	.8124	.8313	.8487	.8648	.8795	.8931	.9054	.9166
4	.5381	.5681	.5973	.6258	.6533	.6799	.7053	.7296	.7528	.7747
5	.3032	.3308	.3590	.3876	.4167	.4459	.4751	.5043	.5332	.5618
6	.1343	.1521	.1711	.1913	.2127	.2352	.2588	.2833	.3087	.3348
7	.0458	.0540	.0632	.0734	.0846	.0970	.1106	.1253	.1411	.1582
8	.0118	.0144	.0176	.0213	.0255	.0304	.0359	.0422	.0493	.0573
9	.0022	.0028	.0036	.0045	.0056	.0070	.0086	.0104	.0127	.0153
10	.0003	.0004	.0005	.0007	.0008	.0011	.0014	.0018	.0022	.0028
11	.0000	.0000	.0000	.0001	.0001	.0001	.0001	.0002	.0002	.0003

x	.41	.42	.43	.44	.45	.46	.47	.48	.49	.50
1	.9982	.9986	.9988	.9990	.9992	.9994	.9995	.9996	.9997	.9998
2	.9834	.9860	.9882	.9901	.9917	.9931	.9943	.9953	.9961	.9968
3	.9267	.9358	.9440	.9513	.9579	.9637	.9688	.9733	.9773	.9807
4	.7953	.8147	.8329	.8498	.8655	.8801	.8934	.9057	.9168	.9270
5	.5899	.6175	.6443	.6704	.6956	.7198	.7430	.7652	.7862	.8062
6	.3616	.3889	.4167	.4448	.4731	.5014	.5297	.5577	.5855	.6128
7	.1765	.1959	.2164	.2380	.2607	.2843	.3089	.3343	.3604	.3872
8	.0662	.0760	.0869	.0988	.1117	.1258	.1411	.1575	.1751	.1938
9	.0183	.0218	.0258	.0304	.0356	.0415	.0481	.0555	.0638	.0730
10	.0035	.0043	.0053	.0065	.0079	.0095	.0114	.0137	.0163	.0193
11	.0004	.0005	.0007	.0009	.0011	.0014	.0017	.0021	.0026	.0032
12	.0000	.0000	.0000	.0001	.0001	.0001	.0001	.0001	.0002	.0002

(*Table C continued*)

$n = 13$

x \ p	.01	.02	.03	.04	.05	.06	.07	.08	.09	.10
1	.1225	.2310	.3270	.4118	.4867	.5526	.6107	.6617	.7065	.7458
2	.0072	.0270	.0564	.0932	.1354	.1814	.2298	.2794	.3293	.3787
3	.0003	.0020	.0062	.0135	.0245	.0392	.0578	.0799	.1054	.1339
4	.0000	.0001	.0005	.0014	.0031	.0060	.0103	.0163	.0242	.0342
5	.0000	.0000	.0000	.0001	.0003	.0007	.0013	.0024	.0041	.0065
6	.0000	.0000	.0000	.0000	.0000	.0001	.0001	.0003	.0005	.0009
7	.0000	.0000	.0000	.0000	.0000	.0000	.0000	.0000	.0001	.0001

x \ p	.11	.12	.13	.14	.15	.16	.17	.18	.19	.20
1	.7802	.8102	.8364	.8592	.8791	.8963	.9113	.9242	.9354	.9450
2	.4270	.4738	.5186	.5614	.6017	.6396	.6751	.7080	.7384	.7664
3	.1651	.1985	.2337	.2704	.3080	.3463	.3848	.4231	.4611	.4983
4	.0464	.0609	.0776	.0967	.1180	.1414	.1667	.1939	.2226	.2527
5	.0097	.0139	.0193	.0260	.0342	.0438	.0551	.0681	.0827	.0991
6	.0015	.0024	.0036	.0053	.0075	.0104	.0139	.0183	.0237	.0300
7	.0002	.0003	.0005	.0008	.0013	.0019	.0027	.0038	.0052	.0070
8	.0000	.0000	.0001	.0001	.0002	.0003	.0004	.0006	.0009	.0012
9	.0000	.0000	.0000	.0000	.0000	.0000	.0000	.0001	.0001	.0002

x \ p	.21	.22	.23	.24	.25	.26	.27	.28	.29	.30
1	.9533	.9604	.9666	.9718	.9762	.9800	.9833	.9860	.9883	.9903
2	.7920	.8154	.8367	.8559	.8733	.8889	.9029	.9154	.9265	.9363
3	.5347	.5699	.6039	.6364	.6674	.6968	.7245	.7505	.7749	.7975
4	.2839	.3161	.3489	.3822	.4157	.4493	.4826	.5155	.5478	.5794
5	.1173	.1371	.1585	.1816	.2060	.2319	.2589	.2870	.3160	.3457
6	.0375	.0462	.0562	.0675	.0802	.0944	.1099	.1270	.1455	.1654
7	.0093	.0120	.0154	.0195	.0243	.0299	.0365	.0440	.0527	.0624
8	.0017	.0024	.0032	.0043	.0056	.0073	.0093	.0118	.0147	.0182
9	.0002	.0004	.0005	.0007	.0010	.0013	.0018	.0024	.0031	.0040
10	.0000	.0000	.0001	.0001	.0001	.0002	.0003	.0004	.0005	.0007
11	.0000	.0000	.0000	.0000	.0000	.0000	.0000	.0000	.0001	.0001

x \ p	.31	.32	.33	.34	.35	.36	.37	.38	.39	.40
1	.9920	.9934	.9945	.9955	.9963	.9970	.9975	.9980	.9984	.9987
2	.9450	.9527	.9594	.9653	.9704	.9749	.9787	.9821	.9849	.9874
3	.8185	.8379	.8557	.8720	.8868	.9003	.9125	.9235	.9333	.9421
4	.6101	.6398	.6683	.6957	.7217	.7464	.7698	.7917	.8123	.8314
5	.3760	.4067	.4376	.4686	.4995	.5301	.5603	.5899	.6188	.6470

(*Table C continued*)

$n = 13$ (Continued)

x \ p	.31	.32	.33	.34	.35	.36	.37	.38	.39	.40
6	.1867	.2093	.2331	.2581	.2841	.3111	.3388	.3673	.3962	.4256
7	.0733	.0854	.0988	.1135	.1295	.1468	.1654	.1853	.2065	.2288
8	.0223	.0271	.0326	.0390	.0462	.0544	.0635	.0738	.0851	.0977
9	.0052	.0065	.0082	.0102	.0126	.0154	.0187	.0225	.0270	.0321
10	.0009	.0012	.0015	.0020	.0025	.0032	.0040	.0051	.0063	.0078
11	.0001	.0001	.0002	.0003	.0003	.0005	.0006	.0008	.0010	.0013
12	.0000	.0000	.0000	.0000	.0000	.0000	.0001	.0001	.0001	.0001

x \ p	.41	.42	.43	.44	.45	.46	.47	.48	.49	.50
1	.9990	.9992	.9993	.9995	.9996	.9997	.9997	.9998	.9998	.9999
2	.9895	.9912	.9928	.9940	.9951	.9960	.9967	.9974	.9979	.9983
3	.9499	.9569	.9630	.9684	.9731	.9772	.9808	.9838	.9865	.9888
4	.8492	.8656	.8807	.8945	.9071	.9185	.9288	.9381	.9464	.9539
5	.6742	.7003	.7254	.7493	.7721	.7935	.8137	.8326	.8502	.8666
6	.4552	.4849	.5146	.5441	.5732	.6019	.6299	.6573	.6838	.7095
7	.2524	.2770	.3025	.3290	.3563	.3842	.4127	.4415	.4707	.5000
8	.1114	.1264	.1426	.1600	.1788	.1988	.2200	.2424	.2659	.2905
9	.0379	.0446	.0520	.0605	.0698	.0803	.0918	.1045	.1183	.1334
10	.0096	.0117	.0141	.0170	.0203	.0242	.0287	.0338	.0396	.0461
11	.0017	.0021	.0027	.0033	.0041	.0051	.0063	.0077	.0093	.0112
12	.0002	.0002	.0003	.0004	.0005	.0007	.0009	.0011	.0014	.0017
13	.0000	.0000	.0000	.0000	.0000	.0000	.0001	.0001	.0001	.0001

$n = 14$

x \ p	.01	.02	.03	.04	.05	.06	.07	.08	.09	.10
1	.1313	.2464	.3472	.4353	.5123	.5795	.6380	.6888	.7330	.7712
2	.0084	.0310	.0645	.1059	.1530	.2037	.2564	.3100	.3632	.4154
3	.0003	.0025	.0077	.0167	.0301	.0478	.0698	.0958	.1255	.1584
4	.0000	.0001	.0006	.0019	.0042	.0080	.0136	.0214	.0315	.0441
5	.0000	.0000	.0000	.0002	.0004	.0010	.0020	.0035	.0059	.0092
6	.0000	.0000	.0000	.0000	.0000	.0001	.0002	.0004	.0008	.0015
7	.0000	.0000	.0000	.0000	.0000	.0000	.0000	.0000	.0001	.0002

x \ p	.11	.12	.13	.14	.15	.16	.17	.18	.19	.20
1	.8044	.8330	.8577	.8789	.8972	.9129	.9264	.9379	.9477	.9560
2	.4658	.5141	.5599	.6031	.6433	.6807	.7152	.7469	.7758	.8021
3	.1938	.2315	.2708	.3111	.3521	.3932	.4341	.4744	.5138	.5519
4	.0594	.0774	.0979	.1210	.1465	.1742	.2038	.2351	.2679	.3018
5	.0137	.0196	.0269	.0359	.0467	.0594	.0741	.0907	.1093	.1298
6	.0024	.0038	.0057	.0082	.0115	.0157	.0209	.0273	.0349	.0439
7	.0003	.0006	.0009	.0015	.0022	.0032	.0046	.0064	.0087	.0116
8	.0000	.0001	.0001	.0002	.0003	.0005	.0008	.0012	.0017	.0024
9	.0000	.0000	.0000	.0000	.0000	.0001	.0001	.0002	.0003	.0004

(*Table C continued*)

n = 14 (Continued)

x \ p	.21	.22	.23	.24	.25	.26	.27	.28	.29	.30
1	.9631	.9691	.9742	.9786	.9822	.9852	.9878	.9899	.9917	.9932
2	.8259	.8473	.8665	.8837	.8990	.9126	.9246	.9352	.9444	.9525
3	.5887	.6239	.6574	.6891	.7189	.7467	.7727	.7967	.8188	.8392
4	.3366	.3719	.4076	.4432	.4787	.5136	.5479	.5813	.6137	.6448
5	.1523	.1765	.2023	.2297	.2585	.2884	.3193	.3509	.3832	.4158
6	.0543	.0662	.0797	.0949	.1117	.1301	.1502	.1718	.1949	.2195
7	.0152	.0196	.0248	.0310	.0383	.0467	.0563	.0673	.0796	.0933
8	.0033	.0045	.0060	.0079	.0103	.0132	.0167	.0208	.0257	.0315
9	.0006	.0008	.0011	.0016	.0022	.0029	.0038	.0050	.0065	.0083
10	.0001	.0001	.0002	.0002	.0003	.0005	.0007	.0009	.0012	.0017
11	.0000	.0000	.0000	.0000	.0000	.0001	.0001	.0001	.0002	.0002

x \ p	.31	.32	.33	.34	.35	.36	.37	.38	.39	.40
1	.9945	.9955	.9963	.9970	.9976	.9981	.9984	.9988	.9990	.9992
2	.9596	.9657	.9710	.9756	.9795	.9828	.9857	.9881	.9902	.9919
3	.8577	.8746	.8899	.9037	.9161	.9271	.9370	.9457	.9534	.9602
4	.6747	.7032	.7301	.7556	.7795	.8018	.8226	.8418	.8595	.8757
5	.4486	.4813	.5138	.5458	.5773	.6080	.6378	.6666	.6943	.7207
6	.2454	.2724	.3006	.3297	.3595	.3899	.4208	.4519	.4831	.5141
7	.1084	.1250	.1431	.1626	.1836	.2059	.2296	.2545	.2805	.3075
8	.0381	.0458	.0545	.0643	.0753	.0876	.1012	.1162	.1325	.1501
9	.0105	.0131	.0163	.0200	.0243	.0294	.0353	.0420	.0497	.0583
10	.0022	.0029	.0037	.0048	.0060	.0076	.0095	.0117	.0144	.0175
11	.0003	.0005	.0006	.0008	.0011	.0014	.0019	.0024	.0031	.0039
12	.0000	.0001	.0001	.0001	.0001	.0002	.0003	.0003	.0005	.0006
13	.0000	.0000	.0000	.0000	.0000	.0000	.0000	.0000	.0000	.0001

x \ p	.41	.42	.43	.44	.45	.46	.47	.48	.49	.50
1	.9994	.9995	.9996	.9997	.9998	.9998	.9999	.9999	.9999	.9999
2	.9934	.9946	.9956	.9964	.9971	.9977	.9981	.9985	.9988	.9991
3	.9661	.9713	.9758	.9797	.9830	.9858	.9883	.9903	.9921	.9935
4	.8905	.9039	.9161	.9270	.9368	.9455	.9532	.9601	.9661	.9713
5	.7459	.7697	.7922	.8132	.8328	.8510	.8678	.8833	.8974	.9102
6	.5450	.5754	.6052	.6344	.6627	.6900	.7163	.7415	.7654	.7880
7	.3355	.3643	.3937	.4236	.4539	.4843	.5148	.5451	.5751	.6047
8	.1692	.1896	.2113	.2344	.2586	.2840	.3105	.3380	.3663	.3953
9	.0680	.0789	.0910	.1043	.1189	.1348	.1520	.1707	.1906	.2120
10	.0212	.0255	.0304	.0361	.0426	.0500	.0583	.0677	.0782	.0898
11	.0049	.0061	.0076	.0093	.0114	.0139	.0168	.0202	.0241	.0287
12	.0008	.0010	.0013	.0017	.0022	.0027	.0034	.0042	.0053	.0065
13	.0001	.0001	.0001	.0002	.0003	.0003	.0004	.0006	.0007	.0009
14	.0000	.0000	.0000	.0000	.0000	.0000	.0000	.0000	.0000	.0001

(*Table C continued*)

$n = 15$

x \ p	.01	.02	.03	.04	.05	.06	.07	.08	.09	.10
1	.1399	.2614	.3667	.4579	.5367	.6047	.6633	.7137	.7570	.7941
2	.0096	.0353	.0730	.1191	.1710	.2262	.2832	.3403	.3965	.4510
3	.0004	.0030	.0094	.0203	.0362	.0571	.0829	.1130	.1469	.1841
4	.0000	.0002	.0008	.0024	.0055	.0104	.0175	.0273	.0399	.0556
5	.0000	.0000	.0001	.0002	.0006	.0014	.0028	.0050	.0082	.0127
6	.0000	.0000	.0000	.0000	.0001	.0001	.0003	.0007	.0013	.0022
7	.0000	.0000	.0000	.0000	.0000	.0000	.0000	.0001	.0002	.0003
	.11	.12	.13	.14	.15	.16	.17	.18	.19	.20
1	.8259	.8530	.8762	.8959	.9126	.9269	.9389	.9490	.9576	.9648
2	.5031	.5524	.5987	.6417	.6814	.7179	.7511	.7813	.8085	.8329
3	.2238	.2654	.3084	.3520	.3958	.4392	.4819	.5234	.5635	.6020
4	.0742	.0959	.1204	.1476	.1773	.2092	.2429	.2782	.3146	.3518
5	.0187	.0265	.0361	.0478	.0617	.0778	.0961	.1167	.1394	.1642
6	.0037	.0057	.0084	.0121	.0168	.0227	.0300	.0387	.0490	.0611
7	.0006	.0010	.0015	.0024	.0036	.0052	.0074	.0102	.0137	.0181
8	.0001	.0001	.0002	.0004	.0006	.0010	.0014	.0021	.0030	.0042
9	.0000	.0000	.0000	.0000	.0001	.0001	.0002	.0003	.0005	.0008
10	.0000	.0000	.0000	.0000	.0000	.0000	.0000	.0000	.0001	.0001
	.21	.22	.23	.24	.25	.26	.27	.28	.29	.30
1	.9709	.9759	.9802	.9837	.9866	.9891	.9911	.9928	.9941	.9953
2	.8547	.8741	.8913	.9065	.9198	.9315	.9417	.9505	.9581	.9647
3	.6385	.6731	.7055	.7358	.7639	.7899	.8137	.8355	.8553	.8732
4	.3895	.4274	.4650	.5022	.5387	.5742	.6086	.6416	.6732	.7031
5	.1910	.2195	.2495	.2810	.3135	.3469	.3810	.4154	.4500	.4845
6	.0748	.0905	.1079	.1272	.1484	.1713	.1958	.2220	.2495	.2784
7	.0234	.0298	.0374	.0463	.0566	.0684	.0817	.0965	.1130	.1311
8	.0058	.0078	.0104	.0135	.0173	.0219	.0274	.0338	.0413	.0500
9	.0011	.0016	.0023	.0031	.0042	.0056	.0073	.0094	.0121	.0152
10	.0002	.0003	.0004	.0006	.0008	.0011	.0015	.0021	.0028	.0037
11	.0000	.0000	.0001	.0001	.0001	.0002	.0002	.0003	.0005	.0007
12	.0000	.0000	.0000	.0000	.0000	.0000	.0000	.0000	.0001	.0001
	.31	.32	.33	.34	.35	.36	.37	.38	.39	.40
1	.9962	.9969	.9975	.9980	.9984	.9988	.9990	.9992	.9994	.9995
2	.9704	.9752	.9794	.9829	.9858	.9883	.9904	.9922	.9936	.9948
3	.8893	.9038	.9167	.9281	.9383	.9472	.9550	.9618	.9678	.9729
4	.7314	.7580	.7829	.8060	.8273	.8469	.8649	.8813	.8961	.9095
5	.5187	.5523	.5852	.6171	.6481	.6778	.7062	.7332	.7587	.7827
6	.3084	.3393	.3709	.4032	.4357	.4684	.5011	.5335	.5654	.5968
7	.1509	.1722	.1951	.2194	.2452	.2722	.3003	.3295	.3595	.3902
8	.0599	.0711	.0837	.0977	.1132	.1302	.1487	.1687	.1902	.2131
9	.0190	.0236	.0289	.0351	.0422	.0504	.0597	.0702	.0820	.0950
10	.0048	.0062	.0079	.0099	.0124	.0154	.0190	.0232	.0281	.0338
11	.0009	.0012	.0016	.0022	.0028	.0037	.0047	.0059	.0075	.0093
12	.0001	.0002	.0003	.0004	.0005	.0006	.0009	.0011	.0015	.0019
13	.0000	.0000	.0000	.0000	.0001	.0001	.0001	.0002	.0002	.0003

(*Table C continued*)

$n = 15$ (Continued)

x \ p	.41	.42	.43	.44	.45	.46	.47	.48	.49	.50
1	.9996	.9997	.9998	.9998	.9999	.9999	.9999	.9999	1.0000	1.0000
2	.9958	.9966	.9973	.9979	.9983	.9987	.9990	.9992	.9994	.9995
3	.9773	.9811	.9843	.9870	.9893	.9913	.9929	.9943	.9954	.9963
4	.9125	.9322	.9417	.9502	.9576	.9641	.9697	.9746	.9788	.9824
5	.8052	.8261	.8454	.8633	.8796	.8945	.9080	.9201	.9310	.9408
6	.6274	.6570	.6856	.7131	.7392	.7641	.7875	.8095	.8301	.8491
7	.4214	.4530	.4847	.5164	.5478	.5789	.6095	.6394	.6684	.6964
8	.2374	.2630	.2898	.3176	.3465	.3762	.4065	.4374	.4686	.5000
9	.1095	.1254	.1427	.1615	.1818	.2034	.2265	.2510	.2767	.3036
10	.0404	.0479	.0565	.0661	.0769	.0890	.1024	.1171	.1333	.1509
11	.0116	.0143	.0174	.0211	.0255	.0305	.0363	.0430	.0506	.0592
12	.0025	.0032	.0040	.0051	.0063	.0079	.0097	.0119	.0145	.0176
13	.0004	.0005	.0007	.0009	.0011	.0015	.0018	.0023	.0029	.0037
14	.0000	.0000	.0001	.0001	.0001	.0002	.0002	.0003	.0004	.0005

$n = 16$

x \ p	.01	.02	.03	.04	.05	.06	.07	.08	.09	.10
1	.1485	.2762	.3857	.4796	.5599	.6284	.6869	.7366	.7789	.8147
2	.0109	.0399	.0818	.1327	.1892	.2489	.3098	.3701	.4289	.4853
3	.0005	.0037	.0113	.0242	.0429	.0673	.0969	.1311	.1694	.2108
4	.0000	.0002	.0011	.0032	.0070	.0132	.0221	.0342	.0496	.0684
5	.0000	.0000	.0001	.0003	.0009	.0019	.0038	.0068	.0111	.0170
6	.0000	.0000	.0000	.0000	.0001	.0002	.0005	.0010	.0019	.0033
7	.0000	.0000	.0000	.0000	.0000	.0000	.0001	.0001	.0003	.0005
8	.0000	.0000	.0000	.0000	.0000	.0000	.0000	.0000	.0000	.0001

	.11	.12	.13	.14	.15	.16	.17	.18	.19	.20
1	.8450	.8707	.8923	.9105	.9257	.9386	.9493	.9582	.9657	.9719
2	.5386	.5885	.6347	.6773	.7161	.7513	.7830	.8115	.8368	.8593
3	.2545	.2999	.3461	.3926	.4386	.4838	.5277	.5698	.6101	.6482
4	.0907	.1162	.1448	.1763	.2101	.2460	.2836	.3223	.3619	.4019
5	.0248	.0348	.0471	.0618	.0791	.0988	.1211	.1458	.1727	.2018
6	.0053	.0082	.0120	.0171	.0235	.0315	.0412	.0527	.0662	.0817
7	.0009	.0015	.0024	.0038	.0056	.0080	.0112	.0153	.0204	.0267
8	.0001	.0002	.0004	.0007	.0011	.0016	.0024	.0036	.0051	.0070
9	.0000	.0000	.0001	.0001	.0002	.0003	.0004	.0007	.0010	.0015
10	.0000	.0000	.0000	.0000	.0000	.0000	.0001	.0001	.0002	.0002

n = 16 (Continued)										
x \ p	.21	.22	.23	.24	.25	.26	.27	.28	.29	.30
1	.9770	.9812	.9847	.9876	.9900	.9919	.9935	.9948	.9958	.9967
2	.8791	.8965	.9117	.9250	.9365	.9465	.9550	.9623	.9686	.9739
3	.6839	.7173	.7483	.7768	.8029	.8267	.8482	.8677	.8851	.9006
4	.4418	.4814	.5203	.5583	.5950	.6303	.6640	.6959	.7260	.7541
5	.2327	.2652	.2991	.3341	.3698	.4060	.4425	.4788	.5147	.5501
6	.0992	.1188	.1405	.1641	.1897	.2169	.2458	.2761	.3077	.3402
7	.0342	.0432	.0536	.0658	.0796	.0951	.1125	.1317	.1526	.1753
8	.0095	.0127	.0166	.0214	.0271	.0340	.0420	.0514	.0621	.0744
9	.0021	.0030	.0041	.0056	.0075	.0098	.0127	.0163	.0206	.0257
10	.0004	.0006	.0008	.0012	.0016	.0023	.0031	.0041	.0055	.0071
11	.0001	.0001	.0001	.0002	.0003	.0004	.0006	.0008	.0011	.0016
12	.0000	.0000	.0000	.0000	.0000	.0001	.0001	.0001	.0002	.0003
	.31	.32	.33	.34	.35	.36	.37	.38	.39	.40
1	.9974	.9979	.9984	.9987	.9990	.9992	.9994	.9995	.9996	.9997
2	.9784	.9822	.9854	.9880	.9902	.9921	.9936	.9948	.9959	.9967
3	.9144	.9266	.9374	.9467	.9549	.9620	.9681	.9734	.9778	.9817
4	.7804	.8047	.8270	.8475	.8661	.8830	.8982	.9119	.9241	.9349
5	.5846	.6181	.6504	.6813	.7108	.7387	.7649	.7895	.8123	.8334
6	.3736	.4074	.4416	.4759	.5100	.5438	.5770	.6094	.6408	.6712
7	.1997	.2257	.2531	.2819	.3119	.3428	.3746	.4070	.4398	.4728
8	.0881	.1035	.1205	.1391	.1594	.1813	.2048	.2298	.2562	.2839
9	.0317	.0388	.0470	.0564	.0671	.0791	.0926	.1076	.1242	.1423
10	.0092	.0117	.0148	.0185	.0229	.0280	.0341	.0411	.0491	.0583
11	.0021	.0028	.0037	.0048	.0062	.0079	.0100	.0125	.0155	.0191
12	.0004	.0005	.0007	.0010	.0013	.0017	.0023	.0030	.0038	.0049
13	.0001	.0001	.0001	.0001	.0002	.0003	.0004	.0005	.0007	.0009
14	.0000	.0000	.0000	.0000	.0000	.0000	.0000	.0001	.0001	.0001
	.41	.42	.43	.44	.45	.46	.47	.48	.49	.50
1	.9998	.9998	.9999	.9999	.9999	.9999	1.0000	1.0000	1.0000	1.0000
2	.9974	.9979	.9984	.9987	.9990	.9992	.9994	.9995	.9997	.9997
3	.9849	.9876	.9899	.9918	.9934	.9947	.9958	.9966	.9973	.9979
4	.9444	.9527	.9600	.9664	.9719	.9766	.9806	.9840	.9869	.9894
5	.8529	.8707	.8869	.9015	.9147	.9265	.9370	.9463	.9544	.9616
6	.7003	.7280	.7543	.7792	.8024	.8241	.8441	.8626	.8795	.8949
7	.5058	.5387	.5711	.6029	.6340	.6641	.6932	.7210	.7476	.7728
8	.3128	.3428	.3736	.4051	.4371	.4694	.5019	.5343	.5665	.5982
9	.1619	.1832	.2060	.2302	.2559	.2829	.3111	.3405	.3707	.4018
10	.0687	.0805	.0936	.1081	.1241	.1416	.1607	.1814	.2036	.2272
11	.0234	.0284	.0342	.0409	.0486	.0574	.0674	.0786	.0911	.1051
12	.0062	.0078	.0098	.0121	.0149	.0183	.0222	.0268	.0322	.0384
13	.0012	.0016	.0021	.0027	.0035	.0044	.0055	.0069	.0086	.0106
14	.0002	.0002	.0003	.0004	.0006	.0007	.0010	.0013	.0016	.0021
15	.0000	.0000	.0000	.0000	.0001	.0001	.0001	.0001	.0002	.0003

(*Table C continued*)

$n = 17$

x \ p	.01	.02	.03	.04	.05	.06	.07	.08	.09	.10
1	.1571	.2907	.4042	.5004	.5819	.6507	.7088	.7577	.7988	.8332
2	.0123	.0446	.0909	.1465	.2078	.2717	.3362	.3995	.4604	.5182
3	.0006	.0044	.0134	.0286	.0503	.0782	.1118	.1503	.1927	.2382
4	.0000	.0003	.0014	.0040	.0088	.0164	.0273	.0419	.0603	.0826
5	.0000	.0000	.0001	.0004	.0012	.0026	.0051	.0090	.0145	.0221
6	.0000	.0000	.0000	.0000	.0001	.0003	.0007	.0015	.0027	.0047
7	.0000	.0000	.0000	.0000	.0000	.0000	.0001	.0002	.0004	.0008
8	.0000	.0000	.0000	.0000	.0000	.0000	.0000	.0000	.0000	.0001

x \ p	.11	.12	.13	.14	.15	.16	.17	.18	.19	.20
1	.8621	.8862	.9063	.9230	.9369	.9484	.9579	.9657	.9722	.9775
2	.5723	.6223	.6682	.7099	.7475	.7813	.8113	.8379	.8613	.8818
3	.2858	.3345	.3836	.4324	.4802	.5266	.5711	.6133	.6532	.6904
4	.1087	.1383	.1710	.2065	.2444	.2841	.3251	.3669	.4091	.4511
5	.0321	.0446	.0598	.0778	.0987	.1224	.1487	.1775	.2087	.2418
6	.0075	.0114	.0166	.0234	.0319	.0423	.0548	.0695	.0864	.1057
7	.0014	.0023	.0037	.0056	.0083	.0118	.0163	.0220	.0291	.0377
8	.0002	.0004	.0007	.0011	.0017	.0027	.0039	.0057	.0080	.0109
9	.0000	.0001	.0001	.0002	.0003	.0005	.0008	.0012	.0018	.0026
10	.0000	.0000	.0000	.0000	.0000	.0001	.0001	.0002	.0003	.0005
11	.0000	.0000	.0000	.0000	.0000	.0000	.0000	.0000	.0000	.0001

x \ p	.21	.22	.23	.24	.25	.26	.27	.28	.29	.30
1	.9818	.9854	.9882	.9906	.9925	.9940	.9953	.9962	.9970	.9977
2	.8996	.9152	.9285	.9400	.9499	.9583	.9654	.9714	.9765	.9807
3	.7249	.7567	.7859	.8123	.8363	.8578	.8771	.8942	.9093	.9226
4	.4927	.5333	.5728	.6107	.6470	.6814	.7137	.7440	.7721	.7981
5	.2766	.3128	.3500	.3879	.4261	.4643	.5023	.5396	.5760	.6113
6	.1273	.1510	.1770	.2049	.2347	.2661	.2989	.3329	.3677	.4032
7	.0479	.0598	.0736	.0894	.1071	.1268	.1485	.1721	.1976	.2248
8	.0147	.0194	.0251	.0320	.0402	.0499	.0611	.0739	.0884	.1046
9	.0037	.0051	.0070	.0094	.0124	.0161	.0206	.0261	.0326	.0403
10	.0007	.0011	.0016	.0022	.0031	.0042	.0057	.0075	.0098	.0127
11	.0001	.0002	.0003	.0004	.0006	.0009	.0013	.0018	.0024	.0032
12	.0000	.0000	.0000	.0001	.0001	.0002	.0002	.0003	.0005	.0007
13	.0000	.0000	.0000	.0000	.0000	.0000	.0000	.0000	.0001	.0001

x \ p	.31	.32	.33	.34	.35	.36	.37	.38	.39	.40
1	.9982	.9986	.9989	.9991	.9993	.9995	.9996	.9997	.9998	.9998
2	.9843	.9872	.9896	.9917	.9933	.9946	.9957	.9966	.9973	.9979
3	.9343	.9444	.9532	.9608	.9673	.9728	.9775	.9815	.9849	.9877
4	.8219	.8437	.8634	.8812	.8972	.9115	.9241	.9353	.9450	.9536
5	.6453	.6778	.7087	.7378	.7652	.7906	.8142	.8360	.8559	.8740
6	.4390	.4749	.5105	.5458	.5803	.6139	.6465	.6778	.7077	.7361
7	.2536	.2838	.3153	.3479	.3812	.4152	.4495	.4839	.5182	.5522
8	.1227	.1426	.1642	.1877	.2128	.2395	.2676	.2971	.3278	.3595
9	.0492	.0595	.0712	.0845	.0994	.1159	.1341	.1541	.1757	.1989
10	.0162	.0204	.0254	.0314	.0383	.0464	.0557	.0664	.0784	.0919

(*Table C continued*)

$n = 17$ (Continued)

x \ p	.31	.32	.33	.34	.35	.36	.37	.38	.39	.40
11	.0043	.0057	.0074	.0095	.0120	.0151	.0189	.0234	.0286	.0348
12	.0009	.0013	.0017	.0023	.0030	.0040	.0051	.0066	.0084	.0106
13	.0002	.0002	.0003	.0004	.0006	.0008	.0011	.0015	.0019	.0025
14	.0000	.0000	.0000	.0001	.0001	.0001	.0002	.0002	.0003	.0005
15	.0000	.0000	.0000	.0000	.0000	.0000	.0000	.0000	.0000	.0001

x \ p	.41	.42	.43	.44	.45	.46	.47	.48	.49	.50
1	.9999	.9999	.9999	.9999	1.0000	1.0000	1.0000	1.0000	1.0000	1.0000
2	.9984	.9987	.9990	.9992	.9994	.9996	.9997	.9998	.9998	.9999
3	.9900	.9920	.9935	.9948	.9959	.9968	.9975	.9980	.9985	.9988
4	.9610	.9674	.9729	.9776	.9816	.9849	.9877	.9901	.9920	.9936
5	.8904	.9051	.9183	.9301	.9404	.9495	.9575	.9644	.9704	.9755
6	.7628	.7879	.8113	.8330	.8529	.8712	.8878	.9028	.9162	.9283
7	.5856	.6182	.6499	.6805	.7098	.7377	.7641	.7890	.8122	.8338
8	.3920	.4250	.4585	.4921	.5257	.5590	.5918	.6239	.6552	.6855
9	.2238	.2502	.2780	.3072	.3374	.3687	.4008	.4335	.4667	.5000
10	.1070	.1236	.1419	.1618	.1834	.2066	.2314	.2577	.2855	.3145
11	.0420	.0503	.0597	.0705	.0826	.0962	.1112	.1279	.1462	.1662
12	.0133	.0165	.0203	.0248	.0301	.0363	.0434	.0517	.0611	.0717
13	.0033	.0042	.0054	.0069	.0086	.0108	.0134	.0165	.0202	.0245
14	.0006	.0008	.0011	.0014	.0019	.0024	.0031	.0040	.0050	.0064
15	.0001	.0001	.0002	.0002	.0003	.0004	.0005	.0007	.0009	.0012
16	.0000	.0000	.0000	.0000	.0000	.0000	.0001	.0001	.0001	.0001

$n = 18$

x \ p	.01	.02	.03	.04	.05	.06	.07	.08	.09	.10
1	.1655	.3049	.4220	.5204	.6028	.6717	.7292	.7771	.8169	.8499
2	.0138	.0495	.1003	.1607	.2265	.2945	.3622	.4281	.4909	.5497
3	.0007	.0052	.0157	.0333	.0581	.0898	.1275	.1702	.2168	.2662
4	.0000	.0004	.0018	.0050	.0109	.0201	.0333	.0506	.0723	.0982
5	.0000	.0000	.0002	.0006	.0015	.0034	.0067	.0116	.0187	.0282
6	.0000	.0000	.0000	.0001	.0002	.0005	.0010	.0021	.0038	.0064
7	.0000	.0000	.0000	.0000	.0000	.0000	.0001	.0003	.0006	.0012
8	.0000	.0000	.0000	.0000	.0000	.0000	.0000	.0000	.0001	.0002

x \ p	.11	.12	.13	.14	.15	.16	.17	.18	.19	.20
1	.8773	.8998	.9185	.9338	.9464	.9566	.9651	.9719	.9775	.9820
2	.6042	.6540	.6992	.7398	.7759	.8080	.8362	.8609	.8824	.9009
3	.3173	.3690	.4206	.4713	.5203	.5673	.6119	.6538	.6927	.7287
4	.1282	.1618	.1986	.2382	.2798	.3229	.3669	.4112	.4554	.4990
5	.0405	.0558	.0743	.0959	.1206	.1482	.1787	.2116	.2467	.2836
6	.0102	.0154	.0222	.0310	.0419	.0551	.0708	.0889	.1097	.1329
7	.0021	.0034	.0054	.0081	.0118	.0167	.0229	.0306	.0400	.0513
8	.0003	.0006	.0011	.0017	.0027	.0041	.0060	.0086	.0120	.0163
9	.0000	.0001	.0002	.0003	.0005	.0008	.0013	.0020	.0030	.0043
10	.0000	.0000	.0000	.0000	.0001	.0001	.0002	.0004	.0006	.0009
11	.0000	.0000	.0000	.0000	.0000	.0000	.0000	.0001	.0001	.0002

(*Table C continued*)

$n = 18$ (Continued)

x \ p	.21	.22	.23	.24	.25	.26	.27	.28	.29	.30
1	.9856	.9886	.9909	.9928	.9944	.9956	.9965	.9973	.9979	.9984
2	.9169	.9306	.9423	.9522	.9605	.9676	.9735	.9784	.9824	.9858
3	.7616	.7916	.8187	.8430	.8647	.8839	.9009	.9158	.9288	.9400
4	.5414	.5825	.6218	.6591	.6943	.7272	.7578	.7860	.8119	.8354
5	.3220	.3613	.4012	.4414	.4813	.5208	.5594	.5968	.6329	.6673
6	.1586	.1866	.2168	.2488	.2825	.3176	.3538	.3907	.4281	.4656
7	.0645	.0799	.0974	.1171	.1390	.1630	.1891	.2171	.2469	.2783
8	.0217	.0283	.0363	.0458	.0569	.0699	.0847	.1014	.1200	.1407
9	.0060	.0083	.0112	.0148	.0193	.0249	.0316	.0395	.0488	.0596
10	.0014	.0020	.0028	.0039	.0054	.0073	.0097	.0127	.0164	.0210
11	.0003	.0004	.0006	.0009	.0012	.0018	.0025	.0034	.0046	.0061
12	.0000	.0001	.0001	.0002	.0002	.0003	.0005	.0007	.0010	.0014
13	.0000	.0000	.0000	.0000	.0000	.0001	.0001	.0001	.0002	.0003

x \ p	.31	.32	.33	.34	.35	.36	.37	.38	.39	.40
1	.9987	.9990	.9993	.9994	.9996	.9997	.9998	.9998	.9999	.9999
2	.9886	.9908	.9927	.9942	.9954	.9964	.9972	.9978	.9983	.9987
3	.9498	.9581	.9652	.9713	.9764	.9807	.9843	.9873	.9897	.9918
4	.8568	.8759	.8931	.9083	.9217	.9335	.9439	.9528	.9606	.9672
5	.7001	.7309	.7598	.7866	.8114	.8341	.8549	.8737	.8907	.9058
6	.5029	.5398	.5759	.6111	.6450	.6776	.7086	.7379	.7655	.7912
7	.3111	.3450	.3797	.4151	.4509	.4867	.5224	.5576	.5921	.6257
8	.1633	.1878	.2141	.2421	.2717	.3027	.3349	.3681	.4021	.4366
9	.0720	.0861	.1019	.1196	.1391	.1604	.1835	.2084	.2350	.2632
10	.0264	.0329	.0405	.0494	.0597	.0714	.0847	.0997	.1163	.1347
11	.0080	.0104	.0133	.0169	.0212	.0264	.0325	.0397	.0480	.0576
12	.0020	.0027	.0036	.0047	.0062	.0080	.0102	.0130	.0163	.0203
13	.0004	.0005	.0008	.0011	.0014	.0019	.0026	.0034	.0044	.0058
14	.0001	.0001	.0001	.0002	.0003	.0004	.0005	.0007	.0010	.0013
15	.0000	.0000	.0000	.0000	.0000	.0001	.0001	.0001	.0002	.0002

x \ p	.41	.42	.43	.44	.45	.46	.47	.48	.49	.50
1	.9999	.9999	1.0000	1.0000	1.0000	1.0000	1.0000	1.0000	1.0000	1.0000
2	.9990	.9992	.9994	.9996	.9997	.9998	.9998	.9999	.9999	.9999
3	.9934	.9948	.9959	.9968	.9975	.9981	.9985	.9989	.9991	.9993
4	.9729	.9777	.9818	.9852	.9880	.9904	.9923	.9939	.9952	.9962
5	.9193	.9313	.9418	.9510	.9589	.9658	.9717	.9767	.9810	.9846
6	.8151	.8372	.8573	.8757	.8923	.9072	.9205	.9324	.9428	.9519
7	.6582	.6895	.7193	.7476	.7742	.7991	.8222	.8436	.8632	.8811
8	.4713	.5062	.5408	.5750	.6085	.6412	.6728	.7032	.7322	.7597
9	.2928	.3236	.3556	.3885	.4222	.4562	.4906	.5249	.5591	.5927
10	.1549	.1768	.2004	.2258	.2527	.2812	.3110	.3421	.3742	.4073
11	.0686	.0811	.0951	.1107	.1280	.1470	.1677	.1902	.2144	.2403
12	.0250	.0307	.0372	.0449	.0537	.0638	.0753	.0883	.1028	.1189
13	.0074	.0094	.0118	.0147	.0183	.0225	.0275	.0334	.0402	.0481
14	.0017	.0022	.0029	.0038	.0049	.0063	.0079	.0100	.0125	.0154
15	.0003	.0004	.0006	.0007	.0010	.0013	.0017	.0023	.0029	.0038
16	.0000	.0001	.0001	.0001	.0001	.0002	.0003	.0004	.0005	.0007
17	.0000	.0000	.0000	.0000	.0000	.0000	.0000	.0000	.0001	.0001

(*Table C continued*)

$n = 19$

x \ p	.01	.02	.03	.04	.05	.06	.07	.08	.09	.10
1	.1738	.3188	.4394	.5396	.6226	.6914	.7481	.7949	.8334	.8649
2	.0153	.0546	.1100	.1751	.2453	.3171	.3879	.4560	.5202	.5797
3	.0009	.0061	.0183	.0384	.0665	.1021	.1439	.1908	.2415	.2946
4	.0000	.0005	.0022	.0061	.0132	.0243	.0398	.0602	.0853	.1150
5	.0000	.0000	.0002	.0007	.0020	.0044	.0085	.0147	.0235	.0352
6	.0000	.0000	.0000	.0001	.0002	.0006	.0014	.0029	.0051	.0086
7	.0000	.0000	.0000	.0000	.0000	.0001	.0002	.0004	.0009	.0017
8	.0000	.0000	.0000	.0000	.0000	.0000	.0000	.0001	.0001	.0003

x	.11	.12	.13	.14	.15	.16	.17	.18	.19	.20
1	.8908	.9119	.9291	.9431	.9544	.9636	.9710	.9770	.9818	.9856
2	.6342	.6835	.7277	.7669	.8015	.8318	.8581	.8809	.9004	.9171
3	.3488	.4032	.4568	.5089	.5587	.6059	.6500	.6910	.7287	.7631
4	.1490	.1867	.2275	.2708	.3159	.3620	.4085	.4549	.5005	.5449
5	.0502	.0685	.0904	.1158	.1444	.1762	.2107	.2476	.2864	.3267
6	.0135	.0202	.0290	.0401	.0537	.0700	.0891	.1110	.1357	.1631
7	.0030	.0048	.0076	.0113	.0163	.0228	.0310	.0411	.0532	.0676
8	.0005	.0009	.0016	.0026	.0041	.0061	.0089	.0126	.0173	.0233
9	.0001	.0002	.0003	.0005	.0008	.0014	.0021	.0032	.0047	.0067
10	.0000	.0000	.0000	.0001	.0001	.0002	.0004	.0007	.0010	.0016
11	.0000	.0000	.0000	.0000	.0000	.0000	.0001	.0001	.0002	.0003
12	.0000	.0000	.0000	.0000	.0000	.0000	.0000	.0000	.0000	.0001

x	.21	.22	.23	.24	.25	.26	.27	.28	.29	.30
1	.9887	.9911	.9930	.9946	.9958	.9967	.9975	.9981	.9985	.9989
2	.9313	.9434	.9535	.9619	.9690	.9749	.9797	.9837	.9869	.9896
3	.7942	.8222	.8471	.8692	.8887	.9057	.9205	.9333	.9443	.9538
4	.5877	.6285	.6671	.7032	.7369	.7680	.7965	.8224	.8458	.8668
5	.3681	.4100	.4520	.4936	.5346	.5744	.6129	.6498	.6848	.7178
6	.1929	.2251	.2592	.2950	.3322	.3705	.4093	.4484	.4875	.5261
7	.0843	.1034	.1249	.1487	.1749	.2032	.2336	.2657	.2995	.3345
8	.0307	.0396	.0503	.0629	.0775	.0941	.1129	.1338	.1568	.1820
9	.0093	.0127	.0169	.0222	.0287	.0366	.0459	.0568	.0694	.0839
10	.0023	.0034	.0047	.0066	.0089	.0119	.0156	.0202	.0258	.0326
11	.0005	.0007	.0011	.0016	.0023	.0032	.0044	.0060	.0080	.0105
12	.0001	.0001	.0002	.0003	.0005	.0007	.0010	.0015	.0021	.0028
13	.0000	.0000	.0000	.0001	.0001	.0001	.0002	.0003	.0004	.0006
14	.0000	.0000	.0000	.0000	.0000	.0000	.0000	.0000	.0001	.0001

(*Table C continued*)

$n = 19$ (Continued)

x \ p	.31	.32	.33	.34	.35	.36	.37	.38	.39	.40
1	.9991	.9993	.9995	.9996	.9997	.9998	.9998	.9999	.9999	.9999
2	.9917	.9935	.9949	.9960	.9969	.9976	.9981	.9986	.9989	.9992
3	.9618	.9686	.9743	.9791	.9830	.9863	.9890	.9913	.9931	.9945
4	.8856	.9022	.9169	.9297	.9409	.9505	.9588	.9659	.9719	.9770
5	.7486	.7773	.8037	.8280	.8500	.8699	.8878	.9038	.9179	.9304
6	.5641	.6010	.6366	.6707	.7032	.7339	.7627	.7895	.8143	.8371
7	.3705	.4073	.4445	.4818	.5188	.5554	.5913	.6261	.6597	.6919
8	.2091	.2381	.2688	.3010	.3344	.3690	.4043	.4401	.4762	.5122
9	.1003	.1186	.1389	.1612	.1855	.2116	.2395	.2691	.3002	.3325
10	.0405	.0499	.0608	.0733	.0875	.1035	.1213	.1410	.1626	.1861
11	.0137	.0176	.0223	.0280	.0347	.0426	.0518	.0625	.0747	.0885
12	.0038	.0051	.0068	.0089	.0114	.0146	.0185	.0231	.0287	.0352
13	.0009	.0012	.0017	.0023	.0031	.0041	.0054	.0070	.0091	.0116
14	.0002	.0002	.0003	.0005	.0007	.0009	.0013	.0017	.0023	.0031
15	.0000	.0000	.0001	.0001	.0001	.0002	.0002	.0003	.0005	.0006
16	.0000	.0000	.0000	.0000	.0000	.0000	.0000	.0000	.0001	.0001

x \ p	.41	.42	.43	.44	.45	.46	.47	.48	.49	.50
1	1.0000	1.0000	1.0000	1.0000	1.0000	1.0000	1.0000	1.0000	1.0000	1.0000
2	.9994	.9995	.9996	.9997	.9998	.9999	.9999	.9999	.9999	1.0000
3	.9957	.9967	.9974	.9980	.9985	.9988	.9991	.9993	.9995	.9996
4	.9813	.9849	.9878	.9903	.9923	.9939	.9952	.9963	.9971	.9978
5	.9413	.9518	.9590	.9660	.9720	.9771	.9814	.9850	.9879	.9904
6	.8579	.8767	.8937	.9088	.9223	.9342	.9446	.9537	.9615	.9682
7	.7226	.7515	.7787	.8039	.8273	.8488	.8684	.8862	.9022	.9165
8	.5480	.5832	.6176	.6509	.6831	.7138	.7430	.7706	.7964	.8204
9	.3660	.4003	.4353	.4706	.5060	.5413	.5762	.6105	.6439	.6762
10	.2114	.2385	.2672	.2974	.3290	.3617	.3954	.4299	.4648	.5000
11	.1040	.1213	.1404	.1613	.1841	.2087	.2351	.2631	.2928	.3238
12	.0429	.0518	.0621	.0738	.0871	.1021	.1187	.1372	.1575	.1796
13	.0146	.0183	.0227	.0280	.0342	.0415	.0500	.0597	.0709	.0835
14	.0040	.0052	.0068	.0086	.0109	.0137	.0171	.0212	.0261	.0318
15	.0009	.0012	.0016	.0021	.0028	.0036	.0046	.0060	.0076	.0096
16	.0001	.0002	.0003	.0004	.0005	.0007	.0010	.0013	.0017	.0022
17	.0000	.0000	.0000	.0001	.0001	.0001	.0001	.0002	.0003	.0004

$n = 20$

x \ p	.01	.02	.03	.04	.05	.06	.07	.08	.09	.10
1	.1821	.3324	.4562	.5580	.6415	.7099	.7658	.8113	.8484	.8784
2	.0169	.0599	.1198	.1897	.2642	.3395	.4131	.4831	.5484	.6083
3	.0010	.0071	.0210	.0439	.0755	.1150	.1610	.2121	.2666	.3231
4	.0000	.0006	.0027	.0074	.0159	.0290	.0471	.0706	.0993	.1330
5	.0000	.0000	.0003	.0010	.0026	.0056	.0107	.0183	.0290	.0432
6	.0000	.0000	.0000	.0001	.0003	.0009	.0019	.0038	.0068	.0113
7	.0000	.0000	.0000	.0000	.0000	.0001	.0003	.0006	.0013	.0024
8	.0000	.0000	.0000	.0000	.0000	.0000	.0000	.0001	.0002	.0004
9	.0000	.0000	.0000	.0000	.0000	.0000	.0000	.0000	.0000	.0001

(*Table C continued*)

$n = 20$ (Continued)

x \ p	.11	.12	.13	.14	.15	.16	.17	.18	.19	.20
1	.9028	.9224	.9383	.9510	.9612	.9694	.9759	.9811	.9852	.9885
2	.6624	.7109	.7539	.7916	.8244	.8529	.8773	.8982	.9159	.9308
3	.3802	.4369	.4920	.5450	.5951	.6420	.6854	.7252	.7614	.7939
4	.1710	.2127	.2573	.3041	.3523	.4010	.4496	.4974	.5439	.5886
5	.0610	.0827	.1083	.1375	.1702	.2059	.2443	.2849	.3271	.3704
6	.0175	.0260	.0370	.0507	.0673	.0870	.1098	.1356	.1643	.1958
7	.0041	.0067	.0103	.0153	.0219	.0304	.0409	.0537	.0689	.0867
8	.0008	.0014	.0024	.0038	.0059	.0088	.0127	.0177	.0241	.0321
9	.0001	.0002	.0005	.0008	.0013	.0021	.0033	.0049	.0071	.0100
10	.0000	.0000	.0001	.0001	.0002	.0004	.0007	.0011	.0017	.0026
11	.0000	.0000	.0000	.0000	.0000	.0001	.0001	.0002	.0004	.0006
12	.0000	.0000	.0000	.0000	.0000	.0000	.0000	.0000	.0001	.0001
	.21	.22	.23	.24	.25	.26	.27	.28	.29	.30
1	.9910	.9931	.9946	.9959	.9968	.9976	.9982	.9986	.9989	.9992
2	.9434	.9539	.9626	.9698	.9757	.9805	.9845	.9877	.9903	.9924
3	.8230	.8488	.8716	.8915	.9087	.9237	.9365	.9474	.9567	.9645
4	.6310	.6711	.7085	.7431	.7748	.8038	.8300	.8534	.8744	.8929
5	.4142	.4580	.5014	.5439	.5852	.6248	.6625	.6981	.7315	.7625
6	.2297	.2657	.3035	.3427	.3828	.4235	.4643	.5048	.5447	.5836
7	.1071	.1301	.1558	.1838	.2142	.2467	.2810	.3169	.3540	.3920
8	.0419	.0536	.0675	.0835	.1018	.1225	.1455	.1707	.1982	.2277
9	.0138	.0186	.0246	.0320	.0409	.0515	.0640	.0784	.0948	.1133
10	.0038	.0054	.0075	.0103	.0139	.0183	.0238	.0305	.0385	.0480
11	.0009	.0013	.0019	.0028	.0039	.0055	.0074	.0100	.0132	.0171
12	.0003	.0003	.0004	.0006	.0009	.0014	.0019	.0027	.0038	.0051
13	.0000	.0000	.0001	.0001	.0002	.0003	.0004	.0006	.0009	.0013
14	.0000	.0000	.0000	.0000	.0000	.0000	.0001	.0001	.0002	.0003
	.31	.32	.33	.34	.35	.36	.37	.38	.39	.40
1	.9994	.9996	.9997	.9998	.9998	.9999	.9999	.9999	.9999	1.0000
2	.9940	.9953	.9964	.9972	.9979	.9984	.9988	.9991	.9993	.9995
3	.9711	.9765	.9811	.9848	.9879	.9904	.9924	.9940	.9953	.9964
4	.9092	.9235	.9358	.9465	.9556	.9634	.9700	.9755	.9802	.9840
5	.7911	.8173	.8411	.8626	.8818	.8989	.9141	.9274	.9390	.9490
6	.6213	.6574	.6918	.7242	.7546	.7829	.8090	.8329	.8547	.8744
7	.4305	.4693	.5079	.5460	.5834	.6197	.6547	.6882	.7200	.7500
8	.2591	.2922	.3268	.3624	.3990	.4361	.4735	.5108	.5478	.5841
9	.1340	.1568	.1818	.2087	.2376	.2683	.3005	.3341	.3688	.4044
10	.0591	.0719	.0866	.1032	.1218	.1424	.1650	.1897	.2163	.2447
11	.0220	.0279	.0350	.0434	.0532	.0645	.0775	.0923	.1090	.1275
12	.0069	.0091	.0119	.0154	.0196	.0247	.0308	.0381	.0466	.0565
13	.0018	.0025	.0034	.0045	.0060	.0079	.0102	.0132	.0167	.0210
14	.0004	.0006	.0008	.0011	.0015	.0021	.0028	.0037	.0049	.0065
15	.0001	.0001	.0001	.0002	.0003	.0004	.0006	.0009	.0012	.0016
16	.0000	.0000	.0000	.0000	.0001	.0001	.0001	.0002	.0002	.0003

(*Table C continued*)

n = 20 (continued)

x \ p	.41	.42	.43	.44	.45	.46	.47	.48	.48	.50
1	1.0000	1.0000	1.0000	1.0000	1.0000	1.0000	1.0000	1.0000	1.0000	1.0000
2	.9996	.9997	.9998	.9998	.9999	.9999	.9999	1.0000	1.0000	1.0000
3	.9972	.9979	.9984	.9988	.9991	.9993	.9995	.9996	.9997	.9998
4	.9872	.9898	.9920	.9937	.9951	.9962	.9971	.9977	.9983	.9987
5	.9577	.9651	.9714	.9767	.9811	.9848	.9879	.9904	.9924	.9941
6	.8921	.9078	.9217	.9340	.9447	.9539	.9619	.9687	.9745	.9793
7	.7780	.8041	.8281	.8501	.8701	.8881	.9042	.9186	.9312	.9423
8	.6196	.6539	.6868	.7183	.7480	.7759	.8020	.8261	.8482	.8684
9	.4406	.4771	.5136	.5499	.5847	.6207	.6546	.6873	.7186	.7483
10	.2748	.3064	.3394	.3736	.4086	.4443	.4804	.5166	.5525	.5881
11	.1480	.1705	.1949	.2212	.2493	.2791	.3104	.3432	.3771	.4119
12	.0679	.0810	.0958	.1123	.1308	.1511	.1734	.1977	.2238	.2517
13	.0262	.0324	.0397	.0482	.0580	.0694	.0823	.0969	.1133	.1316
14	.0084	.0107	.0136	.0172	.0214	.0265	.0326	.0397	.0480	.0577
15	.0022	.0029	.0038	.0050	.0064	.0083	.0105	.0133	.0166	.0207
16	.0004	.0006	.0008	.0011	.0015	.0020	.0027	.0035	.0046	.0059
17	.0001	.0001	.0001	.0002	.0003	.0004	.0005	.0007	.0010	.0013
18	.0000	.0000	.0000	.0000	.0000	.0001	.0001	.0001	.0001	.0002

n = 25

x \ p	.01	.02	.03	.04	.05	.06	.07	.08	.09	.10
1	.2222	.3965	.5330	.6396	.7226	.7871	.8370	.8756	.9054	.9282
2	.0258	.0886	.1720	.2642	.3576	.4473	.5304	.6053	.6714	.7288
3	.0020	.0132	.0380	.0765	.1271	.1871	.2534	.3232	.3937	.4629
4	.0001	.0014	.0062	.0165	.0341	.0598	.0936	.1351	.1831	.2364
5	.0000	.0001	.0008	.0028	.0072	.0150	.0274	.0451	.0686	.0980
6	.0000	.0000	.0001	.0004	.0012	.0031	.0065	.0123	.0210	.0334
7	.0000	.0000	.0000	.0000	.0002	.0005	.0013	.0028	.0054	.0095
8	.0000	.0000	.0000	.0000	.0000	.0001	.0002	.0005	.0011	.0023
9	.0000	.0000	.0000	.0000	.0000	.0000	.0000	.0001	.0002	.0005
10	.0000	.0000	.0000	.0000	.0000	.0000	.0000	.0000	.0000	.0001

x \ p	.11	.12	.13	.14	.15	.16	.17	.18	.19	.20
1	.9457	.9591	.9692	.9770	.9828	.9872	.9905	.9930	.9948	.9962
2	.7779	.8195	.8543	.8832	.9069	.9263	.9420	.9546	.9646	.9726
3	.5291	.5912	.6483	.7000	.7463	.7870	.8226	.8533	.8796	.9018
4	.2934	.3525	.4123	.4714	.5289	.5837	.6352	.6829	.7266	.7660
5	.1331	.1734	.2183	.2668	.3179	.3707	.4241	.4772	.5292	.5793
6	.0499	.0709	.0965	.1268	.1615	.2002	.2425	.2875	.3347	.3833
7	.0156	.0243	.0359	.0509	.0695	.0920	.1185	.1488	.1827	.2200
8	.0041	.0070	.0113	.0173	.0255	.0361	.0495	.0661	.0859	.1091
9	.0009	.0017	.0030	.0050	.0080	.0121	.0178	.0252	.0348	.0468
10	.0002	.0004	.0007	.0013	.0021	.0035	.0055	.0083	.0122	.0173
11	.0000	.0001	.0001	.0003	.0005	.0009	.0015	.0024	.0037	.0056
12	.0000	.0000	.0000	.0000	.0001	.0002	.0003	.0006	.0010	.0015
13	.0000	.0000	.0000	.0000	.0000	.0000	.0001	.0001	.0002	.0004
14	.0000	.0000	.0000	.0000	.0000	.0000	.0000	.0000	.0000	.0001

(*Table C continued*)

n = 25 (Continued)

x \ p	.21	.22	.23	.24	.25	.26	.27	.28	.29	.30
1	.9972	.9980	.9985	.9990	.9992	.9995	.9996	.9997	.9998	.9999
2	.9789	.9838	.9877	.9907	.9930	.9947	.9961	.9971	.9979	.9984
3	.9204	.9360	.9488	.9593	.9679	.9748	.9804	.9848	.9883	.9910
4	.8013	.8324	.8597	.8834	.9038	.9211	.9358	.9481	.9583	.9668
5	.6270	.6718	.7134	.7516	.7863	.8174	.8452	.8696	.8910	.9095
6	.4325	.4816	.5299	.5767	.6217	.6644	.7044	.7415	.7755	.8065
7	.2601	.3027	.3471	.3927	.4389	.4851	.5308	.5753	.6183	.6593
8	.1358	.1658	.1989	.2349	.2735	.3142	.3565	.3999	.4440	.4882
9	.0614	.0788	.0993	.1228	.1494	.1790	.2115	.2465	.2838	.3231
10	.0240	.0325	.0431	.0560	.0713	.0893	.1101	.1338	.1602	.1894
11	.0082	.0117	.0163	.0222	.0297	.0389	.0502	.0636	.0795	.0978
12	.0024	.0036	.0053	.0076	.0107	.0148	.0199	.0264	.0345	.0442
13	.0006	.0010	.0015	.0023	.0034	.0049	.0069	.0096	.0130	.0175
14	.0001	.0002	.0004	.0006	.0009	.0014	.0021	.0030	.0043	.0060
15	.0000	.0000	.0001	.0001	.0002	.0003	.0005	.0008	.0012	.0018
16	.0000	.0000	.0000	.0000	.0000	.0001	.0001	.0002	.0003	.0005
17	.0000	.0000	.0000	.0000	.0000	.0000	.0000	.0000	.0001	.0001

x \ p	.31	.32	.33	.34	.35	.36	.37	.38	.39	.40
1	.9999	.9999	1.0000	1.0000	1.0000	1.0000	1.0000	1.0000	1.0000	1.0000
2	.9989	.9992	.9994	.9996	.9997	.9998	.9998	.9999	.9999	.9999
3	.9932	.9949	.9961	.9971	.9979	.9984	.9989	.9992	.9994	.9996
4	.9737	.9793	.9838	.9874	.9903	.9926	.9944	.9958	.9968	.9976
5	.9254	.9390	.9504	.9600	.9680	.9745	.9799	.9842	.9877	.9905
6	.8344	.8593	.8813	.9006	.9174	.9318	.9441	.9546	.9633	.9706
7	.6981	.7343	.7679	.7987	.8266	.8517	.8742	.8940	.9114	.9264
8	.5319	.5747	.6163	.6561	.6939	.7295	.7626	.7932	.8211	.8464
9	.3639	.4057	.4482	.4908	.5332	.5748	.6152	.6542	.6914	.7265
10	.2213	.2555	.2919	.3300	.3697	.4104	.4517	.4933	.5347	.5754
11	.1188	.1424	.1686	.1975	.2288	.2624	.2981	.3355	.3743	.4142
12	.0560	.0698	.0859	.1044	.1254	.1490	.1751	.2036	.2346	.2677
13	.0230	.0299	.0383	.0485	.0604	.0745	.0907	.1093	.1303	.1538
14	.0083	.0112	.0149	.0196	.0255	.0326	.0412	.0515	.0637	.0778
15	.0026	.0036	.0050	.0069	.0093	.0124	.0163	.0212	.0271	.0344
16	.0007	.0010	.0015	.0021	.0029	.0041	.0056	.0075	.0100	.0132
17	.0002	.0002	.0004	.0005	.0008	.0011	.0016	.0023	.0032	.0043
18	.0000	.0000	.0001	.0001	.0002	.0003	.0004	.0006	.0008	.0012
19	.0000	.0000	.0000	.0000	.0000	.0001	.0001	.0001	.0002	.0003
20	.0000	.0000	.0000	.0000	.0000	.0000	.0000	.0000	.0000	.0001

(*Table C continued*)

n = 25 (Continued)

x \ p	.41	.42	.43	.44	.45	.46	.47	.48	.49	.50
1	1.0000	1.0000	1.0000	1.0000	1.0000	1.0000	1.0000	1.0000	1.0000	1.0000
2	1.0000	1.0000	1.0000	1.0000	1.0000	1.0000	1.0000	1.0000	1.0000	1.0000
3	.9997	.9998	.9998	.9999	.9999	1.0000	1.0000	1.0000	1.0000	1.0000
4	.9983	.9987	.9991	.9993	.9995	.9997	.9998	.9998	.9999	.9999
5	.9927	.9945	.9958	.9969	.9977	.9983	.9988	.9991	.9994	.9995
6	.9767	.9816	.9856	.9888	.9914	.9934	.9950	.9963	.9972	.9980
7	.9394	.9505	.9599	.9677	.9742	.9796	.9840	.9876	.9904	.9927
8	.8692	.8894	.9071	.9227	.9361	.9477	.9575	.9658	.9727	.9784
9	.7593	.7897	.8177	.8431	.8660	.8865	.9046	.9205	.9343	.9461
10	.6151	.6535	.6902	.7250	.7576	.7880	.8160	.8415	.8648	.8852
11	.4548	.4956	.5363	.5765	.6157	.6538	.6902	.7249	.7574	.7878
12	.3029	.3397	.3780	.4174	.4574	.4978	.5382	.5780	.6171	.6550
13	.1797	.2080	.2387	.2715	.3063	.3429	.3808	.4199	.4598	.5000
14	.0941	.1127	.1336	.1569	.1827	.2109	.2413	.2740	.3086	.3450
15	.0431	.0535	.0656	.0797	.0960	.1145	.1353	.1585	.1841	.2122
16	.0171	.0220	.0280	.0353	.0440	.0543	.0663	.0803	.0964	.1148
17	.0058	.0078	.0103	.0134	.0174	.0222	.0281	.0352	.0438	.0539
18	.0017	.0023	.0032	.0044	.0058	.0077	.0102	.0132	.0170	.0216
19	.0004	.0006	.0008	.0012	.0016	.0023	.0031	.0041	.0055	.0073
20	.0001	.0001	.0002	.0003	.0004	.0005	.0008	.0011	.0015	.0020
21	.0000	.0000	.0000	.0000	.0001	.0001	.0002	.0002	.0003	.0005
22	.0000	.0000	.0000	.0000	.0000	.0000	.0000	.0000	.0001	.0001

Table D

Exponential Functions

x	e^x	e^{-x}	x	e^x	e^{-x}
.00	1.000	1.000	3.10	22.198	.045
.10	1.105	.905	3.20	24.533	.041
.20	1.221	.819	3.30	27.113	.037
.30	1.350	.741	3.40	29.964	.033
.40	1.492	.670	3.50	33.115	.030
.50	1.649	.607	3.60	36.598	.027
.60	1.822	.549	3.70	40.447	.025
.70	2.014	.497	3.80	44.701	.022
.80	2.226	.449	3.90	49.402	.020
.90	2.460	.407	4.00	54.598	.018
1.00	2.718	.368	4.10	60.340	.017
1.10	3.004	.333	4.20	66.686	.015
1.20	3.320	.301	4.30	73.700	.014
1.30	3.669	.273	4.40	81.451	.012
1.40	4.055	.247	4.50	90.017	.011
1.50	4.482	.223	4.60	99.484	.010
1.60	4.953	.202	4.70	109.947	.009
1.70	5.474	.183	4.80	121.510	.008
1.80	6.050	.165	4.90	134.290	.007
1.90	6.686	.150	5.00	148.413	.007
2.00	7.389	.135	5.10	164.022	.006
2.10	8.166	.122	5.20	181.272	.006
2.20	9.025	.111	5.30	200.337	.005
2.30	9.974	.100	5.40	221.406	.005
2.40	11.023	.091	5.50	244.692	.004
2.50	12.182	.082	5.60	270.426	.004
2.60	13.464	.074	5.70	298.867	.003
2.70	14.880	.067	5.80	330.300	.003
2.80	16.445	.061	5.90	365.037	.003
2.90	18.174	.055	6.00	403.429	.002
3.00	20.086	.050			

Table E

Cumulative Poisson Distribution

$P(X \geq x|\lambda)$

1000 Times the Probability of x or More Occurrences of Event That Has Average Number of Occurrences Equal to λ

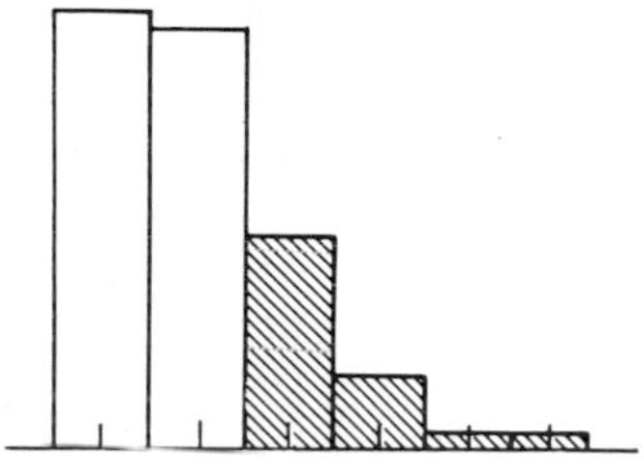

x \ λ	.02	.04	.06	.08	.10	.15	.20	.25
0	1000	1000	1000	1000	1000	1000	1000	1000
1	020	039	058	077	095	139	181	221
2		001	002	003	005	010	018	026
3						001	001	002

x \ λ	.30	.35	.40	.45	.50	.55	.60	.65
0	1000	1000	1000	1000	1000	1000	1000	1000
1	259	295	330	362	393	423	451	478
2	037	049	062	075	090	106	122	139
3	004	006	008	011	014	018	023	028
4			001	001	002	002	003	004
5								001

x \ λ	.70	.75	.80	.85	.90	.95	1.0	1.1
0	1000	1000	1000	1000	1000	1000	1000	1000
1	503	528	551	573	593	613	632	667
2	156	173	191	209	228	246	264	301
3	034	041	047	055	063	071	080	100
4	006	007	009	011	013	016	019	026
5	001	001	001	002	002	003	004	005
6							001	001

x \ λ	1.2	1.3	1.4	1.5	1.6	1.7	1.8	1.9
0	1000	1000	1000	1000	1000	1000	1000	1000
1	699	727	753	777	798	817	835	850
2	337	373	408	442	475	507	537	566
3	121	143	167	191	217	243	269	296
4	034	043	054	066	079	093	109	125
5	008	011	014	019	024	030	036	044
6	002	002	003	004	006	008	010	013
7			001	001	001	002	003	003
8							001	001

(*Table E continued*)

x \ λ	2.0	2.2	2.4	2.6	2.8	3.0	3.2	3.4
0	1000	1000	1000	1000	1000	1000	1000	1000
1	865	889	909	926	939	950	959	967
2	594	645	692	733	769	801	829	853
3	323	377	430	482	531	577	620	660
4	143	181	221	264	308	353	397	442
5	053	072	096	123	152	185	219	256
6	017	025	036	049	065	084	105	129
7	005	007	012	017	024	034	045	058
8	001	002	003	005	008	012	017	023
9			001	001	002	004	006	008
10					001	001	002	003
11								001

x \ λ	3.6	3.8	4.0	4.2	4.4	4.6	4.8	5.0
0	1000	1000	1000	1000	1000	1000	1000	1000
1	973	978	982	985	988	990	992	993
2	874	893	908	922	934	944	952	960
3	697	731	762	790	815	837	857	875
4	485	527	567	605	641	674	706	735
5	294	332	371	410	449	487	524	560
6	156	184	215	247	280	314	349	384
7	073	091	111	133	156	182	209	238
8	031	040	051	064	079	095	113	133
9	012	016	021	028	036	045	056	068
10	004	006	008	011	015	020	025	032
11	001	002	003	004	006	008	010	014
12	001	001	001	001	002	003	004	005
13					001	001	001	002
14								001

x \ λ	5.2	5.4	5.6	5.8	6.0	6.2	6.4	6.6
0	1000	1000	1000	1000	1000	1000	1000	1000
1	994	995	996	997	998	998	998	999
2	966	971	976	979	983	985	988	990
3	891	905	918	928	938	946	954	960
4	762	787	809	830	849	866	881	895
5	594	627	658	687	715	741	765	787
6	419	454	488	522	554	586	616	649
7	268	298	330	362	394	426	458	489
8	155	178	203	229	256	284	313	342
9	082	097	114	133	153	174	197	220
10	040	049	059	071	084	098	114	131
11	018	023	028	035	043	051	061	073
12	007	010	012	016	020	025	031	037
13	003	004	005	007	009	011	014	018
14	001	001	002	003	004	005	006	008
15			001	001	001	002	003	003
16					001	001	001	001
17								001

(*Table E continued*)

x \ λ	6.8	7.0	7.2	7.4	7.6	7.8	8.0	8.5
0	1000	1000	1000	1000	1000			
1	999	999	999	999	999	1000	1000	1000
2	991	993	994	995	996	996	997	998
3	966	970	975	978	981	984	986	991
4	907	918	928	937	945	952	958	970
5	808	827	844	860	875	888	900	926
6	673	699	724	747	769	790	809	850
7	520	550	580	608	635	662	687	744
8	372	401	431	461	490	519	547	614
9	245	271	297	324	352	380	407	477
10	150	170	190	212	235	259	283	347
11	085	099	113	129	146	165	184	237
12	045	053	063	074	085	098	112	151
13	022	027	033	039	046	055	064	091
14	010	013	016	020	024	029	034	051
15	004	006	007	009	011	014	017	027
16	002	002	003	004	005	007	008	014
17	001	001	001	002	002	003	004	007
18			001	001	001	001	002	003
19							001	001
20								001

x \ λ	9.0	9.5	10.0	10.5	11.0	11.5	12.0	12.5
1	1000	1000						
2	999	999	1000	1000	1000	1000	1000	
3	994	996	997	998	999	999	999	1000
4	979	985	990	993	995	997	998	998
5	945	960	971	979	985	989	992	995
6	884	911	933	950	962	972	980	985
7	793	835	870	898	921	940	954	965
8	676	731	780	821	857	886	910	930
9	544	608	667	721	768	809	845	875
10	413	478	542	603	659	711	758	799
11	294	355	417	479	540	598	653	703
12	197	248	303	361	421	480	538	594
13	124	164	208	258	311	367	424	481
14	074	102	136	175	219	267	318	372
15	041	060	083	112	146	185	228	275
16	022	033	049	068	093	122	156	194
17	011	018	027	040	056	076	101	131
18	005	009	014	022	032	046	063	084
19	002	004	007	012	018	026	037	052
20	001	002	003	006	009	014	021	031
21		001	002	003	005	008	012	017
22			001	001	002	004	006	009
23				001	001	002	003	005
24						001	001	002
25							001	001
26								001

(*Table E continued*)

x \ λ	13.0	13.5	14.0	14.5	15	16	17	18
3	1000	1000						
4	999	999	1000	1000	1000			
5	996	997	998	999	999	1000	1000	
6	989	992	994	996	997	999	999	1000
7	974	981	986	990	992	996	998	999
8	946	959	968	976	982	990	995	997
9	900	921	938	952	963	978	987	993
10	834	865	891	912	930	957	974	985
11	748	789	824	855	882	923	951	970
12	647	696	740	780	815	873	915	945
13	537	591	642	689	732	807	865	908
14	427	482	536	587	637	725	799	857
15	325	377	430	482	534	632	719	792
16	236	282	331	381	432	533	629	713
17	165	202	244	289	336	434	532	625
18	110	139	173	210	251	341	436	531
19	070	092	117	147	181	258	345	438
20	043	058	077	099	125	188	264	349
21	025	035	048	064	083	132	195	269
22	014	020	029	040	053	089	139	201
23	008	011	017	024	033	058	095	145
24	004	006	009	014	019	037	063	101
25	002	003	005	008	011	022	041	068
26	001	002	003	004	006	013	025	045
27		001	001	002	003	007	015	028
28			001	001	002	004	009	017
29				001	001	002	005	010
30						001	003	006
31						001	001	003
32							001	002
33								001

x \ λ	19	20	21	22	23	24	25
6	1000						
7	999	1000					
8	998	999	1000	1000			
9	996	998	999	999	1000		
10	991	995	997	998	999	1000	1000
11	982	989	994	996	998	999	999
12	965	979	987	992	996	997	999
13	939	961	975	985	991	995	997
14	902	934	957	972	983	989	994
15	850	895	928	952	969	980	988
16	785	843	889	923	948	966	978
17	708	779	837	883	918	944	962

(*Table E continued*)

x \ λ	19	20	21	22	23	24	25
18	622	703	773	831	877	913	940
19	531	619	698	768	825	872	908
20	439	530	616	694	762	820	866
21	353	441	529	613	690	757	815
22	275	356	442	528	611	686	753
23	207	279	360	444	528	608	682
24	151	213	284	363	445	527	606
25	107	157	218	288	365	446	527
26	073	112	162	223	292	368	447
27	049	078	117	168	228	296	371
28	031	052	083	123	173	232	300
29	020	034	056	087	127	177	237
30	012	022	037	060	092	132	182
31	007	013	024	041	064	096	137
32	004	008	015	027	044	068	100
33	002	005	009	017	029	047	071
34	001	003	006	011	019	031	050
35	001	001	003	006	012	021	034
36		001	002	004	007	013	022
37			001	002	004	008	015
38			001	001	003	005	009
39				001	001	003	006
40					001	002	003
41						001	002
42						001	001
43							001

Table F

Normal Curve Areas
Entries in the Body of the Table Give the Area Under
the Standard Normal Curve from 0 to z.

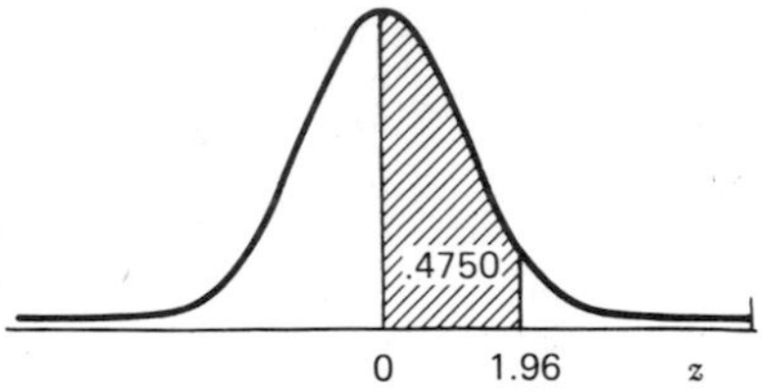

z	.00	.01	.02	.03	.04	.05	.06	.07	.08	.09
.0	.0000	.0040	.0080	.0120	.0160	.0199	.0239	.0279	.0319	.0359
.1	.0398	.0438	.0478	.0517	.0557	.0596	.0636	.0675	.0714	.0753
.2	.0793	.0832	.0871	.0910	.0948	.0987	.1026	.1064	.1103	.1141
.3	.1179	.1217	.1255	.1293	.1331	.1368	.1406	.1443	.1480	.1517
.4	.1554	.1591	.1628	.1664	.1700	.1736	.1772	.1808	.1844	.1879
.5	.1915	.1950	.1985	.2019	.2054	.2088	.2123	.2157	.2190	.2224
.6	.2257	.2291	.2324	.2357	.2389	.2422	.2454	.2486	.2517	.2549
.7	.2580	.2611	.2642	.2673	.2704	.2734	.2764	.2794	.2823	.2852
.8	.2881	.2910	.2939	.2967	.2995	.3023	.3051	.3078	.3106	.3133
.9	.3159	.3186	.3212	.3238	.3264	.3289	.3315	.3340	.3365	.3389
1.0	.3413	.3438	.3461	.3485	.3508	.3531	.3554	.3577	.3599	.3621
1.1	.3643	.3665	.3686	.3708	.3729	.3749	.3770	.3790	.3810	.3830
1.2	.3849	.3869	.3888	.3907	.3925	.3944	.3962	.3980	.3997	.4015
1.3	.4032	.4049	.4066	.4082	.4099	.4115	.4131	.4147	.4162	.4177
1.4	.4192	.4207	.4222	.4236	.4251	.4265	.4279	.4292	.4306	.4319
1.5	.4332	.4345	.4357	.4370	.4382	.4394	.4406	.4418	.4429	.4441
1.6	.4452	.4463	.4474	.4484	.4495	.4505	.4515	.4525	.4535	.4545
1.7	.4554	.4564	.4573	.4582	.4591	.4599	.4608	.4616	.4625	.4633
1.8	.4641	.4649	.4656	.4664	.4671	.4678	.4686	.4693	.4699	.4706
1.9	.4713	.4719	.4726	.4732	.4738	.4744	.4750	.4756	.4761	.4767
2.0	.4772	.4778	.4783	.4788	.4793	.4798	.4803	.4808	.4812	.4817
2.1	.4821	.4826	.4830	.4834	.4838	.4842	.4846	.4850	.4854	.4857
2.2	.4861	.4864	.4868	.4871	.4875	.4878	.4881	.4884	.4887	.4890
2.3	.4893	.4896	.4898	.4901	.4904	.4906	.4909	.4911	.4913	.4916
2.4	.4918	.4920	.4922	.4925	.4927	.4929	.4931	.4932	.4934	.4936
2.5	.4938	.4940	.4941	.4943	.4945	.4946	.4948	.4949	.4951	.4952
2.6	.4953	.4955	.4956	.4957	.4959	.4960	.4961	.4962	.4963	.4964
2.7	.4965	.4966	.4967	.4968	.4969	.4970	.4971	.4972	.4973	.4974
2.8	.4974	.4975	.4976	.4977	.4977	.4978	.4979	.4979	.4980	.4981
2.9	.4981	.4982	.4982	.4983	.4984	.4984	.4985	.4985	.4986	.4986
3.0	.4987	.4987	.4987	.4988	.4988	.4989	.4989	.4989	.4990	.4990

Table G

Random Digits

85967	73152	14511	85285	36009	95892	36962	67835	63314	50162
07483	51453	11649	86348	76431	81594	95848	36738	25014	15460
96283	01898	61414	83525	04231	13604	75339	11730	85423	60698
49174	12074	98551	37895	93547	24769	09404	76548	05393	96770
97366	39941	21225	93629	19574	71565	33413	56087	40875	13351
90474	41469	16812	81542	81652	45554	27931	93994	22375	00953
28599	64109	09497	76235	41383	31555	12639	00619	22909	29563
25254	16210	89717	65997	82667	74624	36348	44018	64732	93589
28785	02760	24359	99410	77319	73408	58993	61098	04393	48245
84725	86576	86944	93296	10081	82454	76810	52975	10324	15457
41059	66456	47679	66810	15941	84602	14493	65515	19251	41642
67434	41045	82830	47617	36932	46728	71183	36345	41404	81110
72766	68816	37643	19959	57550	49620	98480	25640	67257	18671
92079	46784	66125	94932	64451	29275	57669	66658	30818	58353
29187	40350	62533	73603	34075	16451	42885	03448	37390	96328
74220	17612	65522	80607	19184	64164	66962	82310	18163	63495
03786	02407	06098	92917	40434	60602	82175	04470	78754	90775
75085	55558	15520	27038	25471	76107	90832	10819	56797	33751
09161	33015	19155	11715	00551	24909	31894	37774	37953	78837
75707	48992	64998	87080	39333	00767	45637	12538	67439	94914
21333	48660	31288	00086	79889	75532	28704	62844	92337	99695
65626	50061	42539	14812	48895	11196	34335	60492	70650	51108
84380	07389	87891	76255	89604	41372	10837	66992	93183	56920
46479	32072	80083	63868	70930	89654	05359	47196	12452	38234
59847	97197	55147	76639	76971	55928	36441	95141	42333	67483
31416	11231	27904	57383	31852	69137	96667	14315	01007	31929
82066	83436	67914	21465	99605	83114	97885	74440	99622	87912
01850	42782	39202	18582	46214	99228	79541	78298	75404	63648
32315	89276	89582	87138	16165	15984	21466	63830	30475	74729
59388	42703	55198	80380	67067	97155	34160	85019	03527	78140
58089	27632	50987	91373	07736	20436	96130	73483	85332	24384
61705	57285	30392	23660	75841	21931	04295	00875	09114	32101
18914	98982	60199	99275	41967	35208	30357	76772	92656	62318
11965	94089	34803	48941	69709	16784	44642	89761	66864	62803
85251	48111	80936	81781	93248	67877	16498	31924	51315	79921
66121	96986	84844	93873	46352	92183	51152	85878	30490	15974
53972	96642	24199	58080	35450	03482	66953	49521	63719	57615
14509	16594	78883	43222	23093	58645	60257	89250	63266	90858
37700	07688	65533	72126	23611	93993	01848	03910	38552	17472
85466	59392	72722	15473	73295	49759	56157	60477	83284	56367
52969	55863	42312	67842	05673	91878	82738	36563	79540	61935
42744	68315	17514	02878	97291	74851	42725	57894	81434	62041
26140	13336	67726	61876	29971	99294	96664	52817	90039	53211
95589	56319	14563	24071	06916	59555	18195	32280	79357	04224
39113	13217	59999	49952	83021	47709	53105	19295	88318	41626
41392	17622	18994	98283	07249	52289	24209	91139	30715	06604
54684	53645	79246	70183	87731	19185	08541	33519	07223	97413
89442	61001	36658	57444	95388	36682	38052	46719	09428	94012
36751	16778	54888	15357	68003	43564	90976	58904	40512	07725
98159	02564	21416	74944	53049	88749	02865	25772	89853	88714

Table H

Percentiles of the *t* Distribution

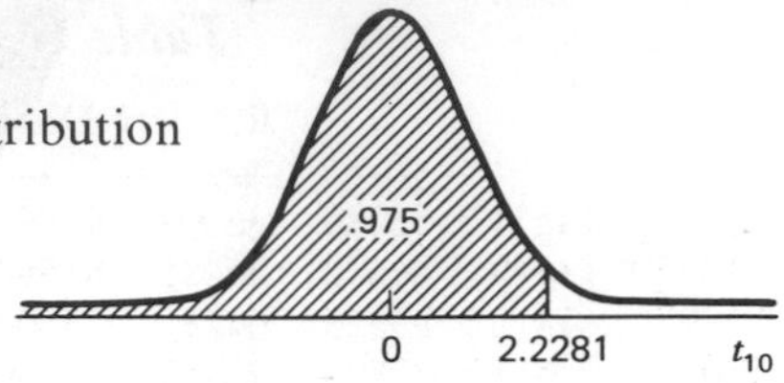

d. f.	$t_{.90}$	$t_{.95}$	$t_{.975}$	$t_{.99}$	$t_{.995}$
1	3.078	6.3138	12.706	31.821	63.657
2	1.886	2.9200	4.3027	6.965	9.9248
3	1.638	2.3534	3.1825	4.541	5.8409
4	1.533	2.1318	2.7764	3.747	4.6041
5	1.476	2.0150	2.5706	3.365	4.0321
6	1.440	1.9432	2.4469	3.143	3.7074
7	1.415	1.8946	2.3646	2.998	3.4995
8	1.397	1.8595	2.3060	2.896	3.3554
9	1.383	1.8331	2.2622	2.821	3.2498
10	1.372	1.8125	2.2281	2.764	3.1693
11	1.363	1.7959	2.2010	2.718	3.1058
12	1.356	1.7823	2.1788	2.681	3.0545
13	1.350	1.7709	2.1604	2.650	3.0123
14	1.345	1.7613	2.1448	2.624	2.9768
15	1.341	1.7530	2.1315	2.602	2.9467
16	1.337	1.7459	2.1199	2.583	2.9208
17	1.333	1.7396	2.1098	2.567	2.8982
18	1.330	1.7341	2.1009	2.552	2.8784
19	1.328	1.7291	2.0930	2.539	2.8609
20	1.325	1.7247	2.0860	2.528	2.8453
21	1.323	1.7207	2.0796	2.518	2.8314
22	1.321	1.7171	2.0739	2.508	2.8188
23	1.319	1.7139	2.0687	2.500	2.8073
24	1.318	1.7109	2.0639	2.492	2.7969
25	1.316	1.7081	2.0595	2.485	2.7874
26	1.315	1.7056	2.0555	2.479	2.7787
27	1.314	1.7033	2.0518	2.473	2.7707
28	1.313	1.7011	2.0484	2.467	2.7633
29	1.311	1.6991	2.0452	2.462	2.7564
30	1.310	1.6973	2.0423	2.457	2.7500
35	1.3062	1.6896	2.0301	2.438	2.7239
40	1.3031	1.6839	2.0211	2.423	2.7045
45	1.3007	1.6794	2.0141	2.412	2.6896
50	1.2987	1.6759	2.0086	2.403	2.6778
60	1.2959	1.6707	2.0003	2.390	2.6603
70	1.2938	1.6669	1.9945	2.381	2.6480
80	1.2922	1.6641	1.9901	2.374	2.6388
90	1.2910	1.6620	1.9867	2.368	2.6316
100	1.2901	1.6602	1.9840	2.364	2.6260
120	1.2887	1.6577	1.9799	2.358	2.6175
140	1.2876	1.6558	1.9771	2.353	2.6114
160	1.2869	1.6545	1.9749	2.350	2.6070
180	1.2863	1.6534	1.9733	2.347	2.6035
200	1.2858	1.6525	1.9719	2.345	2.6006
∞	1.282	1.645	1.96	2.326	2.576

Table I

Percentiles of the Chi-Square Distribution

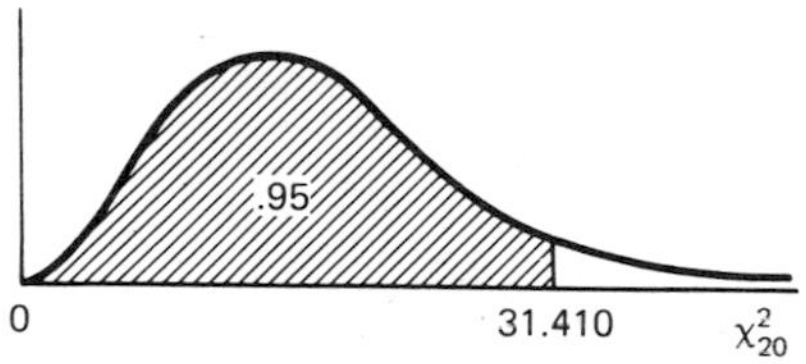

d. f.	$\chi^2_{.005}$	$\chi^2_{.025}$	$\chi^2_{.05}$	$\chi^2_{.90}$	$\chi^2_{.95}$	$\chi^2_{.975}$	$\chi^2_{.99}$	$\chi^2_{.995}$
1	.0000393	.000982	.00393	2.706	3.841	5.024	6.635	7.879
2	.0100	.0506	.103	4.605	5.991	7.378	9.210	10.597
3	.0717	.216	.352	6.251	7.815	9.348	11.345	12.838
4	.207	.484	.711	7.779	9.488	11.143	13.277	14.860
5	.412	.831	1.145	9.236	11.070	12.832	15.086	16.750
6	.676	1.237	1.635	10.645	12.592	14.449	16.812	18.548
7	.989	1.690	2.167	12.017	14.067	16.013	18.475	20.278
8	1.344	2.180	2.733	13.362	15.507	17.535	20.090	21.955
9	1.735	2.700	3.325	14.684	16.919	19.023	21.666	23.589
10	2.156	3.247	3.940	15.987	18.307	20.483	23.209	25.188
11	2.603	3.816	4.575	17.275	19.675	21.920	24.725	26.757
12	3.074	4.404	5.226	18.549	21.026	23.336	26.217	28.300
13	3.565	5.009	5.892	19.812	22.362	24.736	27.688	29.819
14	4.075	5.629	6.571	21.064	23.685	26.119	29.141	31.319
15	4.601	6.262	7.261	22.307	24.996	27.488	30.578	32.801
16	5.142	6.908	7.962	23.542	26.296	28.845	32.000	34.267
17	5.697	7.564	8.672	24.769	27.587	30.191	33.409	35.718
18	6.265	8.231	9.390	25.989	28.869	31.526	34.805	37.156
19	6.844	8.907	10.117	27.204	30.144	32.852	36.191	38.582
20	7.434	9.591	10.851	28.412	31.410	34.170	37.566	39.997
21	8.034	10.283	11.591	29.615	32.671	35.479	38.932	41.401
22	8.643	10.982	12.338	30.813	33.924	36.781	40.289	42.796
23	9.260	11.688	13.091	32.007	35.172	38.076	41.638	44.181
24	9.886	12.401	13.848	33.196	36.415	39.364	42.980	45.558
25	10.520	13.120	14.611	34.382	37.652	40.646	44.314	46.928
26	11.160	13.844	15.379	35.563	38.885	41.923	45.642	48.290
27	11.808	14.573	16.151	36.741	40.113	43.194	46.963	49.645
28	12.461	15.308	16.928	37.916	41.337	44.461	48.278	50.993
29	13.121	16.047	17.708	39.087	42.557	45.722	49.588	52.336
30	13.787	16.791	18.493	40.256	43.773	46.979	50.892	53.672
35	17.192	20.569	22.465	46.059	49.802	53.203	57.342	60.275
40	20.707	24.433	26.509	51.805	55.758	59.342	63.691	66.766
45	24.311	28.366	30.612	57.505	61.656	65.410	69.957	73.166
50	27.991	32.357	34.764	63.167	67.505	71.420	76.154	79.490
60	35.535	40.482	43.188	74.397	79.082	83.298	88.379	91.952
70	43.275	48.758	51.739	85.527	90.531	95.023	100.425	104.215
80	51.172	57.153	60.391	96.578	101.879	106.629	112.329	116.321
90	59.196	65.647	69.126	107.565	113.145	118.136	124.116	128.299
100	67.328	74.222	77.929	118.498	124.342	129.561	135.807	140.169

Table J

Percentiles of the F Distribution

$F_{.995}$

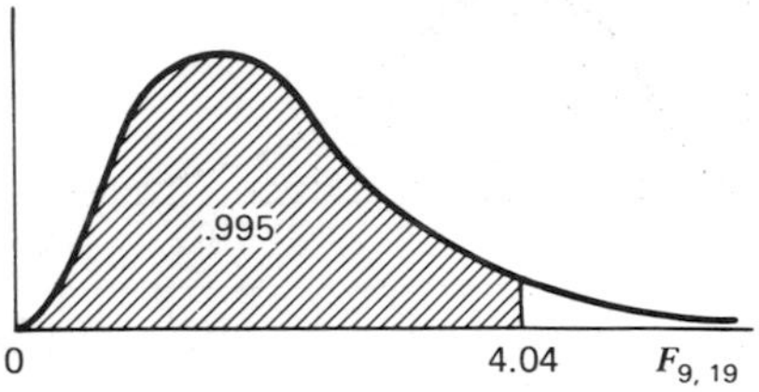

Denominator Degrees of Freedom	Numerator Degrees of Freedom 1	2	3	4	5	6	7	8	9
1	16211	20000	21615	22500	23056	23437	23715	23925	24091
2	198.5	199.0	199.2	199.2	199.3	199.3	199.4	199.4	199.4
3	55.55	49.80	47.47	46.19	45.39	44.84	44.43	44.13	43.88
4	31.33	26.28	24.26	23.15	22.46	21.97	21.62	21.35	21.14
5	22.78	18.31	16.53	15.56	14.94	14.51	14.20	13.96	13.77
6	18.63	14.54	12.92	12.03	11.46	11.07	10.79	10.57	10.39
7	16.24	12.40	10.88	10.05	9.52	9.16	8.89	8.68	8.51
8	14.69	11.04	9.60	8.81	8.30	7.95	7.69	7.50	7.34
9	13.61	10.11	8.72	7.96	7.47	7.13	6.88	6.69	6.54
10	12.83	9.43	8.08	7.34	6.87	6.54	6.30	6.12	5.97
11	12.23	8.91	7.60	6.88	6.42	6.10	5.86	5.68	5.54
12	11.75	8.51	7.23	6.52	6.07	5.76	5.52	5.35	5.20
13	11.37	8.19	6.93	6.23	5.79	5.48	5.25	5.08	4.94
14	11.06	7.92	6.68	6.00	5.56	5.26	5.03	4.86	4.72
15	10.80	7.70	6.48	5.80	5.37	5.07	4.85	4.67	4.54
16	10.58	7.51	6.30	5.64	5.21	4.91	4.69	4.52	4.38
17	10.38	7.35	6.16	5.50	5.07	4.78	4.56	4.39	4.25
18	10.22	7.21	6.03	5.37	4.96	4.66	4.44	4.28	4.14
19	10.07	7.09	5.92	5.27	4.85	4.56	4.34	4.18	4.04
20	9.94	6.99	5.82	5.17	4.76	4.47	4.26	4.09	3.96
21	9.83	6.89	5.73	5.09	4.68	4.39	4.18	4.01	3.88
22	9.73	6.81	5.65	5.02	4.61	4.32	4.11	3.94	3.81
23	9.63	6.73	5.58	4.95	4.54	4.26	4.05	3.88	3.75
24	9.55	6.66	5.52	4.89	4.49	4.20	3.99	3.83	3.69
25	9.48	6.60	5.46	4.84	4.43	4.15	3.94	3.78	3.64
26	9.41	6.54	5.41	4.79	4.38	4.10	3.89	3.73	3.60
27	9.34	6.49	5.36	4.74	4.34	4.06	3.85	3.69	3.56
28	9.28	6.44	5.32	4.70	4.30	4.02	3.81	3.65	3.52
29	9.23	6.40	5.28	4.66	4.26	3.98	3.77	3.61	3.48
30	9.18	6.35	5.24	4.62	4.23	3.95	3.74	3.58	3.45
40	8.83	6.07	4.98	4.37	3.99	3.71	3.51	3.35	3.22
60	8.49	5.79	4.73	4.14	3.76	3.49	3.29	3.13	3.01
120	8.18	5.54	4.50	3.92	3.55	3.28	3.09	2.93	2.81
∞	7.88	5.30	4.28	3.72	3.35	3.09	2.90	2.74	2.62

(*Table J continued*)

Denominator Degrees of Freedom	Numerator Degrees of Freedom 10	12	15	20	24	30	40	60	120	∞
1	24224	24426	24630	24836	24940	25044	25148	25253	25359	25465
2	199.4	199.4	199.4	199.4	199.5	199.5	199.5	199.5	199.5	199.5
3	43.69	43.39	43.08	42.78	42.62	42.47	42.31	42.15	41.99	41.83
4	20.97	20.70	20.44	20.17	20.03	19.89	19.75	19.61	19.47	19.32
5	13.62	13.38	13.15	12.90	12.78	12.66	12.53	12.40	12.27	12.14
6	10.25	10.03	9.81	9.59	9.47	9.36	9.24	9.12	9.00	8.88
7	8.38	8.18	7.97	7.75	7.65	7.53	7.42	7.31	7.19	7.08
8	7.21	7.01	6.81	6.61	6.50	6.40	6.29	6.18	6.06	5.95
9	6.42	6.23	6.03	5.83	5.73	5.62	5.52	5.41	5.30	5.19
10	5.85	5.66	5.47	5.27	5.17	5.07	4.97	4.86	4.75	4.64
11	5.42	5.24	5.05	4.86	4.76	4.65	4.55	4.44	4.34	4.23
12	5.09	4.91	4.72	4.53	4.43	4.33	4.23	4.12	4.01	3.90
13	4.82	4.64	4.46	4.27	4.17	4.07	3.97	3.87	3.76	3.65
14	4.60	4.43	4.25	4.06	3.96	3.86	3.76	3.66	3.55	3.44
15	4.42	4.25	4.07	3.88	3.79	3.69	3.58	3.48	3.37	3.26
16	4.27	4.10	3.92	3.73	3.64	3.54	3.44	3.33	3.22	3.11
17	4.14	3.97	3.79	3.61	3.51	3.41	3.31	3.21	3.10	2.98
18	4.03	3.86	3.68	3.50	3.40	3.30	3.20	3.10	2.99	2.87
19	3.93	3.76	3.59	3.40	3.31	3.21	3.11	3.00	2.89	2.78
20	3.85	3.68	3.50	3.32	3.22	3.12	3.02	2.92	2.81	2.69
21	3.77	3.60	3.43	3.24	3.15	3.05	2.95	2.84	2.73	2.61
22	3.70	3.54	3.36	3.18	3.08	2.98	2.88	2.77	2.66	2.55
23	3.64	3.47	3.30	3.12	3.02	2.92	2.82	2.71	2.60	2.48
24	3.59	3.42	3.25	3.06	2.97	2.87	2.77	2.66	2.55	2.43
25	3.54	3.37	3.20	3.01	2.92	2.82	2.72	2.61	2.50	2.38
26	3.49	3.33	3.15	2.97	2.87	2.77	2.67	2.56	2.45	2.33
27	3.45	3.28	3.11	2.93	2.83	2.73	2.63	2.52	2.41	2.29
28	3.41	3.25	3.07	2.89	2.79	2.69	2.59	2.48	2.37	2.25
29	3.38	3.21	3.04	2.86	2.76	2.66	2.56	2.45	2.33	2.21
30	3.34	3.18	3.01	2.82	2.73	2.63	2.52	2.42	2.30	2.18
40	3.12	2.95	2.78	2.60	2.50	2.40	2.30	2.18	2.06	1.93
60	2.90	2.74	2.57	2.39	2.29	2.19	2.08	1.96	1.83	1.69
120	2.71	2.54	2.37	2.19	2.09	1.98	1.87	1.75	1.61	1.43
∞	2.52	2.36	2.19	2.00	1.90	1.79	1.67	1.53	1.36	1.00

(*Table J continued*)

$F_{.99}$

Denominator Degrees of Freedom	1	2	3	4	5	6	7	8	9
				Numerator Degrees of Freedom					
1	4052	4999.5	5403	5625	5764	5859	5928	5981	6022
2	98.50	99.00	99.17	99.25	99.30	99.33	99.36	99.37	99.39
3	34.12	30.82	29.46	28.71	28.24	27.91	27.67	27.49	27.35
4	21.20	18.00	16.69	15.98	15.52	15.21	14.98	14.80	14.66
5	16.26	13.27	12.06	11.39	10.97	10.67	10.46	10.29	10.16
6	13.75	10.92	9.78	9.15	8.75	8.47	8.26	8.10	7.98
7	12.25	9.55	8.45	7.85	7.46	7.19	6.99	6.84	6.72
8	11.26	8.65	7.59	7.01	6.63	6.37	6.18	6.03	5.91
9	10.56	8.02	6.99	6.42	6.06	5.80	5.61	5.47	5.35
10	10.04	7.56	6.55	5.99	5.64	5.39	5.20	5.06	4.94
11	9.65	7.21	6.22	5.67	5.32	5.07	4.89	4.74	4.63
12	9.33	6.93	5.95	5.41	5.06	4.82	4.64	4.50	4.39
13	9.07	6.70	5.74	5.21	4.86	4.62	4.44	4.30	4.19
14	8.86	6.51	5.56	5.04	4.69	4.46	4.28	4.14	4.03
15	8.68	6.36	5.42	4.89	4.56	4.32	4.14	4.00	3.89
16	8.53	6.23	5.29	4.77	4.44	4.20	4.03	3.89	3.78
17	8.40	6.11	5.18	4.67	4.34	4.10	3.93	3.79	3.68
18	8.29	6.01	5.09	4.58	4.25	4.01	3.84	3.71	3.60
19	8.18	5.93	5.01	4.50	4.17	3.94	3.77	3.63	3.52
20	8.10	5.85	4.94	4.43	4.10	3.87	3.70	3.56	3.46
21	8.02	5.78	4.87	4.37	4.04	3.81	3.64	3.51	3.40
22	7.95	5.72	4.82	4.31	3.99	3.76	3.59	3.45	3.35
23	7.88	5.66	4.76	4.26	3.94	3.71	3.54	3.41	3.30
24	7.82	5.61	4.72	4.22	3.90	3.67	3.50	3.36	3.26
25	7.77	5.57	4.68	4.18	3.85	3.63	3.46	3.32	3.22
26	7.72	5.53	4.64	4.14	3.82	3.59	3.42	3.29	3.18
27	7.68	5.49	4.60	4.11	3.78	3.56	3.39	3.26	3.15
28	7.64	5.45	4.57	4.07	3.75	3.53	3.36	3.23	3.12
29	7.60	5.42	4.54	4.04	3.73	3.50	3.33	3.20	3.09
30	7.56	5.39	4.51	4.02	3.70	3.47	3.30	3.17	3.07
40	7.31	5.18	4.31	3.83	3.51	3.29	3.12	2.99	2.89
60	7.08	4.98	4.13	3.65	3.34	3.12	2.95	2.82	2.72
120	6.85	4.79	3.95	3.48	3.17	2.96	2.79	2.66	2.56
∞	6.63	4.61	3.78	3.32	3.02	2.80	2.64	2.51	2.41

(*Table J continued*)

Denominator Degrees of Freedom	Numerator Degrees of Freedom 10	12	15	20	24	30	40	60	120	∞
1	6056	6106	6157	6209	6235	6261	6287	6313	6339	6366
2	99.40	99.42	99.43	99.45	99.46	99.47	99.47	99.48	99.49	99.50
3	27.23	27.05	26.87	26.69	26.60	26.50	26.41	26.32	26.22	26.13
4	14.55	14.37	14.20	14.02	13.93	13.84	13.75	13.65	13.56	13.46
5	10.05	9.89	9.72	9.55	9.47	9.38	9.29	9.20	9.11	9.02
6	7.87	7.72	7.56	7.40	7.31	7.23	7.14	7.06	6.97	6.88
7	6.62	6.47	6.31	6.16	6.07	5.99	5.91	5.82	5.74	5.65
8	5.81	5.67	5.52	5.36	5.28	5.20	5.12	5.03	4.95	4.86
9	5.26	5.11	4.96	4.81	4.73	4.65	4.57	4.48	4.40	4.31
10	4.85	4.71	4.56	4.41	4.33	4.25	4.17	4.08	4.00	3.91
11	4.54	4.40	4.25	4.10	4.02	3.94	3.86	3.78	3.69	3.60
12	4.30	4.16	4.01	3.86	3.78	3.70	3.62	3.54	3.45	3.36
13	4.10	3.96	3.82	3.66	3.59	3.51	3.43	3.34	3.25	3.17
14	3.94	3.80	3.66	3.51	3.43	3.35	3.27	3.18	3.09	3.00
15	3.80	3.67	3.52	3.37	3.29	3.21	3.13	3.05	2.96	2.87
16	3.69	3.55	3.41	3.26	3.18	3.10	3.02	2.93	2.84	2.75
17	3.59	3.46	3.31	3.16	3.08	3.00	2.92	2.83	2.75	2.65
18	3.51	3.37	3.23	3.08	3.00	2.92	2.84	2.75	2.66	2.57
19	3.43	3.30	3.15	3.00	2.92	2.84	2.76	2.67	2.58	2.49
20	3.37	3.23	3.09	2.94	2.86	2.78	2.69	2.61	2.52	2.42
21	3.31	3.17	3.03	2.88	2.80	2.72	2.64	2.55	2.46	2.36
22	3.26	3.12	2.98	2.83	2.75	2.67	2.58	2.50	2.40	2.31
23	3.21	3.07	2.93	2.78	2.70	2.62	2.54	2.45	2.35	2.26
24	3.17	3.03	2.89	2.74	2.66	2.58	2.49	2.40	2.31	2.21
25	3.13	2.99	2.85	2.70	2.62	2.54	2.45	2.36	2.27	2.17
26	3.09	2.96	2.81	2.66	2.58	2.50	2.42	2.33	2.23	2.13
27	3.06	2.93	2.78	2.63	2.55	2.47	2.38	2.29	2.20	2.10
28	3.03	2.90	2.75	2.60	2.52	2.44	2.35	2.26	2.17	2.06
29	3.00	2.87	2.73	2.57	2.49	2.41	2.33	2.23	2.14	2.03
30	2.98	2.84	2.70	2.55	2.47	2.39	2.30	2.21	2.11	2.01
40	2.80	2.66	2.52	2.37	2.29	2.20	2.11	2.02	1.92	1.80
60	2.63	2.50	2.35	2.20	2.12	2.03	1.94	1.84	1.73	1.60
120	2.47	2.34	2.19	2.03	1.95	1.86	1.76	1.66	1.53	1.38
∞	2.32	2.18	2.04	1.88	1.79	1.70	1.59	1.47	1.32	1.00

(*Table J continued*)

$F_{.975}$

Denominator Degrees of Freedom	Numerator Degrees of Freedom 1	2	3	4	5	6	7	8	9
1	647.8	799.5	864.2	899.6	921.8	937.1	948.2	956.7	963.3
2	38.51	39.00	39.17	39.25	39.30	39.33	39.36	39.37	39.39
3	17.44	16.04	15.44	15.10	14.88	14.73	14.62	14.54	14.47
4	12.22	10.65	9.98	9.60	9.36	9.20	9.07	8.98	8.90
5	10.01	8.43	7.76	7.39	7.15	6.98	6.85	6.76	6.68
6	8.81	7.26	6.60	6.23	5.99	5.82	5.70	5.60	5.52
7	8.07	6.54	5.89	5.52	5.29	5.12	4.99	4.90	4.82
8	7.57	6.06	5.42	5.05	4.82	4.65	4.53	4.43	4.36
9	7.21	5.71	5.08	4.72	4.48	4.32	4.20	4.10	4.03
10	6.94	5.46	4.83	4.47	4.24	4.07	3.95	3.85	3.78
11	6.72	5.26	4.63	4.28	4.04	3.88	3.76	3.66	3.59
12	6.55	5.10	4.47	4.12	3.89	3.73	3.61	3.51	3.44
13	6.41	4.97	4.35	4.00	3.77	3.60	3.48	3.39	3.31
14	6.30	4.86	4.24	3.89	3.66	3.50	3.38	3.29	3.21
15	6.20	4.77	4.15	3.80	3.58	3.41	3.29	3.20	3.12
16	6.12	4.69	4.08	3.73	3.50	3.34	3.22	3.12	3.05
17	6.04	4.62	4.01	3.66	3.44	3.28	3.16	3.06	2.98
18	5.98	4.56	3.95	3.61	3.38	3.22	3.10	3.01	2.93
19	5.92	4.51	3.90	3.56	3.33	3.17	3.05	2.96	2.88
20	5.87	4.46	3.86	3.51	3.29	3.13	3.01	2.91	2.84
21	5.83	4.42	3.82	3.48	3.25	3.09	2.97	2.87	2.80
22	5.79	4.38	3.78	3.44	3.22	3.05	2.93	2.84	2.76
23	5.75	4.35	3.75	3.41	3.18	3.02	2.90	2.81	2.73
24	5.72	4.32	3.72	3.38	3.15	2.99	2.87	2.78	2.70
25	5.69	4.29	3.69	3.35	3.13	2.97	2.85	2.75	2.68
26	5.66	4.27	3.67	3.33	3.10	2.94	2.82	2.73	2.65
27	5.63	4.24	3.65	3.31	3.08	2.92	2.80	2.71	2.63
28	5.61	4.22	3.63	3.29	3.06	2.90	2.78	2.69	2.61
29	5.59	4.20	3.61	3.27	3.04	2.88	2.76	2.67	2.59
30	5.57	4.18	3.59	3.25	3.03	2.87	2.75	2.65	2.57
40	5.42	4.05	3.46	3.13	2.90	2.74	2.62	2.53	2.45
60	5.29	3.93	3.34	3.01	2.79	2.63	2.51	2.41	2.33
120	5.15	3.80	3.23	2.89	2.67	2.52	2.39	2.30	2.22
∞	5.02	3.69	3.12	2.79	2.57	2.41	2.29	2.19	2.11

(*Table J continued*)

Denominator Degrees of Freedom	Numerator Degrees of Freedom 10	12	15	20	24	30	40	60	120	∞
1	968.6	976.7	984.9	993.1	997.2	1001	1006	1010	1014	1018
2	39.40	39.41	39.43	39.45	39.46	39.46	39.47	39.48	39.49	39.50
3	14.42	14.34	14.25	14.17	14.12	14.08	14.04	13.99	13.95	13.90
4	8.84	8.75	8.66	8.56	8.51	8.46	8.41	8.36	8.31	8.26
5	6.62	6.52	6.43	6.33	6.28	6.23	6.18	6.12	6.07	6.02
6	5.46	5.37	5.27	5.17	5.12	5.07	5.01	4.96	4.90	4.85
7	4.76	4.67	4.57	4.47	4.42	4.36	4.31	4.25	4.20	4.14
8	4.30	4.20	4.10	4.00	3.95	3.89	3.84	3.78	3.73	3.67
9	3.96	3.87	3.77	3.67	3.61	3.56	3.51	3.45	3.39	3.33
10	3.72	3.62	3.52	3.42	3.37	3.31	3.26	3.20	3.14	3.08
11	3.53	3.43	3.33	3.23	3.17	3.12	3.06	3.00	2.94	2.88
12	3.37	3.28	3.18	3.07	3.02	2.96	2.91	2.85	2.79	2.72
13	3.25	3.15	3.05	2.95	2.89	2.84	2.78	2.72	2.66	2.60
14	3.15	3.05	2.95	2.84	2.79	2.73	2.67	2.61	2.55	2.49
15	3.06	2.96	2.86	2.76	2.70	2.64	2.59	2.52	2.46	2.40
16	2.99	2.89	2.79	2.68	2.63	2.57	2.51	2.45	2.38	2.32
17	2.92	2.82	2.72	2.62	2.56	2.50	2.44	2.38	2.32	2.25
18	2.87	2.77	2.67	2.56	2.50	2.44	2.38	2.32	2.26	2.19
19	2.82	2.72	2.62	2.51	2.45	2.39	2.33	2.27	2.20	2.13
20	2.77	2.68	2.57	2.46	2.41	2.35	2.29	2.22	2.16	2.09
21	2.73	2.64	2.53	2.42	2.37	2.31	2.25	2.18	2.11	2.04
22	2.70	2.60	2.50	2.39	2.33	2.27	2.21	2.14	2.08	2.00
23	2.67	2.57	2.47	2.36	2.30	2.24	2.18	2.11	2.04	1.97
24	2.64	2.54	2.44	2.33	2.27	2.21	2.15	2.08	2.01	1.94
25	2.61	2.51	2.41	2.30	2.24	2.18	2.12	2.05	1.98	1.91
26	2.59	2.49	2.39	2.28	2.22	2.16	2.09	2.03	1.95	1.88
27	2.57	2.47	2.36	2.25	2.19	2.13	2.07	2.00	1.93	1.85
28	2.55	2.45	2.34	2.23	2.17	2.11	2.05	1.98	1.91	1.83
29	2.53	2.43	2.32	2.21	2.15	2.09	2.03	1.96	1.89	1.81
30	2.51	2.41	2.31	2.20	2.14	2.07	2.01	1.94	1.87	1.79
40	2.39	2.29	2.18	2.07	2.01	1.94	1.88	1.80	1.72	1.64
60	2.27	2.17	2.06	1.94	1.88	1.82	1.74	1.67	1.58	1.48
120	2.16	2.05	1.94	1.82	1.76	1.69	1.61	1.53	1.43	1.31
∞	2.05	1.94	1.83	1.71	1.64	1.57	1.48	1.39	1.27	1.00

(*Table J continued*)

$F_{.95}$

Denominator Degrees of Freedom	Numerator Degrees of Freedom 1	2	3	4	5	6	7	8	9
1	161.4	199.5	215.7	224.6	230.2	234.0	236.8	238.9	240.5
2	18.51	19.00	19.16	19.25	19.30	19.33	19.35	19.37	19.38
3	10.13	9.55	9.28	9.12	9.01	8.94	8.89	8.85	8.81
4	7.71	6.94	6.59	6.39	6.26	6.16	6.09	6.04	6.00
5	6.61	5.79	5.41	5.19	5.05	4.95	4.88	4.82	4.77
6	5.99	5.14	4.76	4.53	4.39	4.28	4.21	4.15	4.10
7	5.59	4.74	4.35	4.12	3.97	3.87	3.79	3.73	3.68
8	5.32	4.46	4.07	3.84	3.69	3.58	3.50	3.44	3.39
9	5.12	4.26	3.86	3.63	3.48	3.37	3.29	3.23	3.18
10	4.96	4.10	3.71	3.48	3.33	3.22	3.14	3.07	3.02
11	4.84	3.98	3.59	3.36	3.20	3.09	3.01	2.95	2.90
12	4.75	3.89	3.49	3.26	3.11	3.00	2.91	2.85	2.80
13	4.67	3.81	3.41	3.18	3.03	2.92	2.83	2.77	2.71
14	4.60	3.74	3.34	3.11	2.96	2.85	2.76	2.70	2.65
15	4.54	3.68	3.29	3.06	2.90	2.79	2.71	2.64	2.59
16	4.49	3.63	3.24	3.01	2.85	2.74	2.66	2.59	2.54
17	4.45	3.59	3.20	2.96	2.81	2.70	2.61	2.55	2.49
18	4.41	3.55	3.16	2.93	2.77	2.66	2.58	2.51	2.46
19	4.38	3.52	3.13	2.90	2.74	2.63	2.54	2.48	2.42
20	4.35	3.49	3.10	2.87	2.71	2.60	2.51	2.45	2.39
21	4.32	3.47	3.07	2.84	2.68	2.57	2.49	2.42	2.37
22	4.30	3.44	3.05	2.82	2.66	2.55	2.46	2.40	2.34
23	4.28	3.42	3.03	2.80	2.64	2.53	2.44	2.37	2.32
24	4.26	3.40	3.01	2.78	2.62	2.51	2.42	2.36	2.30
25	4.24	3.39	2.99	2.76	2.60	2.49	2.40	2.34	2.28
26	4.23	3.37	2.98	2.74	2.59	2.47	2.39	2.32	2.27
27	4.21	3.35	2.96	2.73	2.57	2.46	2.37	2.31	2.25
28	4.20	3.34	2.95	2.71	2.56	2.45	2.36	2.29	2.24
29	4.18	3.33	2.93	2.70	2.55	2.43	2.35	2.28	2.22
30	4.17	3.32	2.92	2.69	2.53	2.42	2.33	2.27	2.21
40	4.08	3.23	2.84	2.61	2.45	2.34	2.25	2.18	2.12
60	4.00	3.15	2.76	2.53	2.37	2.25	2.17	2.10	2.04
120	3.92	3.07	2.68	2.45	2.29	2.17	2.09	2.02	1.96
∞	3.84	3.00	2.60	2.37	2.21	2.10	2.01	1.94	1.88

(*Table J continued*)

Denominator Degrees of Freedom	Numerator Degrees of Freedom 10	12	15	20	24	30	40	60	120	∞
1	241.9	243.9	245.9	248.0	249.1	250.1	251.1	252.2	253.3	254.3
2	19.40	19.41	19.43	19.45	19.45	19.46	19.47	19.48	19.49	19.50
3	8.79	8.74	8.70	8.66	8.64	8.62	8.59	8.57	8.55	8.53
4	5.96	5.91	5.86	5.80	5.77	5.75	5.72	5.69	5.66	5.63
5	4.74	4.68	4.62	4.56	4.53	4.50	4.46	4.43	4.40	4.36
6	4.06	4.00	3.94	3.87	3.84	3.81	3.77	3.74	3.70	3.67
7	3.64	3.57	3.51	3.44	3.41	3.38	3.34	3.30	3.27	3.23
8	3.35	3.28	3.22	3.15	3.12	3.08	3.04	3.01	2.97	2.93
9	3.14	3.07	3.01	2.94	2.90	2.86	2.83	2.79	2.75	2.71
10	2.98	2.91	2.85	2.77	2.74	2.70	2.66	2.62	2.58	2.54
11	2.85	2.79	2.72	2.65	2.61	2.57	2.53	2.49	2.45	2.40
12	2.75	2.69	2.62	2.54	2.51	2.47	2.43	2.38	2.34	2.30
13	2.67	2.60	2.53	2.46	2.42	2.38	2.34	2.30	2.25	2.21
14	2.60	2.53	2.46	2.39	2.35	2.31	2.27	2.22	2.18	2.13
15	2.54	2.48	2.40	2.33	2.29	2.25	2.20	2.16	2.11	2.07
16	2.49	2.42	2.35	2.28	2.24	2.19	2.15	2.11	2.06	2.01
17	2.45	2.38	2.31	2.23	2.19	2.15	2.10	2.06	2.01	1.96
18	2.41	2.34	2.27	2.19	2.15	2.11	2.06	2.02	1.97	1.92
19	2.38	2.31	2.23	2.16	2.11	2.07	2.03	1.98	1.93	1.88
20	2.35	2.28	2.20	2.12	2.08	2.04	1.99	1.95	1.90	1.84
21	2.32	2.25	2.18	2.10	2.05	2.01	1.96	1.92	1.87	1.81
22	2.30	2.23	2.15	2.07	2.03	1.98	1.94	1.89	1.84	1.78
23	2.27	2.20	2.13	2.05	2.01	1.96	1.91	1.86	1.81	1.76
24	2.25	2.18	2.11	2.03	1.98	1.94	1.89	1.84	1.79	1.73
25	2.24	2.16	2.09	2.01	1.96	1.92	1.87	1.82	1.77	1.71
26	2.22	2.15	2.07	1.99	1.95	1.90	1.85	1.80	1.75	1.69
27	2.20	2.13	2.06	1.97	1.93	1.88	1.84	1.79	1.73	1.67
28	2.19	2.12	2.04	1.96	1.91	1.87	1.82	1.77	1.71	1.65
29	2.18	2.10	2.03	1.94	1.90	1.85	1.81	1.75	1.70	1.64
30	2.16	2.09	2.01	1.93	1.89	1.84	1.79	1.74	1.68	1.62
40	2.08	2.00	1.92	1.84	1.79	1.74	1.69	1.64	1.58	1.51
60	1.99	1.92	1.84	1.75	1.70	1.65	1.59	1.53	1.47	1.39
120	1.91	1.83	1.75	1.66	1.61	1.55	1.50	1.43	1.35	1.25
∞	1.83	1.75	1.67	1.57	1.52	1.46	1.39	1.32	1.22	1.00

(*Table J continued*)

	F_{90}								
Denominator degrees of Freedom	Numerator degrees of freedom 1	2	3	4	5	6	7	8	9
1	39.86	49.50	53.59	55.83	57.24	58.20	58.91	59.44	59.86
2	8.53	9.00	9.16	9.24	9.29	9.33	9.35	9.37	9.38
3	5.54	5.46	5.39	5.34	5.31	5.28	5.27	5.25	5.24
4	4.54	4.32	4.19	4.11	4.05	4.01	3.98	3.95	3.94
5	4.06	3.78	3.62	3.52	3.45	3.40	3.37	3.34	3.32
6	3.78	3.46	3.29	3.18	3.11	3.05	3.01	2.98	2.96
7	3.59	3.26	3.07	2.96	2.88	2.83	2.78	2.75	2.72
8	3.46	3.11	2.92	2.81	2.73	2.67	2.62	2.59	2.56
9	3.36	3.01	2.81	2.69	2.61	2.55	2.51	2.47	2.44
10	3.29	2.92	2.73	2.61	2.52	2.46	2.41	2.38	2.35
11	3.23	2.86	2.66	2.54	2.45	2.39	2.34	2.30	2.27
12	3.18	2.81	2.61	2.48	2.39	2.33	2.28	2.24	2.21
13	3.14	2.76	2.56	2.43	2.35	2.28	2.23	2.20	2.16
14	3.10	2.73	2.52	2.39	2.31	2.24	2.19	2.15	2.12
15	3.07	2.70	2.49	2.36	2.27	2.21	2.16	2.12	2.09
16	3.05	2.67	2.46	2.33	2.24	2.18	2.13	2.09	2.06
17	3.03	2.64	2.44	2.31	2.22	2.15	2.10	2.06	2.03
18	3.01	2.62	2.42	2.29	2.20	2.13	2.08	2.04	2.00
19	2.99	2.61	2.40	2.27	2.18	2.11	2.06	2.02	1.98
20	2.97	2.59	2.38	2.25	2.16	2.09	2.04	2.00	1.96
21	2.96	2.57	2.36	2.23	2.14	2.08	2.02	1.98	1.95
22	2.95	2.56	2.35	2.22	2.13	2.06	2.01	1.97	1.93
23	2.94	2.55	2.34	2.21	2.11	2.05	1.99	1.95	1.92
24	2.93	2.54	2.33	2.19	2.10	2.04	1.98	1.94	1.91
25	2.92	2.53	2.32	2.18	2.09	2.02	1.97	1.93	1.89
26	2.91	2.52	2.31	2.17	2.08	2.01	1.96	1.92	1.88
27	2.90	2.51	2.30	2.17	2.07	2.00	1.95	1.91	1.87
28	2.89	2.50	2.29	2.16	2.06	2.00	1.94	1.90	1.87
29	2.89	2.50	2.28	2.15	2.06	1.99	1.93	1.89	1.86
30	2.88	2.49	2.28	2.14	2.05	1.98	1.93	1.88	1.85
40	2.84	2.44	2.23	2.09	2.00	1.93	1.87	1.83	1.79
60	2.79	2.39	2.18	2.04	1.95	1.87	1.82	1.77	1.74
120	2.75	2.35	2.13	1.99	1.90	1.82	1.77	1.72	1.68
∞	2.71	2.30	2.08	1.94	1.85	1.77	1.72	1.67	1.63

(*Table J continued*)

Denominator degrees of freedom	Numerator degrees of freedom 10	12	15	20	24	30	40	60	120	∞
1	60.19	60.71	61.22	61.74	62.00	62.26	62.53	62.79	63.06	63.33
2	9.39	9.41	9.42	9.44	9.45	9.46	9.47	9.47	9.48	9.49
3	5.23	5.22	5.20	5.18	5.18	5.17	5.16	5.15	5.14	5.13
4	3.92	3.90	3.87	3.84	3.83	3.82	3.80	3.79	3.78	3.76
5	3.30	3.27	3.24	3.21	3.19	3.17	3.16	3.14	3.12	3.10
6	2.94	2.90	2.87	2.84	2.82	2.80	2.78	2.76	2.74	2.72
7	2.70	2.67	2.63	2.59	2.58	2.56	2.54	2.51	2.49	2.47
8	2.54	2.50	2.46	2.42	2.40	2.38	2.36	2.34	2.32	2.29
9	2.42	2.38	2.34	2.30	2.28	2.25	2.23	2.21	2.18	2.16
10	2.32	2.28	2.24	2.20	2.18	2.16	2.13	2.11	2.08	2.06
11	2.25	2.21	2.17	2.12	2.10	2.08	2.05	2.03	2.00	1.97
12	2.19	2.15	2.10	2.06	2.04	2.01	1.99	1.96	1.93	1.90
13	2.14	2.10	2.05	2.01	1.98	1.96	1.93	1.90	1.88	1.85
14	2.10	2.05	2.01	1.96	1.94	1.91	1.89	1.86	1.83	1.80
15	2.06	2.02	1.97	1.92	1.90	1.87	1.85	1.82	1.79	1.76
16	2.03	1.99	1.94	1.89	1.87	1.84	1.81	1.78	1.75	1.72
17	2.00	1.96	1.91	1.86	1.84	1.81	1.78	1.75	1.72	1.69
18	1.98	1.93	1.89	1.84	1.81	1.78	1.75	1.72	1.69	1.66
19	1.96	1.91	1.86	1.81	1.79	1.76	1.73	1.70	1.67	1.63
20	1.94	1.89	1.84	1.79	1.77	1.74	1.71	1.68	1.64	1.61
21	1.92	1.87	1.83	1.78	1.75	1.72	1.69	1.66	1.62	1.59
22	1.90	1.86	1.81	1.76	1.73	1.70	1.67	1.64	1.60	1.57
23	1.89	1.84	1.80	1.74	1.72	1.69	1.66	1.62	1.59	1.55
24	1.88	1.83	1.78	1.73	1.70	1.67	1.64	1.61	1.57	1.53
25	1.87	1.82	1.77	1.72	1.69	1.66	1.63	1.59	1.56	1.52
26	1.86	1.81	1.76	1.71	1.68	1.65	1.61	1.58	1.54	1.50
27	1.85	1.80	1.75	1.70	1.67	1.64	1.60	1.57	1.53	1.49
28	1.84	1.79	1.74	1.69	1.66	1.63	1.59	1.56	1.52	1.48
29	1.83	1.78	1.73	1.68	1.65	1.62	1.58	1.55	1.51	1.47
30	1.82	1.77	1.72	1.67	1.64	1.61	1.57	1.54	1.50	1.46
40	1.76	1.71	1.66	1.61	1.57	1.54	1.51	1.47	1.42	1.38
60	1.71	1.66	1.60	1.54	1.51	1.48	1.44	1.40	1.35	1.29
120	1.65	1.60	1.55	1.48	1.45	1.41	1.37	1.32	1.26	1.19
∞	1.60	1.55	1.49	1.42	1.38	1.34	1.30	1.24	1.17	1.00

Table K

Percentage Points of the Studentized Range for 2 through 20 Treatments
Upper 5% points

Error df	2	3	4	5	6	7	8	9	10
1	17.97	26.98	32.82	37.08	40.41	43.12	45.40	47.36	49.07
2	6.08	8.33	9.80	10.88	11.74	12.44	13.03	13.54	13.99
3	4.50	5.91	6.82	7.50	8.04	8.48	8.85	9.18	9.46
4	3.93	5.04	5.76	6.29	6.71	7.05	7.35	7.60	7.83
5	3.64	4.60	5.22	5.67	6.03	6.33	6.58	6.80	6.99
6	3.46	4.34	4.90	5.30	5.63	5.90	6.12	6.32	6.49
7	3.34	4.16	4.68	5.06	5.36	5.61	5.82	6.00	6.16
8	3.26	4.04	4.53	4.89	5.17	5.40	5.60	5.77	5.92
9	3.20	3.95	4.41	4.76	5.02	5.24	5.43	5.59	5.74
10	3.15	3.88	4.33	4.65	4.91	5.12	5.30	5.46	5.60
11	3.11	3.82	4.26	4.57	4.82	5.03	5.20	5.35	5.49
12	3.08	3.77	4.20	4.51	4.75	4.95	5.12	5.27	5.39
13	3.06	3.73	4.15	4.45	4.69	4.88	5.05	5.19	5.32
14	3.03	3.70	4.11	4.41	4.64	4.83	4.99	5.13	5.25
15	3.01	3.67	4.08	4.37	4.59	4.78	4.94	5.08	5.20
16	3.00	3.65	4.05	4.33	4.56	4.74	4.90	5.03	5.15
17	2.98	3.63	4.02	4.30	4.52	4.70	4.86	4.99	5.11
18	2.97	3.61	4.00	4.28	4.49	4.67	4.82	4.96	5.07
19	2.96	3.59	3.98	4.25	4.47	4.65	4.79	4.92	5.04
20	2.95	3.58	3.96	4.23	4.45	4.62	4.77	4.90	5.01
24	2.92	3.53	3.90	4.17	4.37	4.54	4.68	4.81	4.92
30	2.89	3.49	3.85	4.10	4.30	4.46	4.60	4.72	4.82
40	2.86	3.44	3.79	4.04	4.23	4.39	4.52	4.63	4.73
60	2.83	3.40	3.74	3.98	4.16	4.31	4.44	4.55	4.65
120	2.80	3.36	3.68	3.92	4.10	4.24	4.36	4.47	4.56
∞	2.77	3.31	3.63	3.86	4.03	4.17	4.29	4.39	4.47

Error df	11	12	13	14	15	16	17	18	19	20
1	50.59	51.96	53.20	54.33	55.36	56.32	57.22	58.04	58.83	59.56
2	14.39	14.75	15.08	15.38	15.65	15.91	16.14	16.37	16.57	16.77
3	9.72	9.95	10.15	10.35	10.52	10.69	10.84	10.98	11.11	11.24
4	8.03	8.21	8.37	8.52	8.66	8.79	8.91	9.03	9.13	9.23
5	7.17	7.32	7.47	7.60	7.72	7.83	7.93	8.03	8.12	8.21
6	6.65	6.79	6.92	7.03	7.14	7.24	7.34	7.43	7.51	7.59
7	6.30	6.43	6.55	6.66	6.76	6.85	6.94	7.02	7.10	7.17
8	6.05	6.18	6.29	6.39	6.48	6.57	6.65	6.73	6.80	6.87
9	5.87	5.98	6.09	6.19	6.28	6.36	6.44	6.51	6.58	6.64
10	5.72	5.83	5.93	6.03	6.11	6.19	6.27	6.34	6.40	6.47
11	5.61	5.71	5.81	5.90	5.98	6.06	6.13	6.20	6.27	6.33
12	5.51	5.61	5.71	5.80	5.88	5.95	6.02	6.09	6.15	6.21
13	5.43	5.53	5.63	5.71	5.79	5.86	5.93	5.99	6.05	6.11
14	5.36	5.46	5.55	5.64	5.71	5.79	5.85	5.91	5.97	6.03
15	5.31	5.40	5.49	5.57	5.65	5.72	5.78	5.85	5.90	5.96

(*Table K continued*)

Error df	11	12	13	14	15	16	17	18	19	20
16	5.26	5.35	5.44	5.52	5.59	5.66	5.73	5.79	5.84	5.90
17	5.21	5.31	5.39	5.47	5.54	5.61	5.67	5.73	5.79	5.84
18	5.17	5.27	5.35	5.43	5.50	5.57	5.63	5.69	5.74	5.79
19	5.14	5.23	5.31	5.39	5.46	5.53	5.59	5.65	5.70	5.75
20	5.11	5.20	5.28	5.36	5.43	5.49	5.55	5.61	5.66	5.71
24	5.01	5.10	5.18	5.25	5.32	5.38	5.44	5.49	5.55	5.59
30	4.92	5.00	5.08	5.15	5.21	5.27	5.33	5.38	5.43	5.47
40	4.82	4.90	4.98	5.04	5.11	5.16	5.22	5.27	5.31	5.36
60	4.73	4.81	4.88	4.94	5.00	5.06	5.11	5.15	5.20	5.24
120	4.64	4.71	4.78	4.84	4.90	4.95	5.00	5.04	5.09	5.13
∞	4.55	4.62	4.68	4.74	4.80	4.85	4.89	4.93	4.97	5.01

Upper 1% Points

Error df	2	3	4	5	6	7	8	9	10
1	90.03	135.0	164.3	185.6	202.2	215.8	227.2	237.0	245.6
2	14.04	19.02	22.29	24.72	26.63	28.20	29.53	30.68	31.69
3	8.26	10.62	12.17	13.33	14.24	15.00	15.64	16.20	16.69
4	6.51	8.12	9.17	9.96	10.58	11.10	11.55	11.93	12.27
5	5.70	6.98	7.80	8.42	8.91	9.32	9.67	9.97	10.24
6	5.24	6.33	7.03	7.56	7.97	8.32	8.61	8.87	9.10
7	4.95	5.92	6.54	7.01	7.37	7.68	7.94	8.17	8.37
8	4.75	5.64	6.20	6.62	6.96	7.24	7.47	7.68	7.86
9	4.60	5.43	5.96	6.35	6.66	6.91	7.13	7.33	7.49
10	4.48	5.27	5.77	6.14	6.43	6.67	6.87	7.05	7.21
11	4.39	5.15	5.62	5.97	6.25	6.48	6.67	6.84	6.99
12	4.32	5.05	5.50	5.84	6.10	6.32	6.51	6.67	6.81
13	4.26	4.96	5.40	5.73	5.98	6.19	6.37	6.53	6.67
14	4.21	4.89	5.32	5.63	5.88	6.08	6.26	6.41	6.54
15	4.17	4.84	5.25	5.56	5.80	5.99	6.16	6.31	6.44
16	4.13	4.79	5.19	5.49	5.72	5.92	6.08	6.22	6.35
17	4.10	4.74	5.14	5.43	5.66	5.85	6.01	6.15	6.27
18	4.07	4.70	5.09	5.38	5.60	5.79	5.94	6.08	6.20
19	4.05	4.67	5.05	5.33	5.55	5.73	5.89	6.02	6.14
20	4.02	4.64	5.02	5.29	5.51	5.69	5.84	5.97	6.09
24	3.96	4.55	4.91	5.17	5.37	5.54	5.69	5.81	5.92
30	3.89	4.45	4.80	5.05	5.24	5.40	5.54	5.65	5.76
40	3.82	4.37	4.70	4.93	5.11	5.26	5.39	5.50	5.60
60	3.76	4.28	4.59	4.82	4.99	5.13	5.25	5.36	5.45
120	3.70	4.20	4.50	4.71	4.87	5.01	5.12	5.21	5.30
∞	3.64	4.12	4.40	4.60	4.76	4.88	4.99	5.08	5.16

(*Table K continued*)

Error df	11	12	13	14	15	16	17	18	19	20
1	253.2	260.0	266.2	271.8	277.0	281.8	286.3	290.4	294.3	298.0
2	32.59	33.40	34.13	34.81	35.43	36.00	36.53	37.03	37.50	37.95
3	17.13	17.53	17.89	18.22	18.52	18.81	19.07	19.32	19.55	19.77
4	12.57	12.84	13.09	13.32	13.53	13.73	13.91	14.08	14.24	14.40
5	10.48	10.70	10.89	11.08	11.24	11.40	11.55	11.68	11.81	11.93
6	9.30	9.48	9.65	9.81	9.95	10.08	10.21	10.32	10.43	10.54
7	8.55	8.71	8.86	9.00	9.12	9.24	9.35	9.46	9.55	9.65
8	8.03	8.18	8.31	8.44	8.55	8.66	8.76	8.85	8.94	9.03
9	7.65	7.78	7.91	8.03	8.13	8.23	8.33	8.41	8.49	8.57
10	7.36	7.49	7.60	7.71	7.81	7.91	7.99	8.08	8.15	8.23
11	7.13	7.25	7.36	7.46	7.56	7.65	7.73	7.81	7.88	7.95
12	6.94	7.06	7.17	7.26	7.36	7.44	7.52	7.59	7.66	7.73
13	6.79	6.90	7.01	7.10	7.19	7.27	7.35	7.42	7.48	7.55
14	6.66	6.77	6.87	6.96	7.05	7.13	7.20	7.27	7.33	7.39
15	6.55	6.66	6.76	6.84	6.93	7.00	7.07	7.14	7.20	7.26
16	6.46	6.56	6.66	6.74	6.82	6.90	6.97	7.03	7.09	7.15
17	6.38	6.48	6.57	6.66	6.73	6.81	6.87	6.94	7.00	7.05
18	6.31	6.41	6.50	6.58	6.65	6.73	6.79	6.85	6.91	6.97
19	6.25	6.34	6.43	6.51	6.58	6.65	6.72	6.78	6.84	6.89
20	6.19	6.28	6.37	6.45	6.52	6.59	6.65	6.71	6.77	6.82
24	6.02	6.11	6.19	6.26	6.33	6.39	6.45	6.51	6.56	6.61
30	5.85	5.93	6.01	6.08	6.14	6.20	6.26	6.31	6.36	6.41
40	5.69	5.76	5.83	5.90	5.96	6.02	6.07	6.12	6.16	6.21
60	5.53	5.60	5.67	5.73	5.78	5.84	5.89	5.93	5.97	6.01
120	5.37	5.44	5.50	5.56	5.61	5.66	5.71	5.75	5.79	5.83
∞	5.23	5.29	5.35	5.40	5.45	5.49	5.54	5.57	5.61	5.65

Table L

Transformation of r to z
The Body of the Table Contains Values of $z = .5[\ln(1 + r)/(1 - r)] = \tanh^{-1} r$
for Corresponding Values of r, the Correlation Coefficient.

r	.00	.01	.02	.03	.04	.05	.06	.07	.08	.09
.0	.00000	.01000	.02000	.03001	.04002	.05004	.06007	.07012	.08017	.09024
.1	.10034	.11045	.12058	.13074	.14093	.15114	.16139	.17167	.18198	.19234
.2	.20273	.21317	.22366	.23419	.24477	.25541	.26611	.27686	.28768	.29857
.3	.30952	.32055	.33165	.34283	.35409	.36544	.37689	.38842	.40006	.41180
.4	.42365	.43561	.44769	.45990	.47223	.48470	.49731	.51007	.52298	.53606
.5	.54931	.56273	.57634	.59014	.60415	.61838	.63283	.64752	.66246	.67767
.6	.69315	.70892	.72500	.74142	.75817	.77530	.79281	.81074	.82911	.84795
.7	.86730	.88718	.90764	.92873	.95048	.97295	.99621	1.02033	1.04537	1.07143
.8	1.09861	1.12703	1.15682	1.18813	1.22117	1.25615	1.29334	1.33308	1.37577	1.42192
.9	1.47222	1.52752	1.58902	1.65839	1.73805	1.83178	1.94591	2.09229	2.29756	2.64665

Table M

Quantiles of the Kolmogorov Test Statistic

One-Sided Test $p = .90$	.95	.975	.99	.995
Two-Sided Test $p = .80$	.90	.95	.98	.99
$n =$ 1 .900	.950	.975	.990	.995
2 .684	.776	.842	.900	.929
3 .565	.636	.708	.785	.829
4 .493	.565	.624	.689	.734
5 .447	.509	.563	.627	.669
6 .410	.468	.519	.577	.617
7 .381	.436	.483	.538	.576
8 .358	.410	.454	.507	.542
9 .339	.387	.430	.480	.513
10 .323	.369	.409	.457	.489
11 .308	.352	.391	.437	.468
12 .296	.338	.375	.419	.449
13 .285	.325	.361	.404	.432
14 .275	.314	.349	.390	.418
15 .266	.304	.338	.377	.404
16 .258	.295	.327	.366	.392
17 .250	.286	.318	.355	.381
18 .244	.279	.309	.346	.371
19 .237	.271	.301	.337	.361
20 .232	.265	.294	.329	.352
21 .226	.259	.287	.321	.344
22 .221	.253	.281	.314	.337
23 .216	.247	.275	.307	.330
24 .212	.242	.269	.301	.323
25 .208	.238	.264	.295	.317
26 .204	.233	.259	.290	.311
27 .200	.229	.254	.284	.305
28 .197	.225	.250	.279	.300
29 .193	.221	.246	.275	.295
30 .190	.218	.242	.270	.290
31 .187	.214	.238	.266	.285
32 .184	.211	.234	.262	.281
33 .182	.208	.231	.258	.277
34 .179	.205	.227	.254	.273
35 .177	.202	.224	.251	.269
36 .174	.199	.221	.247	.265
37 .172	.196	.218	.244	.262
38 .170	.194	.215	.241	.258
39 .168	.191	.213	.238	.255
40 .165	.189	.210	.235	.252
Approximation for $n > 40$ $\frac{1.07}{\sqrt{n}}$	$\frac{1.22}{\sqrt{n}}$	$\frac{1.36}{\sqrt{n}}$	$\frac{1.52}{\sqrt{n}}$	$\frac{1.63}{\sqrt{n}}$

Table N

Critical Values of the Kruskal-Wallis Test Statistic

Sample Sizes			Critical Value	α
n_1	n_2	n_3		
2	1	1	2.7000	.500
2	2	1	3.6000	.200
2	2	2	4.5714	.067
			3.7143	.200
3	1	1	3.2000	.300
3	2	1	4.2857	.100
			3.8571	.133
3	2	2	5.3572	.029
			4.7143	.048
			4.5000	.067
			4.4643	.105
3	3	1	5.1429	.043
			4.5714	.100
			4.0000	.129
3	3	2	6.2500	.011
			5.3611	.032
			5.1389	.061
			4.5556	.100
			4.2500	.121
3	3	3	7.2000	.004
			6.4889	.011
			5.6889	.029
			5.6000	.050
			5.0667	.086
			4.6222	.100
4	1	1	3.5714	.200
4	2	1	4.8214	.057
			4.5000	.076
			4.0179	.114
4	2	2	6.0000	.014
			5.3333	.033
			5.1250	.052
			4.4583	.100
			4.1667	.105
4	3	1	5.8333	.021
			5.2083	.050
			5.0000	.057
			4.0556	.093
			3.8889	.129

(*Table N continued*)

Sample Sizes			Critical Value	α
n_1	n_2	n_3		
4	3	2	6.4444	.008
			6.3000	.011
			5.4444	.046
			5.4000	.051
			4.5111	.098
			4.4444	.102
4	3	3	6.7455	.010
			6.7091	.013
			5.7909	.046
			5.7273	.050
			4.7091	.092
			4.7000	.101
4	4	1	6.6667	.010
			6.1667	.022
			4.9667	.048
			4.8667	.054
			4.1667	.082
			4.0667	.102
4	4	2	7.0364	.006
			6.8727	.011
			5.4545	.046
			5.2364	.052
			4.5545	.098
			4.4455	.103
4	4	3	7.1439	.010
			7.1364	.011
			5.5985	.049
			5.5758	.051
			4.5455	.099
			4.4773	.102
4	4	4	7.6538	.008
			7.5385	.011
			5.6923	.049
			5.6538	.054
			4.6539	.097
			4.5001	.104
5	1	1	3.8571	.143
5	2	1	5.2500	.036
			5.0000	.048
			4.4500	.071
			4.2000	.095
			4.0500	.119

(***Table N continued***)

Sample Sizes			Critical Value	α
n_1	n_2	n_3		
5	2	2	6.5333	.008
			6.1333	.013
			5.1600	.034
			5.0400	.056
			4.3733	.090
			4.2933	.122
5	3	1	6.4000	.012
			4.9600	.048
			4.8711	.052
			4.0178	.095
			3.8400	.123
5	3	2	6.9091	.009
			6.8218	.010
			5.2509	.049
			5.1055	.052
			4.6509	.091
			4.4945	.101
5	3	3	7.0788	.009
			6.9818	.011
			5.6485	.049
			5.5152	.051
			4.5333	.097
			4.4121	.109
5	4	1	6.9545	.008
			6.8400	.011
			4.9855	.044
			4.8600	.056
			3.9873	.098
			3.9600	.102
5	4	2	7.2045	.009
			7.1182	.010
			5.2727	.049
			5.2682	.050
			4.5409	.098
			4.5182	.101
5	4	3	7.4449	.010
			7.3949	.011
			5.6564	.049
			5.6308	.050

(*Table N continued*)

Sample Sizes			Critical Value	α
n_1	n_2	n_3		
			4.5487	.099
			4.5231	.103
5	4	4	7.7604	.009
			7.7440	.011
			5.6571	.049
			5.6176	.050
			4.6187	.100
			4.5527	.102
5	5	1	7.3091	.009
			6.8364	.011
			5.1273	.046
			4.9091	.053
			4.1091	.086
			4.0364	.105
5	5	2	7.3385	.010
			7.2692	.010
			5.3385	.047
			5.2462	.051
			4.6231	.097
			4.5077	.100
5	5	3	7.5780	.010
			7.5429	.010
			5.7055	.046
			5.6264	.051
			4.5451	.100
			4.5363	.102
5	5	4	7.8229	.010
			7.7914	.010
			5.6657	.049
			5.6429	.050
			4.5229	.099
			4.5200	.101
5	5	5	8.0000	.009
			7.9800	.010
			5.7800	.049
			5.6600	.051
			4.5600	.100
			4.5000	.102

Table Oa

Exact Distribution of χ_r^2 for Tables with from 2 to 9 Sets of Three Ranks
($k = 3$; $n = 2, 3, 4, 5, 6, 7, 8, 9$)
P Is the Probability of Obtaining a Value of χ_r^2 as Great as or Greater than the Corresponding Value of χ_r^2

$n = 2$		$n = 3$		$n = 4$		$n = 5$	
χ_r^2	P	χ_r^2	P	χ_r^2	P	χ_r^2	P
0	1.000	.000	1.000	.0	1.000	.0	1.000
1	.833	0.667	.944	.5	.931	.4	.954
3	.500	2.000	.528	1.5	.653	1.2	.691
4	.167	2.667	.361	2.0	.431	1.6	.522
		4.667	1.94	3.5	.273	2.8	.367
		6.000	.028	4.5	.125	3.6	.182
				6.0	.069	4.8	.124
				6.5	.042	5.2	.093
				8.0	.0046	6.4	.039
						7.6	.024
						8.4	.0085
						10.0	.00077

$n = 6$		$n = 7$		$n = 8$		$n = 9$	
.00	1.000	.000	1.000	.00	1.000	.000	1.000
0.33	.956	.286	.964	.25	.967	.222	.971
1.00	.740	.857	.768	.75	.794	.667	.814
1.33	.570	1.143	.620	1.00	.654	.889	.865
2.33	.430	2.000	.486	1.75	.531	1.556	.569
3.00	.252	2.571	.305	2.25	.355	2.000	.398
4.00	.184	3.429	.237	3.00	.285	2.667	.328
4.33	.142	3.714	.192	3.25	.236	2.889	.278
5.33	.072	4.571	.112	4.00	.149	3.556	.187
6.33	.052	5.429	.085	4.75	.120	4.222	.154
7.00	.029	6.000	.052	5.25	.079	4.667	.107
8.33	.012	7.143	.027	6.25	.047	5.556	.069
9.00	.0081	7.714	.021	6.75	.038	6.000	.057
9.33	.0055	8.000	.016	7.00	.030	6.222	.048
10.33	.0017	8.857	.0084	7.75	.018	6.889	.031
12.00	.00013	10.286	.0036	9.00	.0099	8.000	.019
		10.571	.0027	9.25	.0080	8.222	.016
		11.143	.0012	9.75	.0048	8.667	.010
		12.286	.00032	10.75	.0024	9.556	.0060
		14.000	.000021	12.00	.0011	10.667	.0035
				12.25	.00086	10.889	.0029
				13.00	.00026	11.556	.0013
				14.25	.000061	12.667	.00066
				16.00	.0000036	13.556	.00035
						14.000	.00020
						14.222	.000097
						14.889	.000054
						16.222	.000011
						18.000	.0000006

Table Ob

Exact Distribution of χ_r^2 for Tables with from 2 to 4 Sets of Four Ranks ($k = 4$; $n = 2, 3, 4$)

P Is the Probability of Obtaining a Value of χ_r^2 as Great as or Greater than the Corresponding Value of χ_r^2

$n = 2$		$n = 3$		$n = 4$			
χ_r^2	P	χ_r^2	P	χ_r^2	P	χ_r^2	P
.0	1.000	.2	1.000	.0	1.000	5.7	.141
.6	.958	.6	.958	.3	.992	6.0	.105
1.2	.834	1.0	.910	.6	.928	6.3	.094
1.8	.792	1.8	.727	.9	.900	6.6	.077
2.4	.625	2.2	.608	1.2	.800	6.9	.068
3.0	.542	2.6	.524	1.5	.754	7.2	.054
3.6	.458	3.4	.446	1.8	.677	7.5	.052
4.2	.375	3.8	.342	2.1	.649	7.8	.036
4.8	.208	4.2	.300	2.4	.524	8.1	.033
5.4	.167	5.0	.207	2.7	.508	8.4	.019
6.0	.042	5.4	.175	3.0	.432	8.7	.014
		5.8	.148	3.3	.389	9.3	.012
		6.6	.075	3.6	.355	9.6	.0069
		7.0	.054	3.9	.324	9.9	.0062
		7.4	.033	4.5	.242	10.2	.0027
		8.2	.017	4.8	.200	10.8	.0016
		9.0	.0017	5.1	.190	11.1	.00094
				5.4	.158	12.0	.000072

Table P

Critical Values of the Spearman Test Statistic
Approximate Upper-tail Critical Values r_s^*, Where $P(r_s > r_s^*) \leq \alpha$,
$n = 4(1)30$ Significance Level, α.

n	.001	.005	.010	.025	.050	.100
4	—	—	—	—	.8000	.8000
5	—	—	.9000	.9000	.8000	.7000
6	—	.9429	.8857	.8286	.7714	.6000
7	.9643	.8929	.8571	.7450	.6786	.5357
8	.9286	.8571	.8095	.7143	.6190	.5000
9	.9000	.8167	.7667	.6833	.5833	.4667
10	.8667	.7818	.7333	.6364	.5515	.4424
11	.8364	.7545	.7000	.6091	.5273	.4182
12	.8182	.7273	.6713	.5804	.4965	.3986
13	.7912	.6978	.6429	.5549	.4780	.3791
14	.7670	.6747	.6220	.5341	.4593	.3626
15	.7464	.6536	.6000	.5179	.4429	.3500
16	.7265	.6324	.5824	.5000	.4265	.3382
17	.7083	.6152	.5637	.4853	.4118	.3260
18	.6904	.5975	.5480	.4716	.3994	.3148
19	.6737	.5825	.5333	.4579	.3895	.3070
20	.6586	.5684	.5203	.4451	.3789	.2977
21	.6455	.5545	.5078	.4351	.3688	.2909
22	.6318	.5426	.4963	.4241	.3597	.2829
23	.6186	.5306	.4852	.4150	.3518	.2767
24	.6070	.5200	.4748	.4061	.3435	.2704
25	.5962	.5100	.4654	.3977	.3362	.2646
26	.5856	.5002	.4564	.3894	.3299	.2588
27	.5757	.4915	.4481	.3822	.3236	.2540
28	.5660	.4828	.4401	.3749	.3175	.2490
29	.5567	.4744	.4320	.3685	.3113	.2443
30	.5479	.4665	.4251	.3620	.3059	.2400

Note: The corresponding lower-tail critical value for r_s is $-r_s^*$.

ACKNOWLEDGMENTS FOR TABLES

C. From Charles T. Clark and Lawrence L. Schkade, *Statistical Methods for Administrative Decisions*, Second Edition, South-Western Publishing Company, Cincinnati, Ohio, 1974. Reprinted by special permission.

F. From John E. Freund and Frank J. Williams, *Elementary Business*

Statistics: The Modern Approach, Second Edition © 1972, p. 473. Reprinted by permission of Prentice-Hall, Inc., Englewood Cliffs, New Jersey.

G. From *A Million Random Digits with 100,000 Normal Deviates* by The Rand Corporation, The Free Press, Glencoe, Illinois, 1955. Reprinted by permission.

H. Reproduced from *Documenta Geigy, Scientific Tables* Seventh Edition, 1970, courtesy of CIBA-Geigy Limited, Basle, Switzerland.

I. From A. Hald and S. A. Sinkbaek, "A Table of Percentage Points of the χ^2 Distribution," *Skandinavisk Aktuarietidskrift, 33* (1950), 168–175. Used by permission.

J. From *Biometrika Tables for Statisticians*, Third Edition, Vol. I, Bentley House, London, 1970. Reprinted by permission.

K. From *Biometrika Tables for Statisticians*, Third Edition, Vol. I, Bentley House, London, 1970. Used by permission.

M. From L. H. Miller, "Table of Percentage Points of Kolmogorov Statistics," *Journal of the American Statistical Association, 51* (1956), 111–121. Reprinted by permission of the American Statistical Association. The table as reprinted here follows the format found in W. J. Conover, *Practical Nonparametric Statistics*, © 1971, by John Wiley & Sons, Inc.

N. From W. H. Kruskal and W. A. Wallis, "Use of Ranks in One Criterion Analysis of Variance," *Journal of the American Statistical Association, 47* (1952), 583–621; errata, ibid., *48* (1953), 907–911. Reprinted by permission of the American Statistical Association.

O. From M. Friedman, "The Use of Ranks to Avoid the Assumption of Normality Implicit in the Analysis of Variance," *Journal of the American Statistical Association, 32* (1937), 675–701. Reprinted by permission.

P. From Gerald J. Glasser and Robert F. Winter, "Critical Values of the Coefficient of Rank Correlation for Testing the Hypothesis of Independence," *Biometrika 48* (1961), 444–448. Used by permission. The table as reprinted here contains corrections given in W. J. Conover, *Practical Nonparametric Statistics*, © 1971, by John Wiley & Sons, Inc.

ANSWERS TO ODD-NUMBERED EXERCISES

Chapter 1

1.4.1. (a) 65.1 (b) 65 (c) 65.

1.4.3. (a) 9.4 (b) 11.

1.4.5. Chicken.

1.5.1. (a) 16 (b) 19.66 (c) 4.4.
1.5.3. (a) 12 (b) 17.83 (c) 4.2 (d) 44.68.
1.6.1. Suggested class intervals: 55–59, 60–64, . . . , 80–84.
1.6.3. Suggested class intervals: 80–89, 90–99, . . . , 140–149.
1.8.1. (a) 66.9 (b) 66.6 (c) 65–69 (d) 46.45 (e) 6.8.
1.8.3. (a) 117.33 (b) 116.46 (c) 110–119 (d) 217.26 (e) 14.7.

Review Exercises

13. $\bar{x} = 23.07$ Median = 22 $s^2 = 54.92$ $s = 7.4$.
15. $\bar{x} = 9.32$ Median = 9.1 $s^2 = 2.89$ $s = 1.7$.
17. $\bar{x} = 35.23$ Median = 36.23 $s^2 = 168.0360$ $s = 12.96$.

Chapter 2

2.4.1. (a) 160 (b) 26 (c) 688 (d) 308 (e) 1025 (f) 263.
2.5.1. (a) 30 (b) 210 (c) 30,240 (d) 15 (e) 35 (f) 252 (g) 56 (h) 126 (i) 10.
2.5.3. 120.
2.5.5. 6.
2.5.7. 4.
2.5.9. 560.
2.6.1. (a) .16 (b) .03 (c) .67 (d) .30 (e) .995 (f) .26.
2.6.3. (a) .45 (b) .41 (c) .10 (d) .04.
2.6.5. .95.

Review Exercises

11. (a) 30 (b) 54 (c) 33 (d) 85 (e) 100 (f) 77 (g) 7 (h) 80.
13. .64.
15. .49.

Chapter 3

3.3.1. (a) .1484 (b) .8915 (c) .1085 (d) .2012.
3.3.3. (a) .9729 (b) .9095 (c) .7827 (d) .0271.
3.4.1. (a) .176 (b) .384 (c) .440 (d) .427.
3.4.3. (a) .105 (b) .032 (c) .007 (d) .440.
3.6.1. .4236
3.6.3. .2912.
3.6.5. .0099.
3.6.7. .95.
3.6.9. .901.
3.6.11. (a) .6826 (b) .6915 (c) .5675.

3.6.13. (a) .3446 (b) .3446 (c) .5762.
3.6.15. (a) .3413 (b) .1056 (c) .0062 (d) .3830.

Review Exercises

15. .1719.
17. (a) .0916 (b) .0905 (c) .9095 (d) .1845 (e) .2502.
19. (a) .762 (b).238 (c) .065
21. (a) 1.5 (b) .6247 (c) .6826.
23. (a) .0013 (b) .0668 (c) .8931.
25. 57.10.

Chapter 4

4.4.1. (a) .9772 (b) .9544 (c) .0082 (d) .0082.
4.4.3. (a) .1814 (b) .8016 (c) .0643.
4.4.5. (a) .5 (b) .7333 (c) .9772.
4.5.1. .1379.
4.5.3. .0038.
4.6.1. (a) .0808 (b) .8384 (c) .2005.
4.6.3. .0823.
4.6.5. (a) .1539 (b) .3409 (c) .5230.
4.7.1. .008.

Review Exercises

13. .8664.
15. .9989.
17. .0082.
19. .8882.
21. .0019.

Chapter 5

5.2.1. (a) 88, 92 (b) 87, 93 (c) 86, 94.
5.2.3. (a) 7.63, 8.87 (b) 7.51, 8.99 (c) 7.28, 9.22.
5.3.1. (a) -2.0, 13.0 (b) -3.5, 14.5 (c) -6.3, 17.3.
5.3.3. (a) 4, 10 (b) 3.5, 10.5 (c) 2.3, 11.7.
5.4.1. .04, .12; .03, .13; .01, .15.
5.4.3. .14, .34; .12, .36; .08, .40.
5.5.1. $-.02$, .10; $-.03$, .11; $-.06$, .14.
5.5.3. $-.07$, .19; $-.09$, .21; $-.14$, .26.
5.6.1. 5.76, 8.24; 5.46, 8.54; 4.76, 9.24.
5.6.3. 69.58, 76.42; 68.87, 77.13; 67.41, 78.59.

5.6.5. $-4.33, 7.33; -5.50, 8.50; -7.86, 10.86$. Use 40 df.
5.6.7. 2.1, 4.5; 1.8, 4.8; 1.3, 4.8.
5.6.9. d.f. ≈ 26; 24.7, 33.3.
5.7.1. 27, 16.
5.7.3. 19.
5.8.1. 683, 1068.
5.8.3. 385, 289.
5.9.1. $8.40 < \sigma^2 < 18.54$; $2.90 < \sigma < 4.31$.
5.9.3. $630{,}307.86 < \sigma^2 < 1{,}878{,}027.08$; $793.92 < \sigma < 1{,}370.41$.
5.9.5. $1.37 < \sigma^2 < 4.35$; $1.17 < \sigma < 2.09$.
5.10.1. $1.48 < (\sigma_2{}^2/\sigma_1{}^2) < 9.76$.
5.10.3. $.49 < (\sigma_1{}^2/\sigma_2{}^2) < 2.95$.
5.10.5. $.90 < (\sigma_1{}^2/\sigma_2{}^2) < 3.52$.

Review Exercises

13. $\bar{x} = 79.87$ $s^2 = 28.1238$ $s = 5.30$ 76.93, 82.81.
15. $\tilde{p} = .30$ .19, .41.
17. $\tilde{p}_1 = .20$ $\tilde{p}_2 = .54$ .26, .42.
19. $\tilde{p} = .90$ .87, .93.
21. $\bar{x} = 19.23$ $s^2 = 20.2268$ 16.01, 22.45.

Chapter 6

6.2.1. Yes, $z = 3$ $p = .5 - .4987 = .0013$.
6.2.3. Yes, $z = 2.67$ $p = .5 - .4962 = .0038$
6.2.5. Yes, $z = -5.73$ $p < .5 - .4990 = .0010$
6.2.7. No, $t = -1.5$ $.05 < p < .10$
6.2.9. Yes, $z = 3.08$ $p = .5 - .4990 = .0010$
6.3.1. Yes, $z = -11.91$ $p \approx 0$
6.3.3. $s_p{}^2 = 29.30$, $t = -3.62$ Reject H_0 $p < 2(.005) = .01$.
6.3.5. Do not reject H_0 $z = 1.40$ $p = 2(.5 - .4192) = 2(.0808) = .1616$.
6.3.7. $s_p{}^2 = 5421.25$ $t = -6.66$ Reject H_0 $p < 2(.005) = .010$.
6.3.9. $z = 3.39$ Reject H_0 $p < 2(.5 - .4990) = .0020$.
6.4.1. Yes, $t = 16.63$ $p < .005$.
6.4.3. Reject H_0 $t = -3.45$; $-.5, -.1$ $p < 2(.005) = .010$.
6.5.1. Reject H_0 $z = 3.26$ $p < .5 - .4990 = .0010$.
6.5.3. Yes, $z = -8.94$ $p < .5 - .4990 = .0010$.
6.6.1. $\bar{p} = .66$ $z = 2.45$ Reject H_0
$p = 2(.5 - .4929) = 2(.0071) = .0142$.
6.6.3. $\bar{p} = .27$ $z = 2.90$ Reject H_0
$p = 2(.5 - .4981) = 2(.0019) = .0038$.

6.7.1. Yes, $\chi^2 = 54 \quad p < .005$.
6.7.3. $\chi^2 = 6.75$ Do not reject $H_0 \quad p > .05$ (two-sided test).
6.7.5. $\chi^2 = 28.8$ Do not reject $H_0 \quad p > .10$.
6.8.1. No V. R. = 2.08 $p > .10$.
6.8.3. No V. R. = 1.83 $p > .10$.
6.8.5. Reject H_0 V. R. = 4 $.01 < p < .025$.

Review Exercises

19. $\bar{d} = .40 \quad s_d^2 = .2871 \quad s_d = .54 \quad t = 2.869 \quad .005 < p < .01$.
21. $z = 1.095 \quad 1379 > p > .1357$.
23. $t = 3.873 \quad p < .005$.
25. $\bar{d} = 11.49 \quad s_d^2 = 256.6790 \quad s_d = 16.02 \quad t = 2.485 \quad .025 > p > .01$.

Chapter 7

7.2.1. Yes V. R. = 6.03 $p < .005$.
7.2.3. Yes V. R. = 67.80 $p < .005$.
7.2.5. No V. R. = 4.70 $.025 > p > .01$.
7.2.7. $\bar{x}_A - \bar{x}_C$ and $\bar{x}_B - \bar{x}_C$ are significant.
7.2.9. $\bar{x}_D - \bar{x}_E$ and $\bar{x}_A - \bar{x}_E$ are significant.
7.3.1. Yes V. R. = 13.17 $p < .005$.
7.3.3. Yes V. R. = 30.22 $p < .005$.
7.3.5. V. R. = 276.64 $p < .005$.
7.4.1. (a) V. R. (A) = 38.78, V. R. (B) = 21.57, V. R. (AB) = 2.24
(b) $\alpha < .03 \quad p(A) < .005 \quad p(B) < .005 \quad .10 > p(AB) > .05$.
7.4.3. V. R. (A) = 5.84, V. R. (B) = 44.34, V. R. (AB) = 30.09 $\alpha < .07$
$.05 < p(A) < .10 \quad p(B) < .005 \quad p(AB) < .005$.

Review Exercises

3. V. R. = 8.042 Reject $H_0 \quad p < .005$.
5. V. R. = .825 Do not reject $H_0 \quad p > .10$.
7. V. R. (A) = 6.325 $.005 < p(A) < .01 \quad p(B) < .005$
$.01 > p(AB) > .005$; V. R. (B) = 38.856; V. R. (AB) = 4.970.

Chapter 8

8.3.1. $y_c = 7.05 + 4.09x$.
8.3.3. $y_c = 1.36 - .008x$.
8.3.5. $y_c = 106.67 - 1.54x$.
8.4.1. (a) .90 (b) V. R. = 103.41 ($p < .005$) (c) $t = 10.17$ ($p < .01$)
(f) 3.21, 4.97.

8.4.3. (a) .94 (b) V. R. = 152.42 ($p < .005$) (c) $t = -12.29$ ($p < .01$) (f) $-.009$, $-.007$.

8.4.5. (a) .78 (b) V. R. = 28.91 ($p < .005$) (c) $t = -5.38$ ($p < .01$) (f) -2.2, $-.88$.

8.5.1. (a) $15.23 \pm (2.2010)(1.3558)(.2774)$
(b) $15.23 \pm (2.2010)(1.3558)(1.0377)$.

8.5.3. (a) $.96 \pm (2.2622)(.0341)(.3162)$
(b) $.96 \pm (2.2622)(.0341)(1.0488)$.

8.5.5. (a) $98.97 \pm (2.3060)(2.6004)(.3210)$
(b) $98.97 \pm (2.3060)(2.6004)(1.0503)$.

8.7.1. (b) .90 (c) $t = 7.44$ ($p < .01$) .719, .966.
(Linear interpolation used.)

8.7.3. (b) .93 (c) $t = 7.16$ ($p < .01$) .725, .983.
(Linear interpolation used.)

8.7.5. (b) .54 (c) $t = 3.08$ ($p < .01$) .184, .771.
(Linear interpolation used.)

Review Exercises

17. $r = -.74$ $t = -4.67$

19. $y_c = 19.41 + .9895x$ $r^2 = .9994$ $t = 144.89$.

Source	*SS*	d. f.	MS	V. R.
Regression	1364.4880	1	1364.4880	20,992.123
Residual	.8453	13	.0650	
Total	1365.3333	14		

21. $y_c = 1.2714 + .8533$ $r^2 = .6878$ $t = 5.35$.

Source	*SS*	d. f.	MS	V. R.
Regression	1.6498	1	1.6498	28.64
Residual	.7489	13	.0576	
Total	2.3987	14		

Chapter 9

9.3.1. $y_c = 4639.56 - 244.43x_1 - 422.93x_2$.

9.3.3. $y_c = 13.45 + 4.02x_1 + 2.81x_2$.

9.3.5. $y_c = -422.00 + 11.17x_1 - .63x_2$.

9.4.1. (a) .93.

(b)

Source	SS	d. f.	MS	V. R.	p
Regression	8,247,389.5	2	4,123,694.80	49.57	$<.005$
Residual	582,308.5	7	83,186.93		
Total	8,829,698.0	9			

(c) $t(b_1) = -3.45$, $t(b_2) = -3.22$ ($.01 < p < .02$ for both tests.)

9.4.3. (a) .67.

(b)

Source	SS	d. f.	MS	V. R.	p
Regression	452.56	2	226.28	7.05	$.01 < p < .025$
Residual	224.70	7	32.10		
Total	677.26	9			

(c) $t(b_1) = 3.75$; ($p < .01$); $t(b_2) = 2.04$, ($.05 < p < .10$)

9.4.5. (a) .31.

(b)

Source	SS	d. f.	MS	V. R	p
Regression	17,023.01	2	8,511.505	4.89	$.01 < p < .025$
Residual	38,276.99	22	1,739.86		
Total	55,300.00	24			

(c) $t(b_1) = 3.05$, ($p < .01$); $t(b_2) = -.67$, ($p > .20$).

9.5.1. (a) $2148.62 \pm (2.3646)(288.42) \times \sqrt{\frac{1}{10} + (.060319)(.8)^2 + (.207378)(-.7)^2 + 2(-.086740)(.8)(-.7)}$.

(b) Add 1 under the radical.

9.5.3. (a) $50.41 \pm (2.3646)(5.67) \times \sqrt{\frac{1}{10} + (.035757)(-1.99)^2 + (.059206)(.44)^2 + 2(.022857)(-1.99)(.44)}$.

(b) Add 1 under the radical.

9.5.5. (a) $532.90 \pm 2.0739(41.71) \times \sqrt{\frac{1}{25} + (.007678)(-.52)^2 + (.000506)(-2.12)^2 + 2(-.000002)(-.52)(-2.12)}$.

(b) Add 1 under the radical.

9.6.1. (a) $b_0 = 36.5323$, $b_1 = 6.4758$, $b_2 = -.5749$, $R_{y.12} = .9976$,
$F = 933$ ($p < .005$)
(b) $r_{y1.2} = .505$, $t = 1.755$ ($.20 > p > .10$)
$r_{y2.1} = -.084$, $t = -.253$ ($p > .20$)
$r_{12.y} = .902$, $t = 6.268$ ($p < .01$).

9.6.3. (a) $b_0 = -422.00$, $b_1 = 11.17$, $b_2 = -.63$, $R_{y.12} = .5548$
$F = 4.89$ ($.01 < p < .025$)
(b) $r_{y1.2} = .546$, $t = 3.056$ ($p < .01$)
$r_{y2.1} = -.142$, $t = -.673$ ($p > .20$)
$r_{12.y} = .078$, $t = .367$ ($p > .20$).

Review Exercises

7. $R = .3496$ $F = .83$ ($p > .10$).

9. (a) $y_c = 11.43 + 1.26x_1 + 3.11x_2$
(b) $R^2 = .92$.

(c)

Source	*SS*	d. f.	MS	V. R.	*p*
Regression	1827.004659	2	913.50	69.048	<.005
Residual	158.728641	12	13.23		
	1985.7333	14			

(d) $y_c = 11.43 + 1.26(10) + 3.11(5) = 39.56$.

Chapter 10

10.3.1. $X^2 = 2.072$ $p > .995$.
10.3.3. $X^2 = 3.417$ $p > .10$.
10.3.5. $X^2 = 2.21$ $p > .10$.
10.4.1. $X^2 = 27.272$ $p < .005$.
10.4.3. $X^2 = .765$ $p > .10$.
10.4.5. $X^2 = 42.579$ $p < .005$.
10.5.1. $X^2 = 65.855$ $p < .005$.
10.5.3. $X^2 = 32.754$ $p < .005$.

Review Exercises

11. $X^2 = 10.7827$ $p < .005$.
13. $X^2 = 3.4505$ $p > .10$.
15. $X^2 = 8.1667$ $p < .005$.
17. $X^2 = 67.8015$ $p < .005$.

19. $X^2 = 7.2577$ $.05 > p > .025$.
21. Independence.
23. Homogeneity.

Chapter 11

11.3.1. $P = .3036$ $p = .3036$.
11.4.1. $X^2 = 16.13$ $p < .005$.
11.5.1. $D = .3241$ $p < .01$.
11.5.3. $D = .1057$ $p > .20$.
11.6.1. $H = 19.55$ $p < .005$.
11.6.3. $H = 30.97$ $p < .005$.
11.6.5. $H = 13.86$ $p < .005$.
11.6.7. $H = 14.75$ $.01 > p > .005$.
11.7.1. $\chi_r^2 = 8.67$ $p = .01$.
11.7.3. $\chi_r^2 = 13.74$ $p < .005$.
11.7.5. $\chi_r^2 = 11.1$ $p = .00094$.
11.7.7. $\chi_r^2 = 7.28$ $p \approx .054$.
11.8.1. $r_s = -0.07$ $p > .20$.
11.8.3. r_s(corrected for ties) $= .95$. $p < .002$.
11.8.5. $r_s = .99$ $p < .001$.

Review Exercises

9. $P(X \leq 1 | 10, .5) = 1 - .9893 = .0107$ $p = .0107$.
11. $\chi_r^2 = 16.2$ $p < .005$.
13. $\bar{x} = 44.06$ $s = 11.85$ $D = .1539$ $p > .20$.

Chapter 12

12.2.1. (a) 10.4 (b) 10.1, 11.0 (c) 16.1 (d) 21.5 (e) 16.9 (f) 47.6 (g) 15.2, 27.3.
12.3.1. (a) 97.0, 165.4, 125.0, 62.4, 25.8, 3.5.
(b) 2413 (c) 485; 1312; 1937; 2249; 2378; 2413.
(d) 76.5.

INDEX